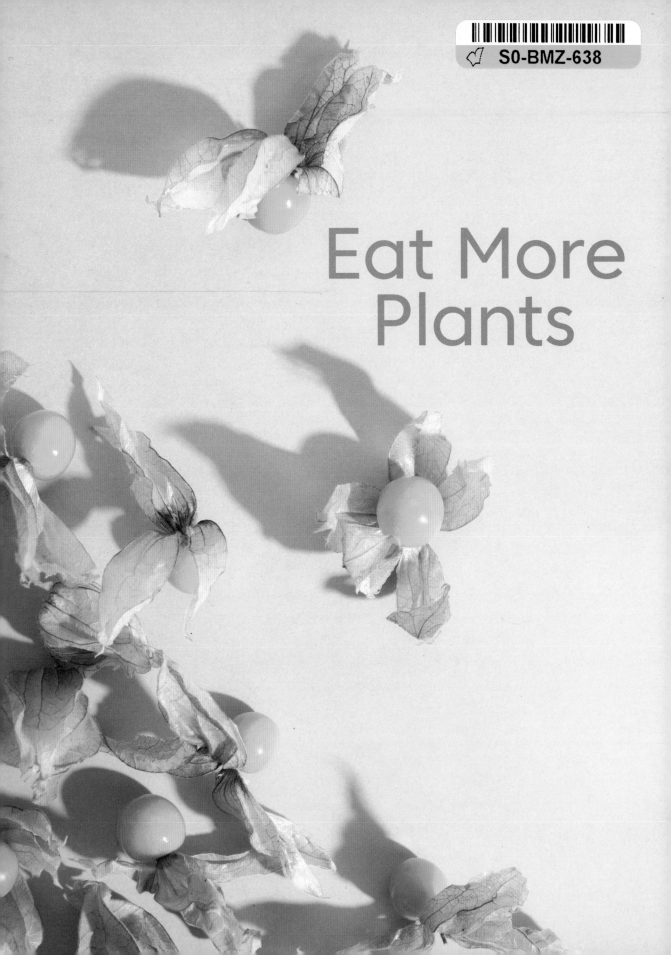

# Eat More Plants

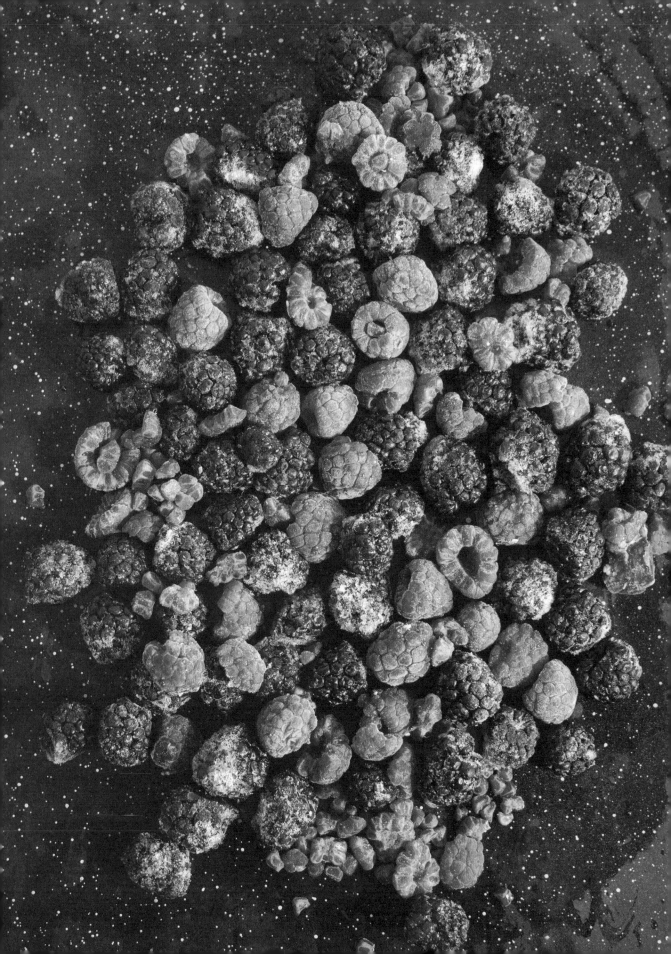

# Eat More Plants

## Over 100 ANTI-INFLAMMATORY, Plant-Based Recipes for Vibrant Living

### DESIREE NIELSEN, RD

PENGUIN

an imprint of Penguin Canada, a division of Penguin Random House Canada Limited

Canada • USA • UK • Ireland • Australia • New Zealand • India • South Africa • China

First published 2019

www.penguinrandomhouse.ca


LIBRARY AND ARCHIVES CANADA CATALOGUING IN PUBLICATION

Nielsen, Desiree, author
    Eat more plants : over 100 anti-inflammatory, plant-based recipes for vibrant living / Desiree Nielsen.

Issued in print and electronic formats.
ISBN 978-0-7352-3571-7 (softcover).—ISBN 978-0-7352-3572-4 (electronic)

    1. Inflammation—Diet therapy—Recipes.  2. Vegetarian cooking.
3. Cookbooks.  I. Title.

RB131.N54 2019  6              41.5'63            C2018-905424-7
                                                  C2018-905425-5


Cover and interior design by Andrew Roberts
Photography by Janis Nicolay
Prop and food styling by Sophie McKenzie


Printed and bound in China


10 9 8 7 6 5 4 3 2 1

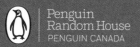

Penguin
Random House
PENGUIN CANADA

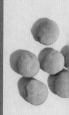

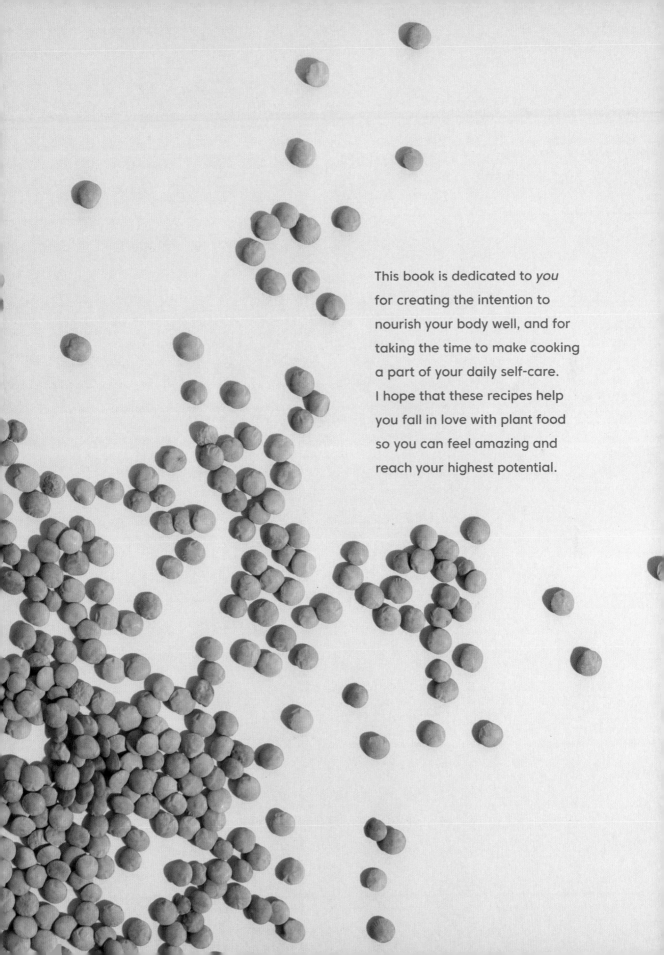

This book is dedicated to *you* for creating the intention to nourish your body well, and for taking the time to make cooking a part of your daily self-care. I hope that these recipes help you fall in love with plant food so you can feel amazing and reach your highest potential.

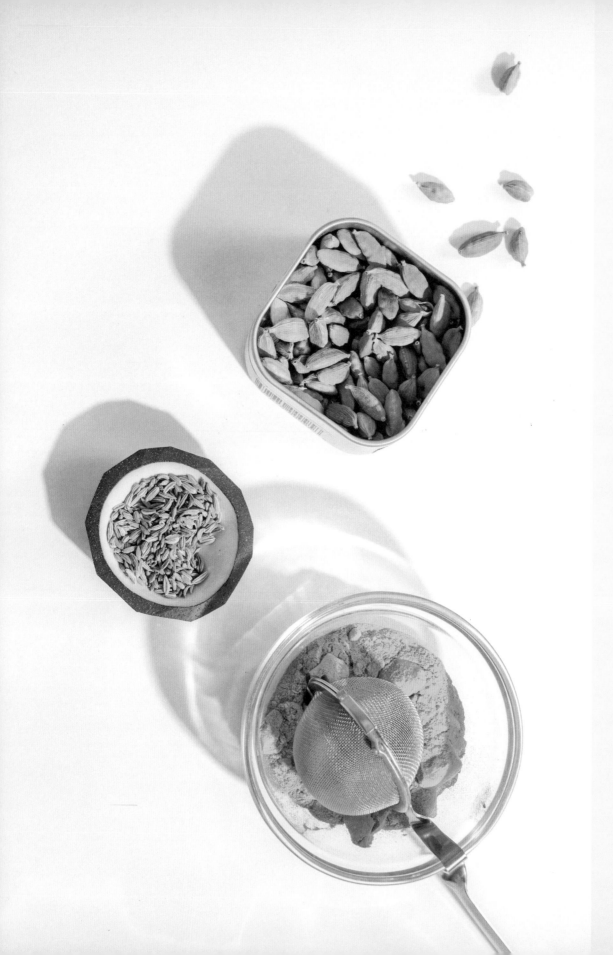

# Contents

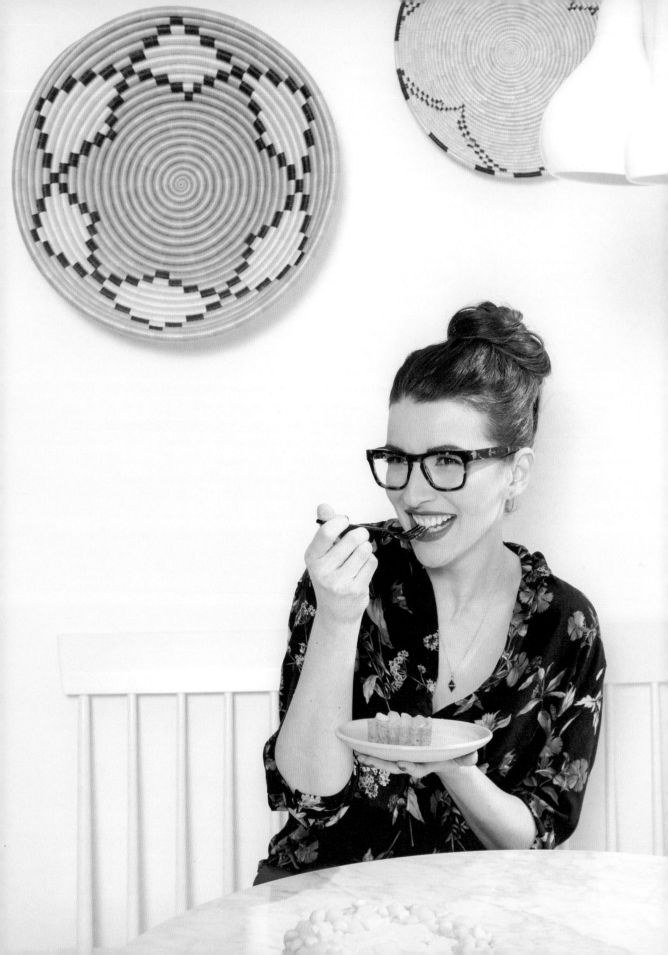

# Introduction

I really like to eat. I also like to cook, so I can eat the food I enjoy the most—healthy, energizing, and so delicious that there is no talk of compromise.

I have been a vegetarian for twenty years. I wish I could say I had noble intentions around making the change, but really, I did it to impress a boy I liked! True story. It is funny how life works; that short-lived teenage crush was the origin of a transformative shift for me. Becoming vegetarian led to a lifelong love of mindfulness, yoga, and of course, nutrition. Back then, I thought mac and cheese was the height of sophistication and health. Vegetarian eating meant no meat, but that did not necessarily equate to eating many whole plant foods.

Shortly after I became vegetarian, I tried a brief and somewhat disastrous stint with totally plant-based eating that left me hungry because I did not really know how to craft a nutritious plant-based meal. But times have changed. I am now a plant-based eater, but I did not get here overnight. It was a slow transition that felt positive and joyful at every step. Moving toward a more plant-based, anti-inflammatory eating plan is probably one of the most transformative actions you can take for your health. It will help you feel more energized and resilient in your everyday life. It will also help you prevent chronic illness and support you in healing.

It takes time to unlearn the hyper-processed eating pattern that is so common in our world. When you break rank with the status quo and dip your toe into plant-based living, it might feel foreign. It might even taste foreign (which is ironic, since by definition artificial sweeteners and colours are the foreign ingredients). However, when you explore it with a sense of play—free of absolutes—you will discover that this plant stuff is actually delicious. Of course, it is all in the approach. Go ahead and add a bit of extra salt or maple syrup to your meal if you need it to help you transition your taste buds. Have fun exploring plant-based versions of your favourite meals. Do not force yourself to eat foods you hate or attempt to cook tofu for the first time without a recipe, or you may think this healthy eating stuff isn't worth the price of admission.

By putting this book in your hands, you are on the right track. When you cook and eat these recipes, you may feel a bit peppier and want to feel that way again. It does not matter if you want nachos on a Friday night (and I have a queso recipe to help with that!). Just eat plants the rest of the time.

Plant-based eating is not about demonizing food or paying penance for indulgence. It is all about the *yum* and feeling good. Ignoring our bodies' needs is not the right way to go. The same goes for demonizing large swaths of edibles. Describing all the things your diet is *free of* is kind of missing the point. Of course, if you are allergic to peanuts, there is a very critical point to their restriction. Someone with celiac disease is going to feel 100 percent better by ditching gluten. For the rest of us? Obviously, there is a middle way. In addition, what tends to define plant-based eating is an attitude of *more*, not less. If you want to eat well, forget the dogma and just focus on cooking the recipes in this book as often as you can. The more you do, the better you will feel.

As a dietitian, I want you to enjoy the act of cooking and eating, and to *crave* healthy foods. This is a major shift for many of us: it is unlikely that you will consume enough vegetables when you are forcing yourself to eat baby carrots at your desk and diving into big bowls of pasta the rest of the time. My intention with this book is to help you shake up your *healthy* food rut. To show you how delicious it is to adopt a more anti-inflammatory, plant-based diet so you can feel incredible. In addition, to give you recipes so doable you will actually make them.

## How We Got Here: Unlearning Nutritionism

I totally understand if nutrition seems a bit confusing at times. Our collective desire to be healthier leads us to seek an enormous amount of food and nutrition information, and there are so many voices with differing opinions. So, how did we get here? To learn that, you have to take a deeper look at how nutrition evolves and how our food system uses nutrition to its own ends.

Food and nutrition are interconnected at the most basic level. We eat food, which contains nutrients, to nourish our bodies; nutrition is the study and application of how nutrients in food affect the body. However, the relationship between the two is not always harmonious.

The hyper-processed food choices we make today sometimes have very little in common with the food that grows out of the ground. Clever food manufacturers have figured out how to make hyper-processed foods taste as delicious and decadent as possible by including giant amounts of salt, sugar, and fat so you will eat more. Our knowledge of what excites taste buds, and what will entice us to eat more and buy more often, means that most coffee shop menus resemble dessert menus. Thanks to the wonders of modern food chemistry, some foods are so intoxicatingly easy to overeat that it becomes almost impossible to put them down, even if they seem born of the lab and not the kitchen. If you have looked at the ingredient list on a bag of neon-orange Cheetos, you know what I mean.

From its foodie roots in home economics class, the science of nutrition gained credibility by dissecting the human diet into the study of single, isolated nutrients. This was an important step; understanding how nutrients affect the human body has allowed us to move toward therapeutic approaches to nutrition that bring true healing. It is because of this research that I can share how certain isolated nutrients—and combinations of nutrients—might influence inflammation in the body.

However, when we study isolated nutrients such as vitamin C or saturated fats, applying that research to real life can get a bit messy. Most of us consume a variety of foods with a complex mix of nutrients, sometimes making it difficult to tease out the true impact of any one substance. However, this kind of research does help food manufacturers influence our purchasing decisions. They can make Cheetos fat-free if that is what we are worried about as consumers. And they can add prebiotics to fruit snacks, but adding fibre to candy does not change the fact that it is candy.

You may be thinking, *Can anyone just tell me if it is okay to eat coconut oil?* If you ask ten health professionals, you will probably get ten different answers based on their interpretation of the research and clinical experience. To make matters worse, every day there is a new headline about what will or will not harm you if you eat it. It is confusing and counterproductive.

We eat *food*, not nutrients. It is the *pattern* of how you eat over time that matters more than a single meal or food choice. Therefore, until the science catches up, most of us might be better off focusing on the *type* of food we eat instead of squinting at the nutrition label for sodium or fibre content. Instead, focus on whole foods and just try to eat more plants.

## Why Pick Plants?

Modern life stretches our bodies and minds to their limits. We demand more of ourselves than ever before, and our bodies are erupting in exhaustion, gut issues, and chronic disease. Nearly one third of Canadians have diabetes or a pre-diabetic metabolism. Autoimmunity is on the rise. So is digestive disease: about 15 percent of us have irritable bowel syndrome. The connection? A chronic inflammatory response and the underlying factors driving it, such as poor diet, stress, and an unbalanced gut flora.

Inflammation is supposed to help protect us from infection or injury; however, the less we sleep, the more stressed we are, and the less we nourish our bodies with whole foods, the more our *lifestyle* becomes the source of injury. This injury occurs on the cellular level and affects every system of your body. In chronic inflammation, your immune system loses its delicate balance between tolerance and action. However, this imbalance can be restored. Make no mistake, your body has the remarkable capacity to heal if you provide it with the tools it needs.

To thrive in today's world, our bodies need nutrient-dense plant foods that supercharge our batteries. I have lived this shift: early in my twenties, I could get away with a diet filled with french fries and still feel good. In my thirties, the hormonal shifts of pregnancy—and the sleepless nights and stressful days that followed—initiated me into the realities of digestive trouble and chronic inflammation. As life ramped up with each passing year, I found that I felt lethargic, foggy, and unmotivated when eating a typical healthy diet. Then I got serious about a whole food, plant-based diet. I created meals with nutrient-dense plants, started to lose my taste for hyper-processed snacks, and began craving *my kind of food*. When I pile on the plants, I feel vibrant, positive, and well even though, technically, I have inflammatory issues. In fact, eating this way helps me minimize the impact that digestive troubles have on my life so that most of the time I do not really notice them.

All that I have learned on my own health journey has helped me deepen my role as a guide for others on their road to wellness. I know what it feels like to be unwell. To feel like there are not enough hours in the day. In addition, I have learned how to make feeding myself well a priority, no matter what.

I am a registered dietitian with an active private practice, and I find that most of my clients come to me already very informed about nutrition. They know the difference between flaxseed and chia seeds, and yet there is often something missing. Sometimes it is cooking more instead of grabbing takeout food or adding more protein to their plates. Often, what is missing is a commitment to putting a bounty of plants on their plates in place of the usual starch-heavy meal or sugary snacks. When you begin to make this shift, it is incredible how good you can feel.

What makes plants so powerful? Their physical structure, packed with water and fibre, along with their unique density of anti-inflammatory compounds nourishes your body and minimizes the damaging effects of daily life. Whole plant foods help you fight inflammation in a number of ways by:

- Increasing your intake of anti-inflammatory compounds like omega-3 fatty acids, flavonoids, and fibre
- Helping you move away from the high-sugar, high–saturated fat, low-fibre eating pattern that is tied to chronic inflammation and disease
- Helping you find a comfortable and healthful weight and support stable blood sugars

- Promoting the growth of beneficial gut microbes that help keep inflammation at bay and help your digestive system to function optimally

Your body is designed to eat an abundance of whole plant foods. By giving your body what it needs, it will do a better job of healing. You will subject your cells to less diet-induced oxidative stress. Nutrient-dense plants will support your body's own natural antioxidant and detoxification pathways. An anti-inflammatory lifestyle will support your immune system and help restore balance within your inflammatory response. Instead of taking handfuls of supplements to try to make up for a less-than-ideal diet, make food your medicine and load your plate with plants.

## Just Eat More Plants

There are few absolutes in nutrition, but every single one of us can benefit from eating more plants. Regardless of how you choose to eat, this is the one rule we all need to live by. If you love bacon, have a little less and be sure to eat more plants. If you eat a vegan diet, watch the cookies and be sure to eat more plants.

Although the dietary tribes will not always admit this, what they have in common *is* plants. A truly Paleo plate? A little bit of animal protein and 75 percent plants. A whole food vegan diet? All plants. Even ketogenic diets, when done well, can include many low-carbohydrate plants.

Life demands more from us than ever before. Stress, poor food choices, and inactivity are all too common, and they are saddling us with chronic inflammatory issues like metabolic syndrome, digestive trouble, and autoimmunity. Food is often a big part of our ills . . . and anti-inflammatory, plant-based eating is a big part of the solution. However, what that looks like for you is your decision.

If you want to go fully plant-based, good on you. I am all for it! It is an incredible way to live, and I have a chapter that will help guide you through the transition. However, if you cannot imagine a life without a burger, do not think that a *plant-centred* life is not for you. The more we pile our plate with plants, the better it is for our bodies, our ecosystem, and our pocketbooks. Eat the recipes in this book as often as you can. Start slowly and see where it takes you.

Wherever you are in your wellness journey, adopting a more plant-based, anti-inflammatory diet will help you get to where you are going. Stay open-minded and be gentle with yourself, as making change is never a straight line. There is no right or wrong here. Have fun in the kitchen and enjoy what you eat! I am honoured that you have chosen this book to help you eat more plants.

## Vibrant Living

True wellness, particularly when your intention is to calm inflammation, is a way of living as much as it is a way of eating. The thoughts we think and the way we move our bodies have just as much of an impact as how we choose to eat. As you explore preparing more anti-inflammatory meals for yourself, consider how the following principles can help guide you in building a truly vibrant life.

### LISTEN TO YOUR BODY

There is no one right way to eat; we all need to find the way of eating that helps us feel our best. You can do that by observing how the food you eat makes you feel: physically, emotionally, and psychologically.

### GET PLANT POWERED

Plant-based foods are nature's nutrient-dense gift to you. Eating more plants is a way of nourishing your body, respecting the impact that your food choices have on others, and treading more lightly on the planet.

### PRACTISE SELF-LOVE

Perfection is a myth; be gentle with your intentions to eat well and give yourself the flexibility to choose foods that nourish your soul as well as your body. There is no right or wrong. Work toward disconnecting your self-worth from your food choices. At the end of the day, it is just food.

### EMBRACE AN ATTITUDE OF MORE, NOT LESS

Focusing on eating less, or choosing certain foods less often, leads to a sense of deprivation, loss, and anxiety. Instead, focus on what to do *more* often. Eat more plants. Drink more water. Cook more often. Make eating well a positive, joyful process.

### CREATE SPACE FOR CHANGE

Making change takes effort. Create the space in your life to allow it to happen. Release commitments that are not important to you so you can shop and cook. Spend time moving your body. Carve out time for stillness and be mindful. Unplug from your screens daily and let your mind wander and be at rest. Make sleep a priority.

### KEEP IT SIMPLE

Choose single-ingredient foods more often—eat real food, not hyper-processed approximations of it. Instead of ordering takeout, get your hands dirty in the kitchen. Reconnect to where your food comes from and grow something on a windowsill or patio or in your backyard. Spend as much time outside as humanly possible and breathe deeply.

## FIND YOUR INNER STRENGTH

Your body has the remarkable capacity to repair and rebuild. This ability is sewn into your DNA and is an integral component of life itself. Know that no matter where you are starting from, you can support your body in healing and find a new vitality. Nourishing yourself well will help you tap into your potential in other aspects of your life with a newfound energy.

## About This Book

I hope that *Eat More Plants* will inspire you to cook more plant-based meals and help you understand just how powerful plant-based living can be in fighting inflammation and feeling more energized every day. The easiest way to start is to simply head into the kitchen and get cooking! If you are looking to immerse yourself in anti-inflammatory living, I have created a 21-day meal plan (page 64) to help provide a little structure in your food choices. It is a great way to guide your exploration of plant-based living or to help accelerate healing when you are new to this lifestyle.

Our knowledge of the intricacies of chronic inflammation and its connection to diet continue to evolve. Therefore, *Eat More Plants* begins with a reminder of how prevalent chronic inflammation is in our society, and how food can create change. If this book is part of your transition toward a totally plant-based diet, I have included all the nutrition information and everything else you need to know in Chapter 3 to help make that transition as smooth as possible.

When you are ready to dive in and start playing in the kitchen, I encourage you to do a big shop so that you will have all the basics at hand. Stock your kitchen with healthy plant-based foods and the right tools and you will find that cooking is a breeze. Chapter 4 will show you exactly which tools and staples I keep in my home kitchen.

All of the recipes in *Eat More Plants* are vegan and gluten-free. That means there is no meat, fish, dairy, eggs, and wheat—not even a bit of honey. Why? So that as many people as possible can benefit from the recipes I have created. No matter what kind of eating plan you follow, there is food in this book to help you make your life more deliciously vibrant. *Eat More Plants* is designed for real life. I hope that it will inspire you to get cooking with plants in new, creative ways that will make eating your vegetables a joy. Rabbit food this is *not*.

Life is busy. You do not need to spend hours in the kitchen to create nourishing meals. As an entrepreneur and a mom of two children, I do not have all day to make dinner happen. Keeping in mind how busy we all are these days, most recipes in *Eat More Plants* can be made in thirty to forty-five minutes. As much as I love to cook, feeding my family on a weekday is all about getting it done. Therefore, to save you time, you will not see a lot of roasted ingredients or casseroles in these recipes.

Of course, the first time you make a new recipe, it will always take a bit longer. I love exploring new recipes on the weekend to decide whether I want them in my weeknight rotation. Moreover, I am not going to lie—eating many vegetables means a lot of chopping, but it is well worth it. When time is tight in the evening, a bit of weekend chopping can help you streamline meal prep, making many of the meals in this book ring in at the twenty-minute mark. You can also find many presliced and prechopped veggies at the supermarket these days; they are a great way to save a bit of extra time.

If you are new to cooking, it is worth following the recipes to the letter at first. Otherwise, consider these recipes a guide. Most of them can be adapted to account for any intolerances or preferences you might have. If you do not love kale, spinach can work. Allergic to peanuts? Try almond butter or sunflower seed butter. Baking recipes will be a bit more difficult to adapt, since each flour and milk alternative behaves differently, but my bread recipe is a great place to explore different flour options.

If you do not follow a gluten-free diet, you can substitute gluten-containing ingredients like soy sauce or regular whole-grain bread in the recipes, but I encourage you to explore using more gluten-free grains as well. While whole wheat can be healthy if you tolerate it, there is also a world of nutritious grains, nuts, and seeds out there, like millet or almond flour, that we can all benefit from eating more often.

Although these recipes are designed to be as inclusive as possible and are suitable for many therapeutic diets, I felt it was important to avoid nutrition information on the recipes. That may seem like an unusual choice coming from a dietitian, but the whole point of this book is to free you from worrying about the minutiae of nutrition so you can get on with enjoying *life*.

All of these recipes are health promoting. All of the fats are healthy fats, and even the desserts are much lower in sugar than most and are made with nourishing ingredients. A little salt is not an issue in a whole food diet. Most of the sodium in our diets comes from processed, packaged, and restaurant foods. I always cook with unsalted beans and canned tomato products; if using salted versions of these staples, you may want to reduce the salt in the recipe. Rest assured that there is nothing contained within these pages that the average eater should be worried about. However, if you are on a therapeutic diet restriction for insulin use or blood pressure, bring this book to your dietitian and he or she can help you adapt or select the best recipes for your needs.

Otherwise, it is all good.

# Eat like you love your body, not like you hate it.

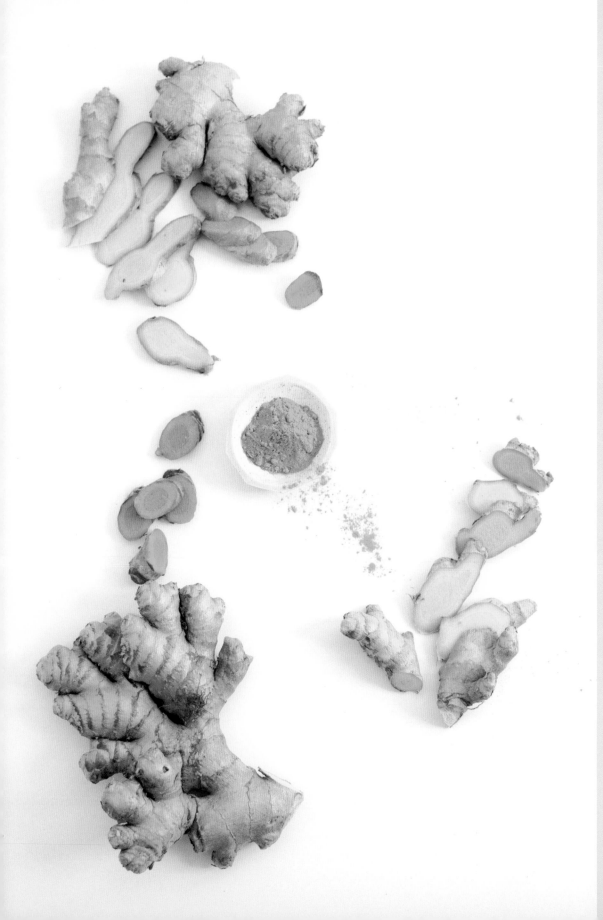

# 1

# Understanding Inflammation and Why It Matters

I have been practising anti-inflammatory nutrition for a decade; what was once a very edgy, controversial topic in wellness is now widely accepted. Hundreds of thousands of studies later, we understand that chronic inflammatory responses are harmful to human health. Because of this, it can be easy to forget that you actually need inflammation. In fact, you cannot live without it. Inflammation is your immune system's first line of defence in the war against infection and injury. If you cut yourself in the kitchen, or hurt your ankle on a run, inflammation is your body's way of healing you.

Unlike the way your immune system makes antibodies that respond to specific threats, inflammation is non-specific and initiated within seconds. That redness on your skin and the heat you feel when you get hurt are your blood vessels dilating. Neutrophils and mast cells—immune cells that are present throughout your body—cause blood vessels to dilate when they sense damage by releasing chemicals like histamines. Histamines also make blood vessels leakier so the immune cells can squeeze through vessel walls to reach your injury. Your immune cells coordinate this dance with expert efficiency, not only cleaning up the damage but also chemically coordinating with fellow mediators of immune function, such as cytokines, to organize the inflammatory defence. Then, just as expertly, when the infection is eradicated and any damage is repaired, the immune system lets the active immune cells die off and the inflammatory response is over.

That is inflammation at its best, a process referred to as *acute* inflammation. You have an injury, inflammation fixes it, and then your immune system returns to its peaceful baseline. Except, sometimes, it does not work that way.

## Acute versus Chronic Inflammation

You might find it surprising, but researchers do not know *exactly* how acute inflammation develops into a prolonged, or *chronic*, response. Without a doubt, inflammation keeps firing because it senses a problem, but how our immune system loses its balance between tolerance and action is not fully understood. The trouble with chronic inflammation is that it further damages the cells and can become a self-perpetuating cycle that is difficult to shift unless you ramp up your anti-inflammatory efforts.

The chronic inflammatory response is generally carried out by different cells from those that operate during acute inflammation, typically macrophages and T lymphocytes. As these immune cells perform their inflammatory functions, they produce enzymes and substances called cytokines that further injure the tissues around them. Therefore, as the immune system fights off some unknown aggressor, it is causing damage that might require its own inflammatory repair response.

Within all of this inflammatory chaos, anti-inflammatory messages are still being produced by the immune system. There just may not be enough of them to oppose the stronger pro-inflammatory response. The million-dollar question? How to amplify anti-inflammatory pathways so the inflammatory response subsides. As it turns out, nutrition is a powerful tool to do just that.

Here is where the science of nutrition has really evolved. Food is so much more than its calories, or the milligrams of sodium it contains. *Food is information*. Every component of the food you eat, or the absence of critical components you should be eating, sends messages to your genes, the energy factories in your cells known as mitochondria, and your immune system.

When I work with clients, I am always looking for places to swap pro-inflammatory choices for anti-inflammatory ones. Clients often come to me with very starch-heavy diets, filled with takeout sandwiches, café muffins, and crackers. Eating a lot of refined flour means few phytochemicals and little fibre to help fight inflammation and feed beneficial gut bacteria. It also means higher blood sugar levels and insulin release, which promotes inflammatory response. I love helping others find nutrient-dense swaps for their everyday staples, such as snacking on kohlrabi instead of crackers, or creating easy homemade muffins that pack in plenty of plants. My clients are always so surprised by how such small, positive shifts can make such a large impact on how they feel.

## How Do I Know If I Have Inflammation?

Since we are not all walking around with our heads on fire, it is not always easy to spot inflammation. Typically, in nutrition practice I will assume some level of inflammation based on the presence of an inflammation-associated condition that can include:

- Obesity and cardiometabolic conditions: type 2 diabetes, heart disease, cancer
- Arthritis and chronic pain conditions: fibromyalgia, rheumatoid arthritis, chronic fatigue syndrome
- Psychological well-being: depression, anxiety
- Autoimmune disease: Hashimoto's thyroiditis, lupus, celiac disease, multiple sclerosis
- Digestive conditions: Crohn's disease, ulcerative colitis, irritable bowel syndrome
- Skin conditions: severe acne, eczema, psoriasis, rosacea

You may have noticed how prevalent these conditions are and, by default, how many of us probably need to do some anti-inflammatory work. If you have any one of these concerns and are not currently feeling well, you are likely battling chronic inflammation. To add fuel to the fire, people under stress will have greater inflammation because cortisol, the hormone of chronic stress, increases inflammatory response. As the inflammatory response gets stronger, it further increases cortisol levels in a nasty feedback loop.

There are tests available to determine your level of chronic inflammation. The best understood is a blood marker called C-reactive protein (CRP). You can ask your family doctor to test your CRP levels. CRP is not specific to one disease, but if your levels are high enough to test positive, you definitely want to start taking nutritional steps aimed at lowering inflammation.

More commonly used in naturopathy or gastroenterology, you can also test for a stool marker called fecal calprotectin, which rises when inflammation is active in the gut. Someone with a flare-up of Crohn's disease, for example, will have high fecal calprotectin levels. Your doctor may also look at liver function or specific inflammatory markers like tumor necrosis factor alpha (TNF-a) if the situation warrants it.

If you are not feeling well, I cannot stress enough how important it is to get a thorough checkup from your doctor to rule out any conditions that are clearly in need of medical treatment. You do not want to fall down the rabbit hole of relying on Google and missing a key diagnosis. Celiac disease is a classic example of this: if you remove gluten from your diet and feel better, you might miss the fact that you have a serious autoimmune disease. Even more, you need to be consistently eating gluten in order for celiac testing to be accurate.

Once your doctor has decided whether there is, or is not, an applicable diagnosis and treatment, you can take matters into your own hands and start working with nutrition. Embrace an active wellness mindset, but do yourself a favour and always get a thorough checkup first.

## Eating Well Is a Lifestyle, Not a Quick Fix

When I review my clients' eating histories, I am more concerned with the pattern of how someone eats than whether that person eats *perfectly* at every meal. It is an important distinction to make, because in our rigid diet mindsets, going off plan for a single meal or day is often considered bad and requires a detox to make up for it.

The good news is that your body does not work that way, even if your brain does. The brain tends to like black-or-white, on-or-off behaviours. It also loves a quick fix, which helps explain why we can get overly concerned with certain superfoods at the expense of how we eat throughout the day. For example, if you eat a diet devoid of fruits and vegetables, you really cannot make up for that with a teaspoon of greens powder in your yogurt. Sorry, but it is just not the same thing.

Similarly, as we strive to further our understanding of the anti-inflammatory components of food, research is calling our previous assumptions into question. Turmeric is a perfect example of this. Turmeric really is the superstar that started this wave of investigation into the anti-inflammatory effects of plant foods. Modern researchers discovered turmeric while noting a decrease in Alzheimer's disease in people living in the Indian subcontinent, where daily turmeric consumption generally outpaces that in the rest of the world. Researchers believed that a molecule called curcumin was the active compound in turmeric spice, launching thousands of studies on curcumin over the years.

In the lab, it seemed at first that curcumin could do no wrong, but human trials have been less certain. How could this be? Turmeric is still one of my favourite spices, and I will always advocate for it in an anti-inflammatory diet. In fact, human trials have shown its effectiveness in osteoarthritis, pain, and metabolic syndrome. However, there is much to learn about how turmeric works in the body and whom it will work for.

A couple of important things are happening here: the first is that we have isolated a component of turmeric, curcumin, that had never been consumed as an isolated compound historically. When making a curry, we use ground or fresh turmeric, not curcumin. In addition, curcumin is not the only active compound in turmeric: there are other related compounds, in addition to essential oils and proteins that might be helpful. The notoriously poor absorption of curcumin, and the speed with which our bodies break it down, has led to conflicting research results. We are learning that curcumin may be having an effect on the immune tissues of the gut itself, instead of being active only once absorbed into the bloodstream. The second issue complicating our understanding of turmeric is that we often expect food to perform in the same way as a drug would. But food and drugs just are not the same. Pharmaceutical drugs contain isolated compounds at concentrations many times greater than those found in plants, so that they will have an immediate effect.

For example, aspirin is an anti-inflammatory medication that evolved from the discovery of salicylic acid in white willow bark.

Just as you would not expect a single plate of broccoli to cure cancer, you cannot expect to eat turmeric once and eliminate inflammation. If you eat meaningful amounts of turmeric daily, as part of a healthy anti-inflammatory diet, you will feel different. Over time, inflammation will subside. Most of my clients have been able to calm their inflammation, at least partially, through diet and lifestyle changes. Does it happen overnight? No, and some clients have to adopt more intensive regimes than others do. Someone whose inflammation is presenting as mild eczema will likely have a much easier time than someone who has suffered from autoimmunity for years.

I genuinely believe that research, as it progresses and is more capable of analyzing the complexity of human nutrition, will come to explain how eating whole foods in specific dietary patterns works. Until then, I am content to eat yummy, nutrient-dense food that makes me feel good. So often, my clients come to me with a great deal of nervousness about which foods will be therapeutic or harmful to their conditions; however, when they start eating a wide variety of nutrient-dense plant foods, they are so surprised at how good they can feel without getting overly rigid in their eating habits. Even if they have an occasional beer or scoop of ice cream. When you are consistently eating whole plant foods, it almost feels as if you are creating greater resiliency within your body that allows you to make the occasional less healthful choice without feeling unwell.

## Should I Take Supplements?

As a dietitian, I believe in a "food first" approach to nutrition. Most of what we need can be supplied by a healthy, whole food diet. Anyone who tells you otherwise probably has some supplements to sell. However, I also believe in the potential of intelligently applied supplementation. At specific life stages (such as pregnancy) or times of stress or disease, certain vitamins, minerals, or other natural compounds are critical to help improve the resilience and strength of your body so you can thrive.

When I am going through a high-intensity period in my life, I ramp up my supplement efforts to help me push through and incorporate adaptogenic herbs and a multivitamin. When all is calm, I prefer a minimal approach to supplementation that includes the following anti-inflammatory basics.

## VITAMIN D3

Vitamin D3 is one of a few supplements that can be recommended for everyone. It is critical to human health and immune function and relatively absent from our food supply, so that even breastfed babies need to supplement. The reason for this is that we make vitamin D in our skin, upon exposure to ultraviolet (UV) light. Living further away from the equator, leading indoor lifestyles, and wearing sunscreen (as we should!) all diminish our body's ability to create vitamin D. Vitamin D insufficiency is rather common; ideally, your physician will test your levels to see how much you need to take. In the absence of individualized guidance, taking 1000 IU of vitamin D3 in the summer and 2000 IU in the winter is a safe, conservative dose for adults.

## OMEGA-3 FATTY ACIDS

If you have significant inflammation, I am also a great believer in adding a plant-based source of long-chain omega-3 fatty acids as a supplement to, not in place of, omega-3-rich plant foods. Because our bodies may not convert alpha-linolenic acid (ALA), the main plant omega-3 found in seeds, to long-chain eicosapentaenoic acid (EPA) or docosahexaenoic acid (DHA) efficiently, consuming EPA and DHA may really give your anti-inflammatory efforts a boost. Plant-based versions of these supplements have come a long way and have much higher potency, and are more affordable, than early versions. See Favourite Suppliers (page 279) for recommendations.

## PROBIOTICS

I am also a big believer in taking quality probiotics when chronic inflammation and digestive trouble exist. Because of the critical role that gut bacteria play in supporting the immune system, and the ability for inflammation to originate in the gut, many of us would benefit from a daily shot of good human-strain bacteria. I have seen the right probiotic literally change guts—and lives—but there is considerable variation in the quality and efficacy of probiotics on the market. See Favourite Suppliers (page 279) for recommendations.

In Chapter 3, I address supplementation for those who follow a 100 percent plant-based diet. For all other supplements, work with an experienced health care practitioner to determine what will benefit you the most. Whereas the right supplement can do a world of good, the wrong one can be a waste of money or even harmful. I would rather you spend your hard-earned money on good food than buy supplements you do not need.

Wellness is not won or lost on a single meal.

## Creating an Anti-Inflammatory Eating Plan

Choosing a more anti-inflammatory way of eating is about choosing a way of eating you can maintain for life. It is both prevention and nutritional therapy, rolled into one. My favourite part of anti-inflammatory eating is that it can be nutritious *and* pleasurable. Most importantly, anti-inflammatory foods should all taste good! Because eating food without enjoyment deprives you of the deep soul nourishment that a good meal can offer.

When I think about designing an anti-inflammatory diet, I focus on five outcomes:

1.  Maintaining blood sugar balance
2.  Improving the quality of fats consumed
3.  Improving intake of antioxidant and anti-inflammatory compounds
4.  Providing nutrition to support your gut–immune system balance
5.  Being mindful of food's impact on gut bacteria

## Blood Sugars: All about Balance

Glucose, a simple, one-molecule sugar, is the energy currency of our body. Whenever we eat carbohydrates, they are broken down into their basic sugars and absorbed into our bloodstream, where they raise our blood sugar levels. When that happens, the pancreas secretes insulin. These basic sugars cannot do much if they remain in our bloodstream; in fact, they can actually cause harm by sticking to proteins and altering their function. This is called glycation, and the resulting molecules are known as advanced glycation end products (AGEs), which may impair metabolic processes, leading to inflammation and tissue damage.

Instead of staying in the bloodstream, you want the sugars to go into your cells so they can be used as a sort of kindling for producing energy. Sugars cannot just waltz into your cells on their own. Insulin is a hormone that works like a key to unlock the cells and let those sweet little sugars in. You *want* this to occur. Without this process, your cells (and you) would starve awash in a sea of food. However, the way in which this sugar delivery happens matters. If you eat a handful of candy or a cinnamon roll, a large amount of sugars enters your bloodstream quite quickly. Having high blood sugar levels is a pro-inflammatory state: it causes acute oxidative stress and increases the expression of pro-inflammatory mediators like TNF-a and interleukin 6 (IL-6). Do this occasionally, and your body can handle it. However, if this is your daily routine, you will increase your levels of chronic inflammation and probably not feel so great.

Therefore, to keep inflammation at bay, we aim to keep blood sugars moderate. How do we do this? By eating more whole plant foods, which by their very definition are not filled with sugar or highly processed, rapidly digested starch. In addition, they are structurally complex and take time to digest and absorb, which further moderates blood sugar rise. Because of this, you do not need to avoid fruit because it contains sugar. Same thing with carbohydrates in general. There is a big biological difference between eating brown rice and a loaf of highly processed rice bread. In some of my recipes, you will find I use small amounts of cane sugar. In a high-fibre, plant-based recipe, a half or one teaspoon of sugar to balance flavours will not spike blood sugars, so you do not need to worry. It is the total effect of the meal that matters most.

Some of us, such as those with type 2 diabetes, may need to lower the amount of carbohydrate we eat to help keep our blood sugars in check; for the rest of us, shifting to whole foods can greatly improve blood sugar stability. Because we are all so individual, interpreting the science of nutrition can be a bit complex; however, no matter what type of eating pattern you favour, my favourite rule still applies. Eat more plants!

## Think Quality, Not Quantity, When It Comes to Fats

It is time to acknowledge that our fear of fats was a big mistake. There was a time when we thought that dietary fats made you fat. In addition, we thought saturated fat was a heart attack waiting to happen. Our shelves were flooded with fat-free versions of our favourite foods: ice cream, cookies, candy, and snacks. We believed that the label "fat-free" meant we could eat with abandon. We did not stop to think about what those foods were actually filled with: refined flours and sugars. This is an example of nutritionism at its worst: we got hung up on a single nutrient and ended up eating fewer nutrient-dense whole foods and getting much sicker as a result.

Nutritional science is not without its flaws. We develop an idea based on observations, test it numerous times in increasingly complex ways, and develop advice based on what the science shows at the time. Of course, as our understanding of the body, and how food affects the body, becomes more sophisticated, we often need to course correct. So yes, we thought fat was bad (so fattening!), but that was a couple of decades ago.

Like so many things in life—from relationships to clothing—quality, not quantity, counts most. This is especially true with respect to inflammation.

Most lipids released by the immune system are derivatives of arachidonic acid. Arachidonic acid is an omega-6 fatty acid that is critical for good health; it is the precursor for both pro- and anti-inflammatory compounds in the body. Interestingly, although preformed arachidonic acid comes from animal products, your body can build arachadonic acid from plant-sourced omega-6 linoleic acid just fine.

It is not possible to create a diet free of omega-6 fats, nor should you want to. This is an important point when we talk about inflammation: it is essential that you consume some omega-6 fatty acids. Because we have associated our excessive omega-6 fat intake as driving pro-inflammatory pathways, it can be easy to assume that all omega-6 fats are bad. However, some omega-6 fatty acids, such as the gamma linolenic acid found in hemp seeds, are thought to be anti-inflammatory, particularly when paired with omega-3 fats. This perfect pairing is one of the reasons why omega-3-rich hemp seeds are one of my favourite anti-inflammatory foods!

Just like life, nutrition is not black or white. It is all about balance.

## Understanding the Balance Between Omega-3 Fatty Acids and Omega-6 Fatty Acids

We should focus our discussion of omega-6 fats on the fact that we typically lack *balance* in our modern diets. It is thought that we evolved on a 1:1 ratio of omega-6 fats to omega-3 fats, and now that ratio hovers closer to 16:1. Eat too many omega-6 fats and you may end up promoting pro-inflammatory pathways fuelled by omega-6 fats instead of anti-inflammatory pathways driven by omega-3 fats. This happens because omega-6 fatty acids compete for the same pathways as omega-3 fatty acids. If you eat a lot of omega-6 fats, the omega-3 fats cannot compete with their numbers.

While research is still debating ideal ratios, few argue with the fact that we greatly overconsume omega-6 fats in comparison to our dietary need for them. In addition, high consumption of omega-6 fats appears to hinder the production of the active forms of omega-3, EPA and DHA, from commonly consumed plant forms of omega-3 fats.

Why is this imbalance so common? Because practically everything we eat in our modern food world is laden with omega-6 fats. Commodity oils like sunflower, soy, and corn that are high in omega-6 fats are inexpensive and used to produce most of the hyper-processed foodstuff we eat instead of eating real home-cooked food. Perfect examples are the muffins you buy as a snack at the coffee shop. The store-bought pizza you grab for a quick dinner. Or the salty snacks you munch on instead of veggies. In addition, our methods of industrial animal production render meat and dairy packed with the inflammatory stuff; where animals were once grass fed, they are now grain fed to help them put on weight more profitably. We typically focus on saturated fat in animal foods, but in fact we should be talking about their omega-6 fat content, too.

Therefore, we have a food system pouring on the omega-6 fats, whereas omega-3 fats are found in just a handful of oily, cold-water fish and seeds. Even with the advent of chia puddings, we have a long way to go!

## Food Sources of Omega-3 Fats and Omega-6 Fats

It is important to note that no food contains just one type of fat; real foods are a complex assortment of nutrients, fats included. However, I typically recommend that you avoid concentrated sources of omega-6 fats and reach for more omega-3-rich foods. Here are the highest sources of both.

### BEST PLANT SOURCES OF OMEGA-3 FATS (EAT MORE)

- Ground flaxseed and cold-pressed flaxseed oil
- Hemp seeds and cold-pressed hemp seed oil
- Chia seeds
- Walnuts
- Microalgae oil (plant-source EPA and DHA available as a supplement)

### PLANT SOURCES OF OMEGA-6 FATS (EAT FEWER)

- Corn oil
- Cottonseed oil
- Peanut oil
- Safflower oil (except high-oleic varieties)
- Sunflower oil (except high-oleic varieties)
- Soybean oil
- Grapeseed oil

Every omega-3-rich plant food also contains some omega-6 fats, as do a host of other healthful whole plant foods such as sunflower and pumpkin seeds, nuts, and even acai berries. Therefore, by removing omega-6-rich cooking oils from your diet in favour of other nutrient-dense whole food sources of omega-6 fats, you will bring the ratio of omega-3 to omega-6 back into better balance. Every nut and seed you consume will also provide a bit of omega-6, so you never need to worry if you are getting enough. Remember, we want some omega-6 fats in our diet . . . we simply need fewer of them than we typically consume.

An anti-inflammatory diet focuses on eating foods that are a good source of omega-3 fats and minimizing concentrated sources of omega-6 fats. I say "concentrated" because I really want you to eat whole soy, nuts, and seeds even though they all have some omega-6 fats, because they are not 100 percent omega-6 fats. These plant foods have balanced nutrition, providing other healthy fats along with minerals, fibre, and protein. Avoiding corn, soy, and seed oils for cooking is easy when there are great alternatives like extra-virgin olive oil and avocado oil.

## The Other Omega: Omega-9 Oleic Acid

I am obsessed with olive oil. It is because of my Mediterranean roots to be sure, but also because the research supports my single-mindedness. The primary fat in olive oil is called oleic acid, which is a monounsaturated fat found in a variety of plant and animal sources. Unlike omega-3 and omega-6 fats, it is not deemed *essential* because the body can produce it. Monounsaturated fat is the prototypical heart-healthy fat; it is also the one fat with almost no controversy surrounding it, even after all these years of research. So, making it a mainstay of your anti-inflammatory diet is a good idea.

If you have heard of omega-9 fats, it is oleic acid being talked about—so ditch the omega-9 supplement and just pour on the olive oil. Oleic acid is thought to be at least inflammation neutral, if not anti-inflammatory. Make extra-virgin olive oil your primary cooking oil and be sure to enjoy these other foods that are rich in healthy omega-9 fats:

- Almonds and almond oil
- Avocados and avocado oil
- Cashews and cashew oil
- Olives

Although it is true that dietary fats have more energy (calories) than proteins or carbohydrates, it is their impact on metabolism that matters most. Importantly, fats do not raise blood sugars, and they help improve the absorption of fat-soluble nutrients, including so many of the anti-inflammatory phytochemicals found in fruits and vegetables. What's more, fat makes food taste good. The reason why restaurant food tastes the way it does is fat and salt. So, embracing a bit more healthy fat in your cooking will ensure that your deeply nourishing meals also taste amazing.

## The Power of Plants: Improving Intake of Anti-Inflammatory Plant Compounds

It is easy to be hung up on what to avoid, so it is worth mentioning all of the amazing compounds, known as phytochemicals, that plant foods contain that can help you fight inflammation. *Phyto* means plant, and *phytochemicals* simply means chemical compounds produced by plants.

You do not have a daily requirement for phytochemicals in the same way you do for vitamin C. However, phytochemicals have known positive impacts on human metabolism, so consuming phytochemical-rich plants daily is in your body's best interest.

Some phytochemicals, like anthocyanins or zeaxanthin, are pigments that give plants their colour. Other phytochemicals *are* nutrients, like beta-carotene, which is a form of vitamin A. Many of these other phytochemicals serve as the plant's immune system. They help defend the plant against infection or disease and can do the same for you.

The name of the phytochemical game is resilience. Your body is designed to mop up damage and repair itself, but modern life can sometimes dole out more than we bargained for. Every day, the act of living, breathing, thinking, and eating creates oxidative and inflammatory damage that phytochemicals help prevent and repair. The more you eat whole plant foods, the more you flood your system with compounds that help protect you against the damage of everyday living and provide powerful information to your body that helps cool chronic inflammation. For example, beets contain phytochemicals called betalains that are thought to inhibit inflammation. In addition, they are a source of beneficial nitrates that can be transformed into nitric oxide in the body. Nitric oxide dilates blood vessels, lowering blood pressure and maybe even improving athletic performance. It may inhibit excessive inflammation and help kill bacteria that the immune system has gobbled up. You will never look at a bowl of borscht in the same way.

An anti-inflammatory eating plan puts whole plant foods, particularly fruits and vegetables, at the centre of your plate. Because this plan is not just about what you are *not* eating, it is about providing an abundance of protective factors that create resilient cells and strong immune systems.

## Top 25 Anti-Inflammatory Plant-Based Foods

I want you to eat a diet with a wide variety of plant foods for better health and vitality. Of course, it does not hurt to play favourites a little. Whether for their concentration of anti-inflammatory compounds or the strength of research behind them, here are my favourite anti-inflammatory plant foods that make up the heart of an anti-inflammatory eating plan.

## FRUITS

### Apples

Key benefits: low glycemic impact, phytochemicals (quercetin, anthocyanins in red varieties, catechins, chlorogenic acid), fibre

How to boost use: grate into porridge or smoothies, bake with spices for a light dessert, chop into salads and enjoy as snacks

### Berries (blackberries, blueberries, strawberries, raspberries) and cherries

Key benefits: low glycemic impact, phytochemicals (anthocyanins, salicylic acid, ellagic acid), fibre

How to boost use: snack on fresh berries, toss on cereals or salads, stir into chia puddings and non-dairy yogurt or blend into smoothies

## VEGETABLES

### Avocados

Key benefits: oleic acid, fibre, phytochemicals (lutein, zeaxanthin, catechins)

How to boost use: blend into creamy dips, add to smoothies, slice into sandwiches, use atop salads and grain bowls

### Beets

Key benefits: phytochemicals (betalains, betaine), minerals (magnesium, manganese, folate)

How to boost use: roast and use as a side dish or atop grain bowls; grate or spiralize into salads; ferment into pickles; purée cooked beets into smoothies, muffins, dips, and hot beverages; add to juicing mix

### Broccoli

Key benefits: vitamins (K, C, B including folate, A), phytochemicals (indole-3-carbinol, sulforaphane), low glycemic impact, fibre

How to boost use: steam or stir-fry, make chopped broccoli salads, layer roasted broccoli into wraps, eat with a dip as a snack, grate into broccoli "rice"

### Fermented vegetables (kimchi, sauerkraut, lacto-fermented vegetables)

Key benefits: beneficial live microorganisms, organic acids, enzymes, L-glutamine in cabbage-based ferments

How to boost use: use as a condiment on sandwiches, grain bowls, and salads; add to savoury pancakes or waffles

### Garlic

Key benefits: phytochemicals (diallyl sulfide, alliin, 1,2-vinyldithiin, thiacremonone), prebiotic fructans

How to boost use: keep roasted garlic on hand to spread on sandwiches and add to dips and sauces; add small amounts of raw garlic to dressings; use in soups, stir-fries, and sautés

### Greens (arugula, beet greens, chard, collard greens, dandelion, kale, purslane)

Key benefits: vitamins (K, C, B including folate, A), phytochemicals (glucosinolates, indole-3-carbinol, sulforaphane, kaempferol, lutein, zeaxanthin, quercetin, chlorophyll)

How to boost use: add to juicing mixes or blend into smoothies; use in salads and sautés or toss with pasta; add to sandwiches; blend into dips and pesto; use collard leaves as sandwich wraps

### Mushrooms (especially wild and Asian varieties)

Key benefits: polysaccharides (beta-glucan, lentinan), vitamin D1, selenium

How to boost use: sauté for sauces, pilafs, and risottos; roast and top pizza, burgers, and sandwiches; use in veggie balls and burgers

### Spinach

Key benefits: phytochemicals (chlorophyll, flavonoids, carotenoids), vitamins (K, A, B including folate), minerals (calcium, magnesium, iron, copper, manganese)

How to boost use: quickly sauté with garlic and red chili peppers as a side dish, toss with pasta, blend into sauces and dips, add to smoothies or juice

### Sweet potatoes

Key benefits: vitamins (A, B, C), minerals (manganese, copper), fibre (when served with skin)

How to boost use: roast as a side dish or add to salads and grain bowls, create a mash or purée into dips or smoothies, slice and toast and top for a non-traditional breakfast "toast"

### Tomatoes

Key benefits: phytochemicals (carotenoids such as lycopene and lutein, flavonoids such as kaempferol and quercetin), vitamins (A, B, C, K), minerals (copper, manganese)

How to boost use: slice fresh tomatoes on salads and sandwiches, roast and toss with pasta, make into a jam to top sandwiches or grain bowls, make fermented ketchup

## GRAINS AND LEGUMES

Beans and lentils (black beans, white beans, kidney beans, chickpeas,
French lentils, green lentils, red lentils)

Key benefits: prebiotic fructan fibres, minerals (iron, zinc, magnesium, copper,
manganese), folate, phytochemicals (anthyocyanins, kaempferol, quercetin)

How to boost use: roast until crispy for a fun snack or salad topper, toss cooked
beans with pasta, purée into dips, add to soups or salads

Oats

Key benefits: soluble beta-glucan fibre, minerals (magnesium, manganese, copper, zinc)

How to boost use: substitute oat flour for part of the flour in pancakes, muffins, and
cookies; enjoy oats as a porridge, homemade granola, or crumble topping for fruit;
use whole oat groats to make a risotto

## NUTS AND SEEDS

Omega-3-rich seeds (hemp seeds, chia seeds, flaxseed)

Key benefits: omega-3 fatty acids, minerals (zinc, iron, magnesium), soluble fibre
(chia, flax), protein (hemp), lignans (flax)

How to boost use: soak for overnight oats or chia puddings, replace eggs with soaked
ground flax or chia, add to smoothies and cereals, blend hemp into creamy sauces
and dressings, bake into muffins or breads

Raw nuts (almonds, cashews, walnuts, macadamia, Brazil nuts) and peanuts

Key benefits: healthy fats (oleic acid, omega-3 fatty acids in walnuts), vitamin E,
minerals (copper, manganese, magnesium, selenium), anti-inflammatory phytochemicals
(phenols), fibre

How to boost use: enjoy raw as a snack, bake into granola or muffins, use as the
base for non-dairy creams or cheese, blend into nut milks or smoothies

## OILS AND FATS

Extra-virgin olive oil

Key benefits: oleic acid, phytochemicals (oleocanthal), vitamins (E, K)

How to boost use: use to sauté vegetables or in place of vegetable oil in
richly flavoured baked goods, use to prepare salad dressings and sauces

## HERBS AND SPICES

**Cocoa powder (raw or non-Dutch processed for highest antioxidant potential)**

Key benefits: phytochemicals (very high in flavonoids)

How to boost use: add to smoothies, blend into a warming drink, add to raw desserts and chia puddings, try adding cocoa nibs to baking and trail mixes or stir into smoothie bowls

**Fresh herbs (basil, cilantro, oregano, mint, parsley, rosemary, thyme)**

Key benefits: phytochemicals (chlorophyll, rosmarinic acid, flavonoids like naringenin), vitamins (K, C), minerals (manganese, copper), volatile oils (thymol in thyme and oregano, carvacrol in oregano)

How to boost use: blend into pesto; toss a handful into salads, pastas, or grain bowls; use in marinades, dips, and dressings

**Ginger**

Key benefits: phytochemicals, volatile oils (gingerols, shogaols, terpenes)

How to boost use: grate into sauces and dressings; sauté with vegetables, stir-fry, or add to curries; add fresh or dried to baking; steep as a tea or blend into smoothies or juice

**Spices (black pepper, cinnamon, cardamom, cayenne, clove, nutmeg)**

Key benefits: phytochemicals (flavonoids like kaempferol), volatile oils (cinnamalde-hyde, eugenol), trace amounts of vitamins and minerals (vitamin K, manganese, copper, calcium)

How to boost use: add to coffee, tea, smoothies, and warm elixirs; add generously to soups, stews, and baked dishes

**Turmeric**

Key benefits: phytochemicals (curcumin, bisdemethoxycurcumin, demethoxycurcumin), volatile oils (tumerone, zingiberene), minerals (manganese, iron)

How to boost use: use to make golden non-dairy milk or chai; add to smoothies or juice fresh turmeric; mix into dressings and sauces; add to curries, stews, and casseroles

## DRINKS

**Fermented drinks (kombucha, kefir)**

Key benefits: beneficial live microorganisms, organic acids, enzymes

How to boost use: sip daily in place of other sweetened beverages (easy to make at home)

**Green tea**
Key benefits: phytochemicals (catechins like epigallocatechin-3-gallate), L-theanine
How to boost use: sip throughout the day hot or cold, enjoy matcha for concentrated benefits, add to smoothies and baking

## Do I Need an Elimination Diet to Calm Inflammation?

An elimination diet is a protocol that eliminates common allergens and gut and immune system irritants, such as egg, dairy, gluten, soy, and alcohol. It is common to see elimination diets recommended for chronic inflammation. The reason is simple: if you are intolerant to a food, your immune system will react with inflammation if you eat it. An elimination protocol allows you to calm your system down and determine which foods are causing the issue during a careful reintroduction phase.

However, I do not always find elimination protocols necessary and think that we are often too quick to jump to the most intensive therapy. To further complicate things, the popularity of elimination protocols has led people to mistakenly believe that soy and gluten are somehow "toxic" foods for all seven billion of us. While it is true that soy is a common allergen, if you are not allergic or intolerant to it, it is a wonderful anti-inflammatory food!

This elimination mindset can lead to a fear of food that has disastrous consequences for our enjoyment of eating and our health. We are missing the nutritional forest for the trees. In fact, sometimes the greatest success of the elimination protocol is that what it really eliminates is all the pro-inflammatory eating patterns we have, such as giant coffee shop muffins for breakfast and candy for dessert.

In my practice, I advocate for the simplest (but no less powerful) solutions *first*. It is better to start your journey simply by consuming a more anti-inflammatory diet. For an overwhelming number of people, this will be more than enough. In fact, it will be life changing. After three to six months of eating this way, if you find you need more, absolutely work with a qualified health professional to guide you through a customized elimination to see if certain foods are compromising your health.

## Nutrition to Support Your Gut–Immune System Balance

It might be news that the health of your gut and your immune system are connected. However, while you may just think of your gut as a boring food tube—if you think of it at all—it is one of the most fascinating places in your body.

Because your gut is continuous with the outside world, it is considered a barrier between you and the great outdoors, just as your skin is. The difference between your gut and your skin is that your gut is just a single cell thick, and as such, it is a far more fragile barrier than your relatively thick skin. Therefore, your immune system, in all its wisdom, places roughly 80 percent of its immune power there.

Yes, your digestive tract is an important site of immune function. Perhaps the most important of them all.

Although it is incredible to think of your gut as an immune organ perhaps for the first time, it might also be surprising to learn that trillions of bacteria are living in your gut, too. These critters live mostly in your colon but also a little bit in your small intestine. Far from passive riders, these bacteria are as critical to your health and the operation of your immune system as any of your other organs are. You can think of your gut bacteria as being critical partners in the business of being a healthy human.

This is big news. One of our greatest advances in understanding inflammation is the knowledge that it can originate in, or be exacerbated by, what is happening with the gut. The gut is an area of the body that is primarily protected by macrophages, which can digest and destroy bacteria. They also produce cytokines that further activate the chronic inflammatory system. So, ensuring that both the gut tissue and the immune system are well nourished is critical to an inflammatory system that functions well.

A healthy, whole food diet that includes many plants is a sure way to support the health of both the gut and the immune system. Vitamin A, found in yellow, orange, and green vegetables, supports immune cell activity and gut barrier function. Vitamin C in kiwis, strawberries, and citrus fruits is critical for multiple immune processes. The only outlier here is vitamin D, a known modulator of the immune response, for which you will have to look to supplements to get a boost.

Minerals are also abundant in plants, typically in greens, nuts, seeds, and legumes. Zinc is a critical mineral for both immune function and gut cell metabolism, including protection of the gut barrier. A woman can get almost half her daily intake of zinc in ¼ cup (60 mL) of pumpkin seeds. Iron is another important mineral for proper immune response; luckily, the combination of vitamin C–rich foods and iron-rich plant foods, such as a good spinach salad, help to improve use of plant-source iron.

Your body is miraculous, and so is your immune system. When it is working well, your immune system is why you get better after you catch a cold and how you survive after an injury. However, immunity requires certain raw materials such as amino acids and minerals to function optimally. Modern living is taking its toll on immunity, and we need to supercharge it with as much supportive nutrition as we can.

The answer is deliciously simple: just eat more plants.

## Be Mindful of How You Feed Your Gut Bacteria

If you are still not convinced that your gut is complex, consider this: there are more bacteria living in your gut than there are stars in the Milky Way galaxy. The presence of trillions of bacteria in your gut helps educate your immune system in a way that encourages balance and tolerance, two very good things with respect to inflammation. Not content to just hang out, gut bacteria (also known as gut flora or microbiota) are in active communication with your immune system and your nervous system. In fact, research tells us that without those bacteria, our immune systems would not work as well as they do. However, a well-functioning immune system is dependent on a *beneficial* mix of gut bacteria doing their good work.

Sometimes, our bacterial community is not as peaceful as we would like it to be. This happens when bad bacteria gain a foothold and start multiplying to a critical mass that allows them to exert their presence within the gut—stress, diet, medication, and travel are common causes. Instead of just causing trouble with other bacteria, in high volumes bad bacteria actually affect our inflammatory status and the integrity of the gut tissue itself.

To help protect the delicate gut cell barrier, a beneficial layer of mucus sits on top of the gut cells. Bad bacteria can degrade this beneficial mucus, get in contact with gut cells, and start to chip away at them. When the gut barrier falters, large molecules that would normally not pass beyond the gut are presented to the immune system, which goes on high alert and starts attacking. However, if the population of bad bacteria is too much for your immune system, that attack goes chronic. The cycle of inflammation, bad bacteria, and a "leaky" gut barrier can progress to the point where bacterial fragments can translocate into places in your body where they should not be. It is thought that this translocation could be part of the link between gut bacteria and conditions of chronic inflammation like depression or rheumatoid arthritis.

Although research is still in its infancy, what you eat has a definite impact on the residents of your colon. Bacteria make a meal out of whatever you do not digest and absorb. We absorb the vast majority of carbohydrate, protein, and fats, but not fibre. Plants contain multiple types of fermentable fibres and indigestible carbohydrates, such as prebiotic inulin, oligosaccharides, and resistant starches. The more you eat high-fibre plant foods like beans, greens, and berries, the more you feed the beneficial bacteria in your colon. Those same plant foods—like berries, cocoa, and turmeric—also contain polyphenols that are thought to boost populations of healthy bacteria.

Bacteria ferment fibres and create short-chain fatty acids that are used to fuel the gut cell, maintain the gut barrier, and help lower inflammation. In fact, those short-chain fatty acids help ensure that good guys have the advantage by lowering the pH of the gut to favour the growth of beneficial bacteria over bad bacteria.

While our gut bacteria respond quickly—within one to two days—of making dietary change, how you eat over time matters far more than the contents of a single meal. Diets high in saturated fat and sugar tend to alter the gut bacterial community for the worse, fostering the growth of potentially disease-causing species such as *E. coli*. Diets high in animal protein can increase the number of methanogens, microbes that—you guessed it—make methane gas that can actually lead to constipation. The fermentation products of protein, such as hydrogen sulfide and ammonia, are potentially harmful to the gut tissue, making the addition of more plant-based proteins a smart move for better gut health.

## Taking a Holistic Approach

Food is a remarkable tool in fighting chronic inflammation; however, it is important to remember than an anti-inflammatory lifestyle is just that: a lifestyle. It is not possible, or desirable, to shun treats forever. Birthdays, holidays, and other celebrations happen, and if you eat well day after day, your body will be resilient enough to handle them. I live by the 80/20 rule. I aim to eat the foods that best serve me 80 percent of the time, so I do not have to worry about the 20 percent. A holiday may look a little more like 60/40, and sometimes you may then require a 90/10 period to feel better after the holiday season or an illness flare-up.

Food is one part—albeit a large part—of the anti-inflammatory equation. I cannot overstate the importance of minimizing the effects of stress on your body. As I stated previously, cortisol triggered in chronic stress increases inflammatory pressures on the body, which in turn amplify cortisol levels in a nasty feedback loop. If releasing daily commitments does not feel doable, finding ways to neutralize stress are critical. I am a big fan of meditation and mindful breath work because it can be done anywhere and anytime. Most people can find five or ten minutes throughout the day to remove distraction and just breathe.

I am also a strong believer in taking time to engage with your senses in the real world, away from screens. Taking time in nature is known to improve mood and reduce stress. I love being outside in my little garden. Even if you have a small patio, you can turn it into an oasis where you can clear your mind after a long day. Taking time to hang out in a nearby park with a good book can be restorative, too.

Even better, move your body outside whenever possible. Exercise is critical to managing the effects of stress and living an anti-inflammatory lifestyle. As a dietitian, I know how critical nutrition is to fostering true wellness; however, nutrition works best as part of a wellness-focused lifestyle.

## Eat More *Medicinal* Plants

I also rely a great deal on adaptogenic herbs and mushrooms when life gets hectic. Adaptogens are herbs that help your body adapt to stress while minimizing the damaging effects of stress on your body. There are many different adaptogenic plants and mushrooms to choose from; here are just a few:

- **Ashwagandha:** A root also known as Indian ginseng, ashwagandha is thought to protect the immune system in times of stress and to relieve anxiety and stress-induced depression.
- **Astragalus:** A flowering plant important to traditional Chinese medicine; the root is used for its anti-inflammatory, immunomodulatory, and neurological benefits.
- **Chaga:** A fungus that grows on birch trees, chaga is known for its beta-glucan content and thought to be anti-inflammatory.
- **Ginseng:** One of the best-researched adaptogens, Panax ginseng is thought to improve cognition and mental well-being in addition to inflammation.
- **Holy basil (tulsi):** The leaves of the holy basil plant are thought to be anti-inflammatory and to support the immune system and ease anxiety.
- **Maca:** A tuber native to Peru that is related to broccoli, maca is traditionally taken for improved stamina and libido.
- **Rhodiola:** A root that is taken to improve fatigue and mental clarity in times of stress.

Adaptogens have a long history of traditional use; however, modern research on them varies widely. My favourite adaptogen, ashwagandha, has a solid evidence base, as does ginseng and astragalus. The evidence on rhodiola is very promising. As with all natural medicines, always check with your health care provider to determine if adaptogens are right for you. Quality formulations count; see Favourite Suppliers (page 279).

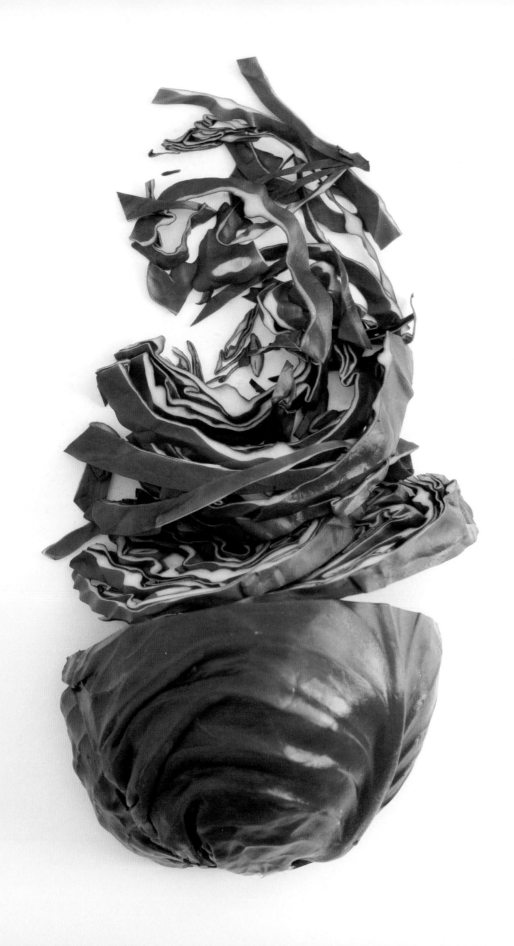

# 2

# The Transformative Power of Plant-Based Foods

**Do you want to be healthier?** Just eat more plants. We have seen how plants help us fight against chronic inflammation, but what about a healthy diet for the rest of life? I advocate for what I call a plant-centred diet, which means exactly what it sounds like: that plants make up the centre of your eating plan.

In a world of too many types of diets, why add another moniker to the mix? Because it is inclusive. It is important to me, as a dietitian, that everyone feel like they can eat this way, even if they do not feel that eating a 100 percent plant-based diet is right for them right now.

It is a powerful way to eat and one that has transformed my own life and the lives of my clients. It is also an approach to eating that is *deceptively* simple, because of how at odds it is with modern living. For example, most of us anchor our plate with starch or protein, using vegetables as a condiment. A little bit of fruit on your pancakes or broccoli in your curry. What I want you to do is flip that so everything else plays a secondary role to fruits, vegetables, nuts, seeds, and legumes.

The underlying reason for this is that, because of our sedentary lives, a typical *energy-dense* diet does not make sense anymore. Most hyper-processed foods contain plenty of calories, but they are largely stripped of their nutrients. In addition, it is nutrients we need to cope with modern life. A fast-paced, high-stress, technology-filled life calls for eating more whole plant foods to shift you into what we call a *nutrient-dense* diet.

## In Praise of Roughage

Fibre is abundant in plant-based foods, but technically our body does not need it. Our body cannot digest and absorb fibres, so they stay in our gut and pass on through. It could be easy to discount fibre, and many of us do, but we should rethink the benefits of eating foods that are high in fibre. In addition to helping us stay regular, fibre fights inflammation by feeding beneficial bacteria in the gut. These bacteria, in turn, fight off more inflammatory strains of bacteria and, as they ferment fibre, produce short-chain fatty acids, which send a message to our immune systems to cool down.

In North America, we still have woefully inadequate intakes of fibre. U.S. data from the 2009–2010 National Health and Nutrition Examination Survey (NHANES) found that women get an average of 15 grams a day and men get 18 grams a day. This does not sound too bad until you realize that women need 25 grams of fibre a day and men need 38 grams.

I know that a dietitian talking fibre does not seem revolutionary, until you understand how transformative fibre can be to your health. A high-fibre, plant-based diet will help you:

- Regulate your appetite and weight
- Balance blood sugars and regulate blood cholesterol
- Optimize elimination
- Support your immune system and digestive tract

## HOW A PLANT-BASED DIET HELPS YOU REGULATE YOUR APPETITE AND WEIGHT

As mentioned in Chapter 1, eating more whole plant foods helps you feel relaxed in your appetite because of physical and chemical interactions between plants and your metabolism. Whole plant foods contain a great deal of water and fibre, two substances that take up space in the stomach and activate stretch receptors that play into hunger-satiety feedback mechanisms in the brain. In addition, their fibrous cell walls take more work for the body to break down, slowing your ability to absorb their nutrients into the bloodstream. This sounds like it could be a negative thing, but it is not. The slower your blood sugars rise, the better controlled your appetite will be.

In addition, high-fibre plant foods may help with appetite regulation via a surprising middle-microbe—the bacteria living in your gut. It is thought that short-chain fatty acids, which are produced when bacteria ferment fibres, may influence appetite. Clinical trials looking at the effect of fibre intake on appetite have been mixed; however, this may be due to the lack of consistency on the type and amount of fibre tested.

Gelling-type soluble fibres like psyllium and beta-glucans in barley and oats may be most efficacious, although the research is far from conclusive. Researchers are still trying to understand how short-chain fatty acids, which by definition are fats and concentrated sources of energy, might relate to lower appetite and weight, but there appears to be a complex interaction between short-chain fatty acids, appetite hormones, and energy metabolism.

Many whole plant foods are lower in energy (measured in calories) than hyper-processed foods, so filling up on plants makes it less likely that you will throw yourself out of energy balance and gain weight. From a behavioural perspective, eating whole plant foods (as opposed to vegan junk food), with their lower levels of sugar and fat, should be less likely to create and reinforce learned reward behaviour that leads to over-eating. High-fat, high-carbohydrate meals lead to bumps in feel-good neurotransmitters called serotonin and dopamine, which over time teach you to self-medicate with food. Serotonin leads to feelings of contentedness, whereas dopamine governs reward and motivation. Subconsciously, you begin to realize that you can lift your spirits through high-fat, high-sugar food choices, and this becomes a tough habit to break.

It is true that people with a 100 percent plant-based diet tend to weigh less than those with an omnivorous diet. Not just calories lead to weight gain. The metabolic effect of those calories matters, too. I find that my plant-based clients who are struggling with their weight often consume a great deal of high-starch and high-sugar choices like bread, pizza, and cookies instead of putting a lot of legumes and vegetables on their plates.

When life gets busy, it is easy to rely on convenience foods. If your breakfast is now the vegan muffin at the coffee shop or if you make a big bowl of pasta tossed with olive oil for dinner so you do not have to go to the store, before you know it you could be eating a lot of starch and sugar that does not fill you up and raises blood sugars, leading to constant hunger and weight gain. This is why taking the time to learn how to compose a balanced plant-based meal is so important, as is building a repertoire of recipes that are easy to make. That way, your busy morning default becomes a simple smoothie at home, with a scoop of protein powder to keep you fuelled all morning.

## HOW PLANTS HELP BALANCE YOUR BLOOD SUGARS AND BLOOD CHOLESTEROL

The effect that a given food has on your blood sugar rise is called its glycemic load. We rarely eat foods in isolation (maybe just at snack time when we eat an apple or a small handful of almonds), so instead of focusing only on specific foods, it is the composition of meals that really has the greatest impact on blood sugar control. The rate at which your body will absorb carbohydrates from foods depends on several factors:

- Fibre, protein, and fat content of the meal
- Acidic components present in the meal (increased acid slows stomach emptying)
- Sugar or starch structure of the carbohydrate-containing food
- Cooking technique (cooking denatures proteins and gelatinizes starches, making them more digestible)

Serotonin and dopamine: technically, the only two things you actually enjoy.

Whole plant foods, with their tough cell walls, take work for the body to break down. When you choose a piece of fruit over juice or consume a seed cracker instead of a white rice bread, you are making choices that will result in better blood sugar balance. Including plant-based proteins such as tempeh or chickpeas and healthy plant fats such as olives or avocado in a meal will further slow the digestion and absorption of nutrients so that blood sugar rise is moderate. It is very common for my clients to create plant-based meals by simply removing the meat from the recipe; however, a healthy plant-based meal requires additional sources of protein, like legumes, *in place of* meat. Adding these sources of protein will improve blood sugar response and appetite.

Why does glycemic load matter? If you are diabetic or have pre-diabetes, there is a simple answer. High blood sugars initiate stronger insulin release, which leads to greater insulin resistance and risk of the complications of diabetes.

But, what if you don't have diabetes? Diabetes does not happen overnight. It takes years, maybe decades, of metabolic dysfunction to develop diabetes. However, the more you consume hyper-processed foods and low-fibre meals anchored by sugar and refined flours, the higher your risk of the disease. This should not scare you into banning birthday cake; remember, it is what you eat *habitually* that matters most.

From an everyday perspective, the more rapidly absorbed carbohydrates you consume, the higher and faster your blood sugar will spike. The steeper the spike, the more dramatic the crash. Ever get "hangry"? That is caused by a blood sugar imbalance, and when that low occurs, it is less likely you are going to reach for some roasted chickpeas. Even though you may have consumed adequate calories to keep you going, once that energy is pulled out of the bloodstream, your body thinks you are starving. In its survivalist wisdom, your body will be driven toward more quick carbohydrates, like the candy on a co-worker's desk or the croissants in the kitchen, creating a vicious cycle of craving.

Eating a diet filled with whole plant foods helps you feel relaxed in your appetite, instead of always feeling hungry and preoccupied with food. If you know what it feels like to struggle with appetite and cravings, you will know what a gift this is. Slow, sustained bumps in blood sugars combined with non-rewarding effects on the brain play into the beneficial impacts on natural hunger-satiety mechanisms—so you can feel less of a battle.

Insulin is a critical hormone to pay attention to, and not just because of diabetes. Insulin has a role to play in managing weight. Insulin is a storage hormone, so the greater your insulin release, the tougher it will be to maintain a stable weight or lose weight. In fact, a common side effect of administering insulin in type 2 diabetes to help get blood sugars under control is weight gain. In addition, chronically high insulin levels (often in the pre-diabetic or diabetic state) have been associated with the progression of diseases beyond diabetes: cancer, polycystic ovary syndrome, and Alzheimer's disease. So, maybe blood sugars should matter to all of us.

## PLANTS, CHOLESTEROL, AND YOUR HEART

It was once common dietary advice to avoid eating cholesterol for fear of hurting your heart, but current research has shown us otherwise. One of the reasons for this is that we have realized that dietary cholesterol (only found in animal foods) does not affect blood cholesterol. In fact, our own body produces far more cholesterol than we consume; it is a key component of vitamin D, hormones, cell membranes, and bile. Although we call them by the same name, the cholesterol we eat and the cholesterol in our blood are not the same thing. At this point, it appears that only those with diabetes might need to be concerned about dietary cholesterol.

However, eating saturated fat does increase your blood cholesterol levels. In addition, while higher cholesterol levels will not guarantee you a heart attack, high levels of certain molecules in the cholesterol family are still associated with risk of cardiovascular disease.

Eating a healthy, plant-based diet, which will have naturally lower levels of saturated fats—even if you do eat some coconut—is a positive first step. It is thought that replacing saturated fats with carbohydrate (particularly refined carbohydrate) may mitigate the benefits, so it is important to make healthy plant fats like avocado, nut butters, and olive oil a mainstay in your diet. However, all that wonderful fibre is also a key player. Soluble fibre, which forms a gel, traps bile salts in the gut and carries them out of the body. What does this have to do with cholesterol? The liver, using cholesterol, makes bile salts. Therefore, if the liver must produce more bile to replace the bile you excreted, it will lower circulating levels of cholesterol in your blood.

## HOW PLANTS OPTIMIZE ELIMINATION

Roughage might be my favourite quirk of the plant world. Fibres, whether soluble or insoluble, fermentable or non-fermentable, are all extremely beneficial for gut health.

Your gut is one long muscular tube; think of fibre as its personal trainer. Insoluble fibres act like a broom, sweeping the gut clean and eliminating waste more expeditiously. Soluble fibres create the gel that binds potentially toxic substances, lowers blood cholesterol, and eases elimination. Both fibres add weight to stools, making them easier to pass in a timely fashion.

Diverticular disease is one of the most common digestive issues that plague us as we get older. Diverticula are little outpouchings of the gut wall; they are essentially thickened, flabby muscle. And those pouches can collect digestive debris and bacteria and get infected. Gross. Why does this happen? Age and Western-style diet contribute; in part, your risk may be higher if the gut has not been in regular fibre training.

Is your bowel sluggish? Constipation is rampant in our society, and it is easy to see why: we do not move our body much, and we do not eat enough high-water, high-fibre plant foods. This affects the gut directly, since you need fibre to move contents through in an appropriate manner. In addition, less body hydration can slow down elimination as the gut attempts to reclaim as much water from the stool as possible.

## HOW PLANTS HELP FEED BENEFICIAL GUT BACTERIA

The benefits of eating more plants are all amazing, but what really gets me pumped is learning more about how plants help feed your gut bacteria, or *microbiota*.

You see, good bugs like plant fibre. The fermentable fibres found in plant foods feed beneficial bacteria so that they can grow well and defend you against more harmful strains. There are bacteria that dig on fats or proteins, but at this point in the research, it would appear that you really do not want too many of those types of critters. Instead, you want to eat a variety of plant foods, with their soluble, insoluble, and prebiotic fibres that beneficial bacteria turn into short-chain fatty acids: namely, acetate, lactate, propionate, and butyrate. Butyrate is quickly becoming the darling of gut research because it appears to be the preferred fuel for the gut cell, meaning that more butyrate leads to a healthier gut. In addition, it may have beneficial effects on immune function, helping to calm inflammation and even positively affecting the nervous system.

## Demystifying Fibre

You are probably thinking, *Is fibre that mysterious?* Of course, when you realize how many different types of fibres there are, you will understand why I chose that title for this section. Some substances can have more than one property (for example, be soluble and prebiotic/fermentable). Many plant foods contain more than one of these categories, which is why eating a varied diet of plant foods is such a good idea.

### SOLUBLE FIBRE

The *soluble* in soluble fibre refers to its solubility in water, meaning that the fibre molecule will hydrate and become gel-like in the gut. Put a spoonful of chia into a glass of water and you will see soluble fibre in action. Soluble fibre is my first choice for those with irritable guts, as it tends to be less irritating than insoluble fibre. It typically slows down the digestion and absorption of nutrients, resulting in better blood sugar balance, while adding weight to the stool to encourage healthy elimination. Less abundant than insoluble fibre, you will find soluble fibre in citrus fruits, okra, eggplant, psyllium, oats, and barley. Pectin, the substance that helps you make jam, is a soluble fibre. Most of the fibres your gut bacteria ferment are soluble, but they can also ferment some insoluble fibres, too.

## INSOLUBLE FIBRE

Insoluble fibre is the roughage of plant cell walls. Your grandma ate bran for a reason, and it was not because it is a culinary delicacy. Unlike soluble fibre, insoluble fibre does not dissolve into a gel; instead, it sweeps through the gut and helps speed up elimination. Lignans, celluloses, and hemicelluloses in nuts, seeds, grains, and vegetables are the most common types of insoluble fibre.

## RESISTANT STARCH

Resistant starches, distinct from insoluble or soluble fibres, are named for their ability to resist digestion. What makes a starch resistant? It might be hard to digest because it is locked behind plant walls, such as eating whole oat groats instead of oat flour. Or the starch granules could be ungelatinized, such as in cooked and cooled grains and potatoes or underripe bananas. Resistant starches are found in many different plant foods, and they travel to the colon where they feed beneficial bacteria and help you fight inflammation.

## PREBIOTIC FIBRE

The definition of prebiotics is changing as we learn more about what fosters the growth of bacteria; however, most of the well-researched prebiotics are indigestible fibres such as fructo-oligosaccharides. Eating prebiotics helps to increase the numbers of beneficial microbes in the gut, helping you fight inflammation and keep your gut healthy. Inulin, a fructo-oligosaccharide or *fructan*, is one of the best-researched prebiotics in existence. It is found in many everyday plant foods, such as:

- Artichokes
- Asparagus
- Bananas
- Barley, wheat, and rye

- Chicory roots
- Jerusalem artichokes (sunchokes)
- Leeks, onion, and garlic

There are other non-inulin fructans and galacto-oligosaccharides in plant foods like legumes, peaches, and figs that also benefit gut health. Pectin, a soluble fibre found in apples, is also prebiotic.

A whole food, plant-based diet is your foundation for a healthier gut. Plant foods, in addition to increasing fibre intake, provide plenty of anti-inflammatory phytochemicals that fight inflammation and help foster a stronger gut bacterial population. Eating plant foods will also help you avoid the hyper-processed, high-fat, high-sugar diet that is associated with an increase in more harmful, pro-inflammatory bacteria.

If you are looking to show your gut bacteria even more love, consider incorporating the following practices into your lifestyle:

1. Eat fermented plant foods, such as sauerkraut, kimchi, kombucha, and miso, daily to introduce small amounts of friendly microbes into your diet.
2. Eat fewer high-sugar treats such as sugar-sweetened beverages and coffee drinks, candy, store-bought dessert, and sweet snack foods. The recipes in this book will show you how to enjoy higher fibre sweets with fewer added sugars.
3. Eat more prebiotic-rich plant foods, such as beans, onions, garlic, asparagus, and artichokes, to feed those beneficial bacteria well.
4. Take time every day to de-stress, as stress can alter your gut flora. Do simple deep breathing or mindfulness meditation, go for a walk, or take the time to read or enjoy a bath.
5. In addition to eating fermented foods, consider a human-strain probiotic to help you heal your gut and fight inflammation. A probiotic contains a higher dose of good bacteria than most fermented foods for accelerated change.

## How Plants Help You Form a More Intuitive Relationship with Food

There are few relationships more intimate than our relationship with food. Your body will break down whatever it can into tiny, absorbable bits that it will use to build and repair your tissues, once it has discarded the useless or potentially harmful bits. What you eat becomes your body, so you literally *are* what you eat!

Without a doubt, food plays a large role in our *disease*. When did food become our enemy, and when did we wrap up our self-worth in the virtuousness of our food choices? We have lost many of the simple pleasures of a good meal while simultaneously using food as taste bud entertainment and self-medication. We agonize over what to eat, deprive ourselves of foods we love, and restrict ourselves unnecessarily as penance for past indulgences.

Food has always been a source of joy in my life, and for my first 15 or so years on earth, I simply ate without thinking about whether a food was healthy or not. Apples, broccoli, or chips: it was all just food. Over time, food became something that was good or bad, healthy or not. How I felt about myself was deeply tied to my food choices and my body shape for a while. Ironically, these types of thoughts led me to make choices that were pro-inflammatory, which left my physical and mental well-being at risk. When I developed irritable bowel syndrome post-pregnancy, connecting food choice to how it made me feel was a powerful tool for repairing my relationship with food. It liberated me to follow a path that led to deep appreciation for the healing power of plants.

When you are experiencing health challenges, it is all too common to have a fraught relationship with food. Particularly if the act of eating is connected to your symptoms, making food choices can bring its own anxiety. Know that no matter where you are starting from, no matter what your food choices have been like in the past, the recipes in these pages will help get you to where you need to be. These are healing foods. Approach them with a curious and playful mindset.

Instead of feeling a need to adopt a 100 percent anti-inflammatory diet overnight, know that each time you choose to make a recipe in this book, you are moving toward a healthier body. You do not *undo* your good work by making a less healthful choice occasionally. Have some ice cream and move on. Maybe then make a yummy salad for dinner.

Our collective relationship with food has become so fraught with judgment that we have lost our natural, intuitive connection to eating. How many of us actually eat when we are hungry and stop when we are pleasantly full? Or, how many of us give ourselves permission to enjoy a celebratory feast without having to "detox" our way out of it? Eating a whole food, plant-based diet has helped me restore a peaceful, joyful relationship with food. Perhaps it will help you, too.

When you eat more whole plant foods, you are eating as nature intended, and it is easier to move toward a more intuitive relationship with food. Without your conscious thought, your body is using finely tuned mechanisms to regulate your food intake and appetite. So, why can you eat a whole bag of chips without batting an eyelash? Because those foods were designed to circumvent these natural appetite mechanisms and light up the reward centres of our brain like fireworks on a summer night. Their physiological effects, including inflammation, lead us to physical and mental states that then lead us to seek more comfort in hyper-processed foods.

Whole plant foods, with their high fibre and water content, fill up the stomach, leading to a physical sensation of fullness that signals your brain to put on the brakes. Plants take time to digest, meaning they lead to a slow, steady rise in blood sugar that keeps energy levels, cravings, and appetite on an even keel. Whole plant foods do not hijack your neural reward pathways to give you a food high that keeps you going back for more. Most potato chips, however, are designed to have the perfect ratio of carbs to salt and fat that keep you eating to get that flavour buzz. They have essentially no fibre to fill up the stomach, so you can eat and eat and eat (can anyone tell that potato chips used to be my vice?). In addition, every time you eat chips, you reinforce the habit and strengthen reward circuitry. Oh, and it changes your taste buds. The more you eat hyper-processed foods, the less you will appreciate naturally occurring flavours. However, that can change—as long as you do not try to wrangle your taste buds overnight.

## Whatever Your Reasons, Plants Are Powerful

Plant foods are an incredible gift; they can help you feel more energized while fighting inflammation and chronic disease. We have seen how plants can feed beneficial bacteria and protect gut health and how a plant-based diet can help support a healthy and comfortable weight. Transitioning from a standard, hyper-processed diet to one filled with whole plant foods may even help you rebuild a healthy relationship with food.

However, a plant-based diet also helps you tread more lightly on the planet. It is thought that adopting a more plant-based diet, particularly one that focuses on eating locally available foods, can help us reduce the water and energy required to produce food and make our food system more sustainable.

Whether for personal, ethical, social, or environmental reasons, eating more plants just makes good sense. Moreover, it is delicious.

You are what you eat. And what your bacteria eat.

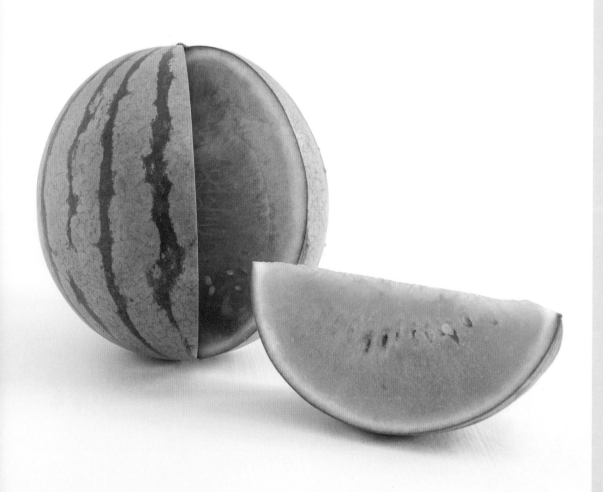

# 3

# Nutrition for a Plant-Based Diet

As a vegetarian for more than twenty years, of course I believe it is an awesome way to eat. However, I have also experienced varying degrees of health as a vegetarian, depending on the quality of my diet. As a teenager, I spent two months in Japan eating almost nothing but plain soba noodles, soy sauce, ice cream, jam, and white bread. That was not a high point. Therefore, it is important to learn about the nutritional benefits of a plant-based diet and how best to incorporate more whole foods in your meals for optimal health.

As a dietitian, I need good-quality research to feel comfortable guiding *you* through the transition toward plant-based living. And luckily, there is. Based on the available evidence, both Dietitians of Canada and the Academy of Nutrition and Dietetics in the United States agree that vegetarian and vegan diets are safe and healthful throughout the lifespan, from birth to kicking ass in your elder years.

If you are transitioning to a plant-based diet, I recommend taking it slow. The reason for this is that you only have so much energy in any given day, and I do not want what should be a positive and enjoyable eating change to cause you stress. The best way to do that? Perhaps focus on one meal at a time, like breakfast. Alternatively, spend a few weeks or months finding new ways to make plant-based versions of your favourite recipes and products. Enjoy including more plants on your plate when you have the option, and if you are visiting relatives for the weekend or on a business trip and it is easier to eat a conventional plate, do it.

If eating a plant-based diet is your goal, transitioning over three to six months will help the change feel less overwhelming and make you more likely to stick with it. I totally understand feeling excited and perhaps wanting to change *tomorrow* . . . but if you give yourself a little room for the official change to occur, I guarantee it will feel awesome! This chapter will give you everything you need to know to make the change healthfully. If you are already there? Consider this chapter a mini nutrition check-in to make sure you are on track. Let us start with the basics.

# Plant-Based Nutrition Cheat Sheet

This plan is something I share with my plant-based clients; it was born out of helping my clients understand what healthy eating looks like in practice. While understanding your nutrient requirements is important for better health, what matters most is knowing how to turn those requirements into an actual meal.

## HOW TO BUILD A PLANT-BASED MEAL

Whenever you compose a meal, try to follow these proportions:

- 50 percent fruits and/or vegetables (aim for no more than three to four pieces of fruit a day)
- 25 percent concentrated protein (non-soy powders, whole organic soy foods, legumes, hemp seeds)
- 25 percent slow-burning whole grains (optional)

Always add 1 to 2 tablespoons (15 to 30 mL) of healthy fats, such as extra-virgin olive oil, nut butters, avocado, or seeds, to every meal. They improve flavour and help with blood sugar balance and absorption of critical fat-soluble nutrients and plant compounds.

Why are whole grains optional at a meal? If you are very sedentary, working to reach a healthy weight, or over age thirty-five, I find that you may not need the extra energy of whole grains at *every* meal. This is particularly true because, hopefully, you are still obtaining nutrient-dense carbohydrates from legumes and vegetables. If you are eating fewer whole grains, be sure to eat larger portions of legumes and a bit of extra healthy fat so you are not hungry.

## FOODS TO EAT DAILY

The Crucifers: Kale, cabbage (all kinds), Brussels sprouts, cauliflower, broccoli, collards, kohlrabi, watercress, arugula

This vegetable family is extremely nutrient-dense, cancer-preventive, and anti-inflammatory. Sulphur-based phytochemicals in the crucifers support liver function, help prevent cancer formation, and foster optimal hormone balance. Eating ½ to 1 cup (125 to 250 mL) a day is beneficial to long-term health.

Nuts and Nut Butters: Cashew, almond, peanut, walnut, macadamia

Nuts are one of the plant foods that provide nutrients found in animal-based foods. They contain healthy fats, protein (peanuts and almonds mostly), and minerals such as zinc and iron that are critical when on a plant-based diet.

### Omega-3 Seeds: Hemp, chia, ground flax

Omega-3 fats fight inflammation, and hemp, chia, and flax are the most concentrated plant sources of omega-3 fats. Chia and flax are high in soluble fibre, and flax provides hormone-supportive lignans. Hemp is higher in protein than most seeds, with 10 grams per 3 tablespoons (45 mL). These seeds are also mineral rich (iron, zinc, magnesium). Always consume flax ground to benefit from the incredible nutrition inside the seed, as the hull is extremely difficult for your body to digest.

### Calcium-Rich Foods: Organic tofu, beans, fortified non-dairy milks, tahini, molasses

Calcium is important for nervous system function and muscular contraction. Life is sustained on very small amounts of calcium circulating in the bloodstream, with the rest stored within your bones. For the first thirty or so years of your life, your body is building bone mass; the more calcium you consume, the stronger your bones will be. After age thirty, bone building declines and getting enough calcium in your diet keeps your blood levels stable so your body does not need to deplete the calcium stored in your bones.

### Legumes and Beans: Organic soybeans, chickpeas, black beans, lentils, white beans, kidney beans

Legumes are richer in protein and minerals (particularly iron) than most other plant foods, so they are a staple of a plant-based diet. While all plants contain a little bit of protein, you should include concentrated sources of protein, such as beans, at each meal to harness their appetite-satisfying and blood sugar–balancing benefits. Organic whole food soy (as opposed to hyper-processed meat substitutes and protein powders) is a healthful food as long as you are not soy-intolerant.

### Alliums: Onions, garlic, leeks, scallions, shallots

Alliums are very anti-inflammatory foods that contain sulphur-based nutrients to help fight cancer. In addition, they have indigestible prebiotic components that feed beneficial bacteria in the gut.


## Nutrients to Be Mindful of on a Plant-Based Diet

Most people are concerned about getting enough protein when eating a plant-based diet, but they should probably be more concerned about adequate nutritional requirements of iron. I have not included detailed information on calcium, vitamin D, or omega-3 fatty acids here because they are a concern for everyone, whether you are vegan or a carnivore (see above, and Chapter 1, for more information on these nutrients). Instead, I focus on what you need to know about iron, zinc, vitamin B12, and iodine when eating fewer or no animal products.

## IRON

Iron is used by the body to form hemoglobin, the molecule in red blood cells that binds oxygen and carries it from our lungs to the rest of our tissues. Low iron can lead to altered red blood cell formation and anemia, which is typically associated with symptoms of exhaustion, brain fog, and lightheadedness.

A plant-based diet can give you all of the iron you need; in fact, evidence suggests that vegetarian diets provide as much, if not more, iron than omnivore diets, but pre-menopausal women may not be getting enough iron because of menstruation losses. The reason why iron is a concern on a plant-based diet is that plant-based sources of iron are typically less well absorbed than animal (haem iron) sources. However, that is not necessarily a bad thing. High haem iron intake is associated with increased risk of certain diseases, such as coronary heart disease. Iron can also be a gut irritant; a diet high in haem iron may contribute to gut-level inflammation and bacterial dysbiosis.

Iron metabolism is also far less clear-cut than you might expect. For example, the body regulates its absorption of iron based on your iron status; so, if you have lower iron stores, your body will typically upregulate absorption. In addition, the body downregulates iron absorption when you are consuming high doses. This is why treating anemia is sometimes very hard. Treatment is usually mega-doses of iron, but if the body does not absorb them, your iron levels will not rise.

In my twenty years of vegetarianism, my iron levels have always been on the low side of normal (which is in line with what we see in the research), but I have had anemia only once. It was in the third trimester of my second pregnancy; I supplemented until it resolved postpartum.

It is worthwhile asking for iron testing (as part of a full medical checkup) after three to six months of adopting a plant-based diet to see how your body is adapting and catch any potential lows early. Adult men need 8 mg of iron daily, and women need 18 mg daily. However, because of absorption issues with non-haem iron, it is often recommended that vegetarians consume 180 percent more. Because this is very difficult to do with food, I typically recommend first aiming to meet your basic iron needs through food, and then increasing intake with supplements only if your iron levels cannot be maintained through diet alone.

Focus on iron-rich plant foods such as legumes, nuts, and seeds at every meal and eat plenty of fruits and vegetables to keep your vitamin C intake high for optimal absorption. If you are struggling with iron levels despite eating plenty of iron-rich foods, keep calcium supplements minimal and drink coffee and tea only between meals because high doses of calcium, coffee, and tea can all hinder iron absorption from food. Consider a supplement if your iron stores are low, but consult your doctor for advice. Often, I find that it is easier for women to take a prenatal vitamin, as the iron content is usually much higher than in the average multivitamin and it will get you closer to that 32 mg (180 percent of 18 mg) for extra support.

## ZINC

Zinc typically follows protein in our food supply, so eliminating animal products from your diet can mean lower zinc intake, unless you are eating plenty of zinc-rich seeds and legumes. Zinc is a mineral that deserves more attention, since it is a critical substrate for the immune system and gut cell metabolism. If you want to live an anti-inflammatory life, you need to focus on zinc—it is always key to my nutritional recommendations with clients.

Like iron, zinc from plant-based foods is typically less bioavailable than animal sources; for that reason, some suggest getting 50 percent more zinc than is typically required. For men, that is 11 mg (or 16 mg), and for women it is 8 mg (or 12 mg). I also recommend first aiming for your basic requirement, and then moving to the 50 percent higher level only if low zinc stores are suspected or diagnosed. What does zinc insufficiency look like? Less specific symptoms include unexplained weight loss or fatigue; clearer signs are changes in your sense of smell or taste and slow healing. If you have any of these symptoms and are concerned that you might have a zinc deficiency, see your doctor and dietitian.

Plant-based foods typically contain 1 to 2 mg of zinc per serving, so I encourage a daily pumpkin seed habit. A ¼ cup (60 mL) of raw pumpkin seeds provides almost 3 mg of zinc. Other wonderful sources of zinc include:

- Legumes (including tofu and green peas): ¾ cup (175 mL), 1.1 to 1.9 mg
- Oatmeal: ¼ cup (60 mL) dry, 1.5 mg
- Hemp seeds: 2 tablespoons (30 mL), 1.8 mg
- Wheat germ: 2 tablespoons (30 mL), 2.4 mg
- Wild rice: ½ cup (125 mL) cooked, 1.2 mg
- Baked beans: ¾ cup (175 mL), 4.3 mg
- Tempeh: ¾ cup (175 mL), 2.4 mg
- Nuts (peanuts, cashews, almonds): ¼ cup (60 mL), 1 to 2 mg
- Tahini: 2 tablespoons (30 mL), 1.4 mg

## VITAMIN B12

Vitamin B12 is the only nutrient found exclusively in animal foods. It is critical for the formation of red blood cells, the formation and repair of DNA, and nervous system function. In fact, severe B12 deficiency can mimic the signs and symptoms of dementia.

B12 absorption depends on the release of intrinsic factor (IF) in the stomach; if you take medication for acid reflux or are over age fifty, you need to supplement with B12. Metformin for diabetes or alcohol use may also inhibit absorption. If you are transitioning to a 100 percent plant-based diet, you also need to take B12 for life.

Adults need a minimum of 2.4 micrograms (mcg) of B12 a day; although it is a water-soluble vitamin, the body actually stores it, so B12 deficiency can take time to manifest. Data from the UK suggests that 11 percent of vegans are B12 deficient, and there are ongoing conversations about the consequences of having inadequate, rather than deficient, levels and actually defining those levels.

Although you can obtain vitamin B12 from food with diligent attention to consuming fortified foods like non-dairy almond or soy milks, nutritional yeast, and meat substitutes such as bean-based burgers and soy-based sausages, I recommend supplementing so your intake is consistent and automatic, particularly when you are new to a plant-based diet.

## IODINE

When was the last time you thought about iodine? Maybe when your grandma put it on your scraped knee as a child, but probably not as a nutrient. Iodine is a mineral that is rarely talked about as part of a plant-based diet but now, particularly with the popularity of natural (non-iodized) salts, it is an issue.

Iodine is used in the production of thyroid hormones, meaning it is critical for metabolic regulation and brain health. You need 150 mcg of iodine per day to protect your thyroid; because much of what you eat is excreted, it is important to consume iodine daily. You can get this by consuming ¼ teaspoon (1 mL) of iodized salt a day. It is that easy.

You might be surprised that I recommend adding refined salts to some diets. Fancy salts are fun, but if you are following a 100 percent plant-based diet, I recommend iodized salt because it contains potassium iodide or iodate, which is a more stable form of iodine. The ocean is our mother source for iodine, but natural iodine sublimes out of salt when it is exposed to humidity and ambient temperatures, so natural salts are an unreliable source.

If you eat animal foods, you will consume more iodine because animals store it in their tissues. So, on a plant-based diet, I recommend good old iodized salt, like our grannies used. Soil content of iodine varies, so most plant foods are not reliable sources. Sea vegetables and soy milk have varying levels of iodine, but in practice, I do not feel that they are a realistic daily source.

If you love fancy salts, save them for finishing a dish before serving.

## Putting It All Together

What does it look like to get all of your critical nutrients in a day on a plant-based diet? It is simpler than you might think. Here, I show you the foods you would need to consume over the course of a day to hit your nutrient targets—all it takes are simple, wholesome plant foods!

| Nutrient | Daily Goal (Adults) | How to Meet Your Goal |
|---|---|---|
| Calcium | 1000 mg | 2 cups (500 mL) fortified non-dairy milk + ¼ cup (60 mL) almonds + ½ cup (125 mL) cooked spinach + ¼ of a 12-ounce (350 g) package tofu = 1000 mg |
| Vitamin D | 600 IU for basic bone health needs | Supplement with 1000 to 2000 IU daily for enhanced gut and immune system support |
| Omega-3 fatty acids (ALA) | Men: 1.6 g  Women: 1.1 g | 1 tablespoon (15 mL) chia seeds, hemp seeds, or ground flaxseed will meet 100 percent of daily needs |
| Iron | Men: 8 to 14 mg  Women: 18 to 32 mg | 1 cup (250 mL) cooked oatmeal + 1 cup (250 mL) lentils + 1 cup (250 mL) cooked spinach = 14.5 mg |
| Zinc | Men: 11 to 16 mg  Women: 8 to 12 mg | ¼ cup (60 mL) pumpkin seeds + 1 cup (250 mL) cooked oatmeal + ½ cup (125 mL) hummus + 1 cup (250 mL) lentils = 10 mg |
| Vitamin B12 | 2.4 mcg | 2 cups (500 mL) fortified non-dairy milk or 1½ teaspoons (7 mL) vitamin B12–fortified nutritional yeast will meet 100 percent of daily needs, or a daily supplement |
| Iodine | 150 mcg | ¼ teaspoon (1 mL) iodized salt used in cooking will meet 100 percent of daily needs |

## What about Kids?

Let's talk about raising vegetarian and vegan kids. Both my kids were ovo-lacto vegetarian from birth, and many of their meals are now 100 percent plant-based. The nutrients of concern for children are the same as for adults; kids just need different dosages.

I find that feeding kids poses two main challenges: with their variable appetites and willingness to eat healthful plant foods, kids can be more at risk for deficiency. I give my kids supplements. They both get omega-3s, vitamin D, and a multivitamin. I had not given them a multivitamin until recently; my young daughter seems to survive on milk and air some days, but now both of my children get a daily dose of "nutrient insurance." I used to be able to send my son to daycare with a half an avocado as a snack. He would eat hummus like it was yogurt—with a spoon! This is one of the reasons why I never worried about his nutrition; that and the fact he grew like a weed! My daughter, while very robust, is still in her picky two-year-old phase. Sometimes she will not even eat baked french fries, instead preferring to eat all the ketchup and calling it a day. Hence the multivitamin.

The second concern is that a high-fibre, plant-based diet can fill up children, making it harder for them to eat enough. The solution? Include more high-energy foods like fats and dried fruits. Your children are little energy furnaces, and they should not be restricted from full-fat foods or concentrated sources of healthy carbohydrates like dried fruit and grains. Add plenty of healthy oils like hemp oil to oats or smoothies. Make chia puddings for snack time, with ground chia seeds for better absorption and full-fat canned coconut milk. Let kids have homemade treats like cookies, with whole-grain flours and a lot of healthy fats.

Childhood nutrition is critical. When on a plant-based diet, we tend to underplay this, if only to quell the tide of others who criticize these choices. However, plant-based families tend to be much more active than others in monitoring nutrition needs. Even an omnivore child who eats little more than jam, toast, and a bit of chicken and milk could be seriously at risk for nutrient deficiencies.

If you are raising a plant-based family, I recommend checking in with a plant-friendly dietitian if you have never done so. In addition, if you are planning to raise a vegan child from birth, seeing a registered dietitian before weaning your child is highly recommended to help ensure that you are set up for success. The current recommendation is to continue with soy-based formula or soy milk as a drink supplement until after age two because most plant-based milk alternatives provide little nutrition compared to dairy milk.

## Giving Your Kids What They Need

| Nutrient | Daily Goal (Children and Teens) | How to Meet Your Goal |
|---|---|---|
| Calcium | Ages 1 to 3: 700 mg<br>Ages 4 to 8: 1000 mg<br>Ages 9 to 18: 1300 mg | 2 cups (500 mL) fortified non-dairy milk + 1 tablespoon (15 mL) blackstrap molasses = 680 mg |
| Vitamin D | Birth to age 1: 400 IU<br>Age 1 to 18: 600 IU | I recommend supplementing with 400 to 600 IU daily until the teenage years |
| Omega-3 fatty acids (ALA) | Ages 1 to 3: 700 mg<br>Ages 4 to 8: 900 mg<br>Ages 9 to 13: 1200 mg (boys), 1000 mg (girls)<br>Ages 14 to 18: 1600 mg (boys), 1100 mg (girls) | ½ to 1 tablespoon (7 to 15 mL) ground flaxseed, chia seeds, or hemp seeds will meet 100 percent of daily needs |
| Iron | Ages 1 to 3: 7 mg<br>Ages 4 to 8: 10 mg<br>Ages 9 to 13: 8 mg<br>Ages 14 to 18: 11 mg (boys), 15 mg (girls) | 1 cup (250 mL) cooked oatmeal + 1 cup (250 mL) lentils + 1 cup (250 mL) cooked spinach = 14.5 mg |
| Zinc | Ages 1 to 3: 3 mg<br>Ages 4 to 8: 5 mg<br>Ages 9 to 13: 8 mg<br>Ages 14 to 18: 11mg (boys), 9 mg (girls) | ¼ cup (60 mL) pumpkin seeds + 1 cup (250 mL) cooked oatmeal + ½ cup (125 mL) hummus + 1 cup (250 mL) lentils = 10 mg |
| Vitamin B12 | Ages 1 to 3: 0.9 mcg<br>Ages 4 to 8: 1.2 mcg<br>Ages 9 to 13: 1.8 mcg<br>Ages 14 to 18: 2.4 mcg | 2 cups (500 mL) fortified non-dairy milk or 1½ teaspoons (7 mL) vitamin B12–fortified nutritional yeast meets teenage needs, or provide a daily vitamin B12 supplement (recommended) |
| Iodine | Ages 1 to 3: 90 mcg<br>Ages 4 to 8: 90 mcg<br>Ages 9 to 13: 120 mcg<br>Ages 14 to 18: 150 mcg | ¼ teaspoon (1 mL) iodized salt used in cooking will meet 100 percent of daily needs |

## Navigating Common Challenges in Changing Your Diet: A Plan for Success

Making dietary change takes effort, even when you are excited about it! The reason for this is that so many of our food behaviours over the course of a day are unconscious, guided by habit and experience.

In trying to make new choices, you will have to consciously guide your food behaviours until they become new habits. The first step is to make a plan. As mentioned, I really like the slow and steady approach. However, if you want to go all in, consider setting a start date one to two months from now to get your nutritional house in order.

How will you spend this time? Here are a few suggestions:

- Start a food journal of everything you eat and drink for one week. Note all the times you eat an animal-source food. Note when you skimp on protein or vegetables at a meal. Sit down with your journal and figure out which foods you will need substitutes for and what kinds of new recipes you will need to replace current favourites. If you are not currently eating a healthful diet, perhaps this is the perfect time to sit down with a plant-friendly registered dietitian for guidance.

- Join a Facebook group for vegetarians or vegans in your city. This can be an invaluable resource for finding local food products, stores, and restaurants to help you supply your new eating plan.

- Scan the menus of your favourite restaurants to see what dishes you can eat on your new eating plan. Looking scarce? Search out the vegetarian and vegan-friendly restaurants in your city using an online resource like Happy Cow. That way, when you are going out you will be able to suggest restaurants that you can enjoy as well.

- Tell friends and family what you are planning to do, and solicit their support. Note that in doing this, you can expect a bit of resistance. Sometimes, when faced with others' dietary changes, it can reflect our own choices and cause guilt and discomfort. For others, giving and receiving food is a way of communicating love, and making different choices may feel like a loss of connection with you. Remain positive, demonstrate enthusiasm, and commit to renewing traditions like cookie exchanges, Super Bowl parties, and Girls Nights in a pro-plant way.

When you give yourself time to plan ahead, it will allow you to feel more relaxed in your new eating plan. In addition, remember that if at the beginning you end up faltering a bit, that is totally okay. Change is a process.

I am sorry for what I said when I was "hangry."

## PLANT-BASED EATING FOR THE NEWBIE
## (AKA THE EFFECTS OF CARB LOADING IN THE NON-ATHLETE)

Many of my clients find that in transitioning to a plant-based diet, they end up eating too many starchy carbs. The result? They feel sluggish, are constantly hungry, and potentially even gain some weight.

Earlier in the chapter, I talked about the role of carbohydrates and blood sugars, so here I will focus on the practical side. Why is it so common to end up eating a ton of starch? Primarily, because it is easy. When navigating a dietary change, at times you can feel like you are not sure about what to eat because you can no longer make your go-to meals (this is also why a plan is so important).

It is so easy to eat toast, some rice, or a bowl of pasta when hungry, or to find those foods on a restaurant menu where tofu scrambles and lentil bowls are scarce. This is fine, but only occasionally. If this becomes the bulk of your diet, you will be on a blood sugar roller coaster without much nutrition. The "hanger," my friends, is real.

Even if you are committed to cooking a lot at home, there is one other slip-up you might not expect. It has to do with an overreliance on vegetables. This might sound strange coming from a dietitian, but we cannot live exclusively on vegetables. For example, I love jackfruit, but it does not contain protein. So, if you eat jackfruit or cauliflower steaks as a meal regularly, you may be missing a lot of opportunities for protein that will keep you full and satisfied. So, to get your required protein, try adding puréed hemp seeds into a gravy for the jackfruit or serving cauliflower steak on a bed of quinoa and hummus.

Eating out can also be a bit of a challenge at first, as often the plant-based meal is simply a meal that has had the meat removed; few mainstream restaurants serve a lot of beans or tofu. If you are vegetarian, it is a bit easier with eggs and cheese, but a lot of cheese is not going to help you feel more satisfied or maintain a healthy weight. Do not be afraid to ask if you can order off the menu or cobble together a meal of sides. If the salmon is served on a bed of lentils, ask if you can have lentils alongside your tomato pasta. Alternatively, scope out the edamame, roasted Brussels sprouts, and quinoa from a sides menu and turn them into a meal.

Here are some quick tips to help you transition to a plant-based diet:

- Always keep canned beans and frozen bags of pre-cooked whole grains such as brown rice or millet on hand. Hungry? A can of chickpeas sautéed with spinach and garlic comes together as fast as boiling pasta.
- If going out to eat, have a high-protein snack first, like some baked tofu or roasted chickpeas, to make up for the most commonly missing portion of the meal.

- Always keep emergency snacks with you, such as a protein-rich energy ball or raw nuts.
- When dining with friends, offer to bring a protein-rich main to supplement the meal.
- Travel with nuts and hemp seeds. It is so easy to add a few tablespoons of hemp seeds to hotel oatmeal for protein.
- If pasta is feeling like a necessary go-to, try one of the bean-based pastas to ramp up your protein intake.
- If your appetite is getting intense, keep a food journal and note where you could be adding extra healthy fats or proteins. If this is not immediately obvious, have a dietitian review what you are eating.
- Eat enough protein: a sprinkle of beans will not be enough. Instead, serve yourself 1 cup (250 mL) of cooked beans or up to half of a 12-ounce (350 g) package of tofu. Make vegetable burgers from beans, not rice. Prioritize protein-containing snacks like nuts and seeds over primarily carbohydrate snacks like fruit or baked goods to help get you full and satisfied.

### ADAPTING TO A HIGH-FIBRE DIET

I meet many clients who are concerned about eating plant foods because of all of the gas they will produce. I am not going to lie: eating a healthy whole foods diet, with all of that roughage, is going to cause gas. Gas is evidence that you are eating fibre (and have bacteria in your gut fermenting that fibre).

Typically, as long as you do not have a diagnosed digestive disease like irritable bowel syndrome or Crohn's disease, the best way to fix gas and bloating issues from plant foods is to double down and keep eating them. This might seem counterintuitive, but your body is remarkably adaptive. Over time, your system—a big part of which is your miraculous, fermenting gut bacteria—will transform in response to your new diet. However, if you ramp up fibre intake quickly, it could feel like your gut is about to explode. So, slow and steady does it. You cannot expect to totally eliminate having gas, but you can expect that it will fall within the spectrum of normal and not cause you distress.

Making the switch to a plant-based diet is an exciting way to refresh your love of food and cooking and to re-energize your body. If you have a pre-existing health condition, always talk to your doctor before making such a big change.

# Seven Steps to Help You Banish the Bloat

1. **DRINK A LOT OF WATER**

   Fibre requires water to do its job; the more fibre you eat, the more water you need to drink. Consume at least 6 cups (1.5 L) a day.

2. **MOVE YOUR BODY TO MOVE YOUR BOWELS**

   Your gut is a muscle. Exercise helps it move its contents along. So, commit to daily movement. Yoga is phenomenal, particularly twists; if the idea of passing gas in yoga class freaks you out, consider a home practice.

3. **EAT FERMENTED FOODS AND PROBIOTICS**

   Live fermented foods contain enzymes and beneficial microbes that aid digestion; in addition, the act of fermenting vegetables makes them easier to digest. A good probiotic will help provide high counts of beneficial bacteria that will encourage a healthy bacterial community. You will be less prone to more troublesome gas.

4. **PREPARE BEANS PROPERLY**

   When using canned beans, thoroughly drain and rinse them. This will remove many of the indigestible carbohydrates, also known as FODMAPs to those with irritable bowel syndrome, that contribute to gas, because they leach into cooking water. When preparing beans from fresh, soak them for at least 12 hours, discard the soaking water, and boil them in fresh water. Then rinse the beans well before you use them.

5. **LIGHTLY COOK VEGETABLES**

   When new to plant-based eating, it can help to consume more of your vegetables cooked instead of raw because cooking will help break down tough cell walls and make them easier to digest.

6. **TRY ENZYMES**

   Beano works, but it is not plant-based. Visit a health food store and look for a vegetarian digestive enzyme mix that contains alpha-galactosidase, the key enzyme in Beano.

7. **EAT GINGER AND FENNEL**

   Ginger and fennel have traditionally been used to "expel wind"; it is common in Indian restaurants to be served a tiny dish of candy-coated fennel seeds at the end of a meal. Try chewing three or four fennel seeds (if your spice jar is looking stale, buy a fresh bag!) or crystallized ginger, or sip teas made from ginger or fennel—both are delicious and soothing to drink as teas.

## Eat More Plants 21-Day Meal Plan

Sometimes, it can be tricky to imagine what eating a 100 percent whole food, plant-based diet looks like. To help you dive into this kind of eating, I created a 21-day meal plan to make it easier to get into the habit of eating more plants.

I realize that we are not always able to cook from scratch three meals a day! For this reason, I make use of repurposed leftovers and lunches you can prepare the night before or batch prep on the weekend.

When starting a meal plan, be sure to honour your hunger signals. If you are hungry in between meals, eat a snack. If you are not hungry, feel free to skip it! I feel the same way about dessert; while many of us have been raised eating daily sweets, it is not always necessary after a filling meal. Where possible, I have made use of snacks and treats that you can prepare on the weekend and eat all week or freeze for later. Therefore, you will always have something on the go when you need it.

### DAY 1
**Breakfast** Ginger Turmeric Smoothie (page 97)
**Lunch** Tomato Jam Tartines (page 210) with smashed chickpeas for added protein
**Dinner** Carrot Tofu Hippie Scramble (page 156)
**Snack** Peanut Butter Energy Fudge (page 233)

### DAY 2
**Breakfast** Tahini Fig Toast (page 103)
**Lunch** Leftover Carrot Tofu Hippie Scramble (page 156)
**Dinner** Sweet Potato Pasta with Mushrooms and Walnut Cream (page 165)
**Snack** Turmeric Chai (page 250)

### DAY 3
**Breakfast** Matcha Mango Chia Pudding (page 91)
**Lunch** Shiitake BLT Sandwich (page 139)
**Dinner** Mayo-Roasted Carrots with Curried Millet (page 182)
**Dessert** Almond Snickerdoodle Cookies (page 222)

### DAY 4
**Breakfast** Moroccan Mint Smoothie (page 95)
**Lunch** Tomato Jam Tartines (page 210) with smashed chickpeas for added protein
**Dinner** Smoky Peanut Corn Chowder (page 145)
**Snack** Leftover Peanut Butter Energy Fudge (page 233)

**DAY 5**

Breakfast Ginger Turmeric Smoothie (page 97)

Lunch Leftover Smoky Peanut Corn Chowder (page 145)

Dinner Edamame Hula Bowl with Almond Miso Sauce (page 181)

Snack Carrot Tahini Granola Bar (page 234)

Dessert Leftover Almond Snickerdoodle Cookies (page 222)

**DAY 6**

Breakfast Golden Milk Porridge (page 92)

Lunch Zucchini Zoodles with Sungold Cherry Tomato Sauce (page 114)

Dinner Mujadara Neat-Balls in Spiced Tomato Sauce (page 177)
served with Real Deal Gluten-Free Bread (page 267)

Dessert Raspberry Cacao Slice (page 238)

**DAY 7**

Breakfast Green Goddess Tofu Scramble (page 100) served with
leftover Real Deal Gluten-Free Bread (page 267)

Lunch Mujadara Neat-Ball Sandwiches (see page 177) served with
Fried Eggplant with Chili and Pomegranate Molasses (page 203)

Dinner Quinoa, Beet, and Kale Salad with Pistachio Butter Dressing (page 124)

Snack Spiced Carrot Dip (page 193) served with sliced vegetables

**DAY 8**

Breakfast Tahini Fig Toast (page 103)

Lunch Sandwich made with Real Deal Gluten-Free Bread (page 267),
Spiced Carrot Dip (page 193), sliced vegetables, and smoked tofu

Dinner Spiced Chickpea, Sundried Tomato, and Spinach Salad (page 119)

Snack Protein-Packed Savoury Tofu Muffins (page 106)

Dessert Raspberry Cacao Slice (page 238)

**DAY 9**

Breakfast Blushing Beet Smoothie Bowl (page 98)

Lunch Leftover Spiced Chickpea, Sundried Tomato, and Spinach Salad (page 119)
served with Spiced Carrot Dip (page 193) and Seedy Crackers (page 265)

Dinner Portuguese Green Bean Stew (page 150) served with a whole grain

Snack Protein-Packed Savoury Tofu Muffins (page 106)

**DAY 10**

Breakfast Ginger Turmeric Smoothie (page 97)

Lunch Leftover Portuguese Green Bean Stew (page 150) served with a whole grain

**Dinner** Whole-grain or bean-based pasta with Beet Pesto (page 262)

**Snack** Cardamom Rose Beet Latte (page 252)

## DAY 11

**Breakfast** Blushing Beet Smoothie Bowl (page 98)

**Lunch** Gluten-free wrap with leftover Beet Pesto (page 262),
Fermented Cashew Cream Cheese (page 271), and sliced vegetables

**Dinner** Channa Masala (page 173) with added spinach and served with a whole grain

**Snack** Protein-Packed Savoury Tofu Muffins (page 106)

## DAY 12

**Breakfast** Matcha Mango Chia Pudding (page 91)

**Lunch** Gluten-free wrap with leftover Channa Masala (page 173)

**Dinner** Grilled Tofu Caprese Salad (page 131)

**Snack** Peanut Butter Energy Fudge (page 233)

## DAY 13

**Breakfast** Golden Milk Porridge (page 92)

**Lunch** Beet Tartare (page 194) served with leftover Fermented Cashew
Cream Cheese (page 271) and Seedy Crackers (page 265)

**Dinner** Jicama Avocado Tacos (page 144) and Mexican Street Corn (page 209)
served with refried black beans and Verdita (page 245) mixed with soda water

**Dessert** Lebanese Turmeric Cake (page 231)

## DAY 14

**Breakfast** Moroccan Mint Smoothie (page 95) and Blackberry Ginger Muffins (page 105)

**Lunch** Green Onion Pancakes with XOXO Sauce (page 207) and
Vietnamese Cucumber Salad with Ginger and Mint (page 128)

**Dinner** Creamy Pasta with Smoked Tofu and Kale (page 159)

**Snack** Peanut Butter Energy Fudge (page 233)

## DAY 15

**Breakfast** Tahini Fig Toast (page 103)

**Lunch** Leftover Green Onion Pancakes with XOXO Sauce (page 207) and
Vietnamese Cucumber Salad with Ginger and Mint (page 128)

**Dinner** Red Grape, Chickpea, and Pine Nut Stew (page 149) served with a whole grain

**Snack** Lebanese Turmeric Cake (page 231)

## DAY 16

**Breakfast** Ginger Turmeric Smoothie (page 97)

**Lunch** Leftover Red Grape, Chickpea, and Pine Nut Stew (page 149) served with a whole grain

Dinner Chili Garlic Brussels Sprouts (page 214) served over Cheesy Lentil Grits (page 216)

Snack Blackberry Ginger Muffins (page 105) and Iced Ginger Vanilla Matcha Latte (page 246)

**DAY 17**

Breakfast Blushing Beet Smoothie Bowl (page 98)

Lunch Shiitake BLT Sandwich (page 139)

Dinner Cauliflower Peperonata Sauté (page 178)

Snack Peanut Butter Energy Fudge (page 233)

Dessert Raspberry Cacao Slice (page 238)

**DAY 18**

Breakfast Ginger Turmeric Smoothie (page 97) and Blackberry Ginger Muffins (page 105)

Lunch Gluten-free wrap with Fermented Cashew Cream Cheese (page 271) and leftover Cauliflower Peperonata Sauté (page 178)

Dinner Green Machine Burgers (page 140) served with Vietnamese Cucumber Salad with Ginger and Mint (page 128)

Snack Lebanese Turmeric Cake (page 231)

**DAY 19**

Breakfast Golden Milk Porridge (page 92)

Lunch Gluten-free wrap with leftover Green Machine Burgers (page 140) and Vietnamese Cucumber Salad with Ginger and Mint (page 128)

Dinner Socca Pizza with Zucchini, Olives, and Basil (page 171) served with Green Pea, Radish, and Date Salad with Apple Miso Dressing (page 132)

Snack Carrot Tahini Granola Bar (page 234)

**DAY 20**

Breakfast Blushing Beet Smoothie Bowl (page 98)

Lunch Pan-Roasted Grape and Arugula Salad with Oat and Walnut Crumble (page 135)

Dinner Truffled Mushroom Pâté (page 189), served with sliced vegetables and Seedy Crackers (page 265), and Lemon Millet Risotto with Roasted Radicchio (page 161)

Dessert Healthy Breakfast Cupcakes with Salted Chocolates Frosting (page 109)

**DAY 21**

Breakfast Peaches and Cream Breakfast Parfait (page 94)

Lunch Leftover Truffled Mushroom Pâté (page 189), served with sliced vegetables and Seedy Crackers (page 265), and Roasted Cauliflower Salad with Creamy Caper-Raisin Dressing (page 117)

Dinner Chickpea Gnocchi with Olive Tomato Sauce (page 166)

Snack Healthy Breakfast Cupcakes with Salted Chocolate Frosting (page 109)

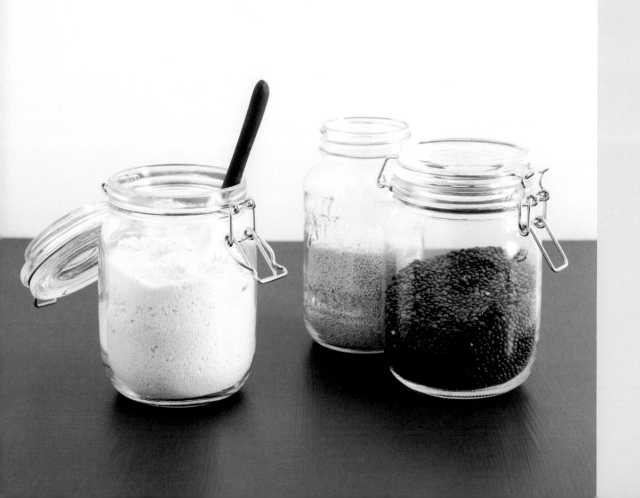

# 4

# Setting Up Your Kitchen and Meal Prep Basics

When you are new to plant-based cooking and eating, it can take time to build up your tools and your pantry. The first kitchen tool I bought when striking out on my own was a sandwich press. Not sure how practical that was. Now, I have more cooking experience, so I want to share all of my tips for getting yourself ready to rock in the kitchen.

The biggest change when putting more plants on your plate is that you will be doing a lot more chopping. Cooking plant-based meals is easy, but a whole food approach to cooking will take a bit more prep time when compared to opening a jar of pasta sauce. Of course, once you get into a rhythm, you will be surprised at how little extra time it takes to make a meal that has a lot of fresh vegetables, grains, and legumes. And, when you start to feel the benefits of eating this way, prep time becomes *you* time. Put on some music, embrace the meditativeness of it all, and get to chopping.

## Kitchen Tools and Equipment

To outfit your kitchen, you might need to do a bit of shopping first. I am a big gadget girl; some have proved useful, others less so. Although I am not a chef, having the proper equipment and tools has really helped me up my game in the kitchen. If you are just starting out, I recommend sticking to the basics so you do not spend too much on gadgets as you begin to transform your diet. Many of us live and cook in smaller spaces, so be mindful of storage and do not overwhelm yourself with too many tools. Once you have your kitchen outfitted with the essentials like knives and cookware, you might want to consider some of the nice-to-have tools, such as a high-speed blender, that would be great additions to your kitchen. The more you cook, the clearer it will be which tools can help make your kitchen life easier.

Wondering how a few extra tools can improve your kitchen game? When you eat the volume of vegetables that I do, the ability to vary textures completely changes your experience of eating. When I was just starting out as a home cook, I used to chop everything in very large chunks to save time. Although my plant-based meals were healthy, all the vegetables had the same consistency and were a chore to chew. As well, it got a bit repetitive.

Embrace new ways of serving your old standbys with fun extras like a spiralizer. Spirals of zucchini make it feel like a very new vegetable, one that my kids will actually eat. Carrots sliced paper-thin on a mandolin have a pleasing crunch without giving your jaw a workout. It really does make a difference!

## KNIVES

Everyone has different knife preferences, but having at least a good-quality 6- to 10-inch (15 to 25 cm) chef's knife and a paring knife is critical. My favourite knife is actually a *mini* chef's knife: a small 4-inch (10 cm) version that is stronger than a paring knife but far more agile than a chef's knife. A serrated bread knife rounds out my minimal collection of four knives.

Sharp knives mean faster cutting with less effort and fewer slips, so be sure to keep them sharp. It is worthwhile to buy the best-quality knives you can comfortably afford and take good care of them. If you do this, your knives will last a long time.

## POTS AND PANS

At a bare minimum, you should have a large skillet, large pot, and saucepan. Nonstick is great for newer cooks, but you need to throw them out as soon as they get scratched because it's unwise to consume particles of nonstick coating. Use only silicone tools and gentle sponges on your nonstick pans to avoid scratching them.

In addition to being relatively nonstick, cast iron pans have the added benefits of being easy to clean and adding iron to your meals.

When you're ready for more of an investment, try a good-quality set of stainless steel pots and pans with a multi-layered base. Your pots and pans will dictate the temperatures at which you cook and how food caramelizes. I use All-Clad stainless steel cookware, with a five-layer base, which retains heat well, so you will notice that most of my recipes are cooked at low and medium temperatures. It took me about three months to get used to them, burning a lot of foods and sticking everything in the process! However, food caramelizes beautifully in stainless steel cookware; you will probably need to increase the heat when using nonstick to get the same effect unless you cook on a gas stove.

I also love my large Le Creuset Dutch oven, which you will need to make the Real Deal Gluten-Free Bread (page 267). If you are going to invest in enameled cast iron cookware (which will literally last forever with Le Creuset's re-enameling service), buy a 7¼-quart (6.9 L) size. Always wash by hand and with a soft sponge.

### RIMMED BAKING SHEETS

A rimmed baking sheet (also called a jellyroll pan or a half sheet pan) is an 11- × 17-inch (28 × 43 cm) metal pan with a 1-inch (2.5 cm) deep lip. I use my rimmed baking sheets for roasting vegetables, toasting nuts, making pizza, or freezing summer produce before storing it in freezer bags. You can buy nonstick baking sheets for ease of use, but be sure to use soft utensils and sponges to protect them. Otherwise, uncoated metal baking sheets from the kitchen supply shop work like a dream for baking and roasting with a protective layer of parchment paper.

### CUTTING BOARDS

To preserve the edge of your knives, and for better food safety, a wood cutting board is best. If you have the counter space to dedicate to a cutting board, I am a big fan of heavy Boos blocks. If, like me, you need all the counter space you can get, I also like Epicurean composite boards that can be easily tucked away when not in use.

### MIXING BOWLS

I often use cereal bowls for mixing small amounts, but a basic set of small, medium, and large glass mixing bowls is an inexpensive and worthwhile addition to your kitchen.

### BASIC UTENSILS

Grab a set of basic cooking utensils for the kitchen. You will also need a full set of measuring spoons and cups. The recipes in this book include both imperial and metric measurements, but take note of what kind of measuring utensils you have or need to buy so you can use the right measurements when cooking.

### VEGETABLE PEELER

A sharp vegetable peeler is a thing of beauty. I do not actually peel a lot of veggies (like carrots) because peels are nutritious, but for vegetables with tough skins (like butternut squash), a good peeler makes quick work of the chore. It can also be used to make vegetable ribbons for salads if you do not have a spiralizer. You can find a great vegetable peeler for less than ten dollars.

### GRATERS

I like the traditional upright box graters, with sides for slicing, coarsely grating vegetables, and finely grating ginger and garlic, as I find them much easier to use. I also have a fine microplane grater that works best for grating ginger, if you want to add another grater to your collection.

## MANDOLIN

My mandolin is my sous chef! It is an affordable tool that makes creating perfectly thin and uniform slices of vegetables almost effortless. In addition, a mandolin makes quick work of slicing, so it is less of a chore. Mandolin blades are extremely sharp, so be sure to always use the hand guard to protect your fingers!

## SPIRALIZER

I am crazy about my spiralizer, an old Japanese version from Benriner that is basic and easy to clean. Creating noodles out of beets, zucchini, carrots, and sweet potatoes makes eating your vegetables way more fun, and kids absolutely love it.

Newer versions of spiralizers are easy to use; look for one with multiple blade thicknesses and suction cups on its feet so it does not travel all over your counter. If your spiralizer does not have suction cups, gently wet a kitchen towel and place it under the spiralizer while you use it.

## SALAD SPINNER

I went years without a salad spinner, but salad is 100 percent more enjoyable when it is properly dried. Dressing coats the leaves properly, making them more flavourful. If you want to up your salad game, spin it. If you do not have a salad spinner, be sure to carefully dry salad greens in a clean kitchen towel.

## COLANDER

A colander makes draining pasta and rinsing vegetables so much easier. I went a while without a colander for space reasons, but it is a well-spent couple of dollars.

## NUT MILK BAG

If you want to make your own nut milk, you need a special cloth bag that will trap all of the pulp (so much easier than using cheesecloth). Nut milk bags are washable and reusable and easily found in health food stores or online. Also, do not throw away the pulp! Dry and freeze all that goodness and add in ½-cup (125 mL) increments to muffins, energy balls, pancakes, and smoothies. See Tip (page 270).

## PARCHMENT PAPER

If you love to cook but hate the cleanup, parchment paper can be a real lifesaver. Put a layer of parchment paper on your baking sheet for a nonstick surface and easy cleanup. And it composts, so bonus!

## IMMERSION BLENDER

One of my first kitchen tools, alongside a sandwich press, was a handheld immersion blender that I bought for forty dollars and still have today. This is a super-versatile workhorse that I would recommend buying before an upright blender. When paired with a large, wide-mouthed cup, an immersion blender actually does a better job of puréeing smaller volumes of most sauces, and even cashew cream, than a blender or food processor. You can also blend smoothies as long as they do not have too many tough leafy greens like kale or frozen chunks of fruit. Before I had a food processor, with a great deal of persistence I even relied on my immersion blender to whip up hummus and black bean brownies.

## FOOD PROCESSOR

It was years before I bought a food processor, but having one makes plant-based cooking a lot easier. You can grate a pound of carrots in about 60 seconds and effortlessly blend tough ingredients like chickpeas, cauliflower, nuts, and herbs. I have a 12-cup (3 L) machine from Breville, an Australian company whose products I find to be very high quality. Mine comes with a small jar for smaller jobs.

## HIGH-SPEED BLENDER

It can feel hard to justify the price of a high-speed blender, but they are significantly more effective than less expensive blenders. For example, they can *liquefy* vegetables into juice. You will never have a kale smoothie that chews like salad again. Cashew creams become silky and light in a way that a food processor cannot match. You might need to replace the plastic jar after five years of heavy use, but the motor should last at least ten years. I use a Blendtec high-speed blender, and I love it.

## Stocking Your Pantry

A well-stocked pantry means that there is always something to eat. Although I typically cook around whatever fresh vegetables are on hand, my pantry is what completes the meal with its endless variety. In addition, in a pinch—usually when I am not feeling up to shopping—I can often craft a healthful meal with everyday basics. Here, I am sharing the staples that I cook with most often so that you can build your anti-inflammatory kitchen with ease.

## FLOURS

When creating an anti-inflammatory meal, one of the most powerful swaps you can make is to include more nutrient-dense flours in your recipe. Refined, low-fibre flours spike blood sugars and are nutrient-poor. The following alternatives make traditionally less healthy recipes truly nutrient-dense.

- Almond Flour

  High in protein, healthy fats, and fibre, almond flour has a sweet, neutral taste that allows your chosen flavours to shine through. The terms *almond flour* and *almond meal* are often used interchangeably; very finely ground almond flour is now available for even lighter textures in your baked goods. You can also make your own almond flour in a high-speed blender from blanched almonds, although it requires sifting and re-blending to gain a uniform texture.

- Brown Rice Flour

  Brown rice flour lightens up the texture of baked goods and has a mild taste with the slightest grit in its texture. I often use it in combination with a heavier flour, like chickpea.

- Chickpea Flour

  One of my favourite flours for its nutritional density, chickpea flour is high fibre, high protein, and mineral rich. It has a deep, savoury flavour that I really enjoy. It absorbs liquid readily and is often soaked before using for easier digestion.

- Gluten-Free All-Purpose Flour

  There is a wide variety of gluten-free all-purpose flour mixes on the market. Many of them are highly refined and not a great fit for anti-inflammatory cooking. For ease, I have created my recipes using the same blend: Bob's Red Mill All Purpose Flour (not the 1-to-1 blend). I have chosen this blend, which is chickpea-based, for nutrient density and because it is widely available in supermarkets and online. If you bake with another blend, your results may vary, as baking is truly an exact science.

## BEANS, LEGUMES, AND TOFU

I often cook beans from scratch and aim to have two to three types of legumes on hand at a time. If I use canned beans, I always choose unsalted so I can control the salt content of my meals. If you use salted beans, start with half of the salt called for in the recipe, then adjust seasoning to your taste.

- Black Beans

  Black beans make an excellent addition to salads, stir-fries, or richly flavoured dips. Their deeply coloured skin is a clue that they contain anti-inflammatory plant pigments.

- Chickpeas

  Chickpeas are the most versatile, crowd-pleasing legume. They can be roasted as a snack, blended as a dip or baking ingredient, and scrambled or mashed into a sandwich filling. Add them whole to just about any meal for a protein boost.

- Edamame

  Edamame are young green soybeans. Because they are high in protein and minerals, I always keep a bag of shelled, non-GMO edamame in the freezer for easy additions to meals.

- Lentils (French, beluga, red, green, and brown)

  Each variety of lentils is unique in texture and flavour. French green lentils are a versatile staple, as they hold their texture well and have a rich flavour. I also love firm beluga black lentils for salads. Red lentils break down readily in cooking, making them excellent for lending a thick texture to soups, stews, and sauces.

- Tofu (pressed, extra firm, and smoked)

  I eat tofu regularly; I always buy organic, which is non-GMO and processed without hexane. Pressed tofu has a meaty texture that holds up well to grilling or stir-frying. Extra-firm tofu can be crumbled, sliced, or cubed. Smoked tofu is a ready-to-eat variety that tastes like smoked mozzarella. I often snack on smoked tofu or slice it into sandwiches.

- White Beans (navy, cannellini, and white kidney)

  White beans are my secret weapon: they have a creamy, buttery texture that I rely on for making dips and creamy, protein-rich sauces. They are delicious when tossed with pasta, and I also love them mashed into a simple sandwich filling.

## CANNED GOODS

Canned and jarred foods have gotten a bad rap from their hyper-processed cousins; these pantry staples add flavour and variety to your plant-based meals.

- Capers

  Capers are pickled flower buds; their briny tang adds a delicious bright spot to salads, pasta, and dips. Wait until you try them fried! Once opened, store capers in the refrigerator.

- Coconut Manna

  Like the coconut version of a nut butter, manna is whole puréed coconut. It is creamy, tastes decadent, and adds a rich and buttery flavour to sauces, smoothies, porridge, and desserts.

- Coconut Milk (light and full fat)

  Coconut milk is a creamy base for smoothies, sauces, baking, and curries. The cream top on full-fat coconut milk can be whipped like whipping cream!

- Young Jackfruit in Brine

  Jackfruit is a large, tropical fruit that is very fibrous and not at all sweet. Its fibrous flesh works well as a "pulled pork"–type texture in tacos, pizzas, and sandwiches. They are typically found in urban supermarkets or Asian food stores, but double-check the package before you buy, as jackfruit is also sold canned in sweet syrup.

- Kalamata Olives

  Olives are my favourite flavour pick-me-up; blended into salty tapenade, they make a delicious spread. Olives add a salty hit to tomato sauce, salads, and vegetable sautés. Store them in the refrigerator once opened.

- Sun-Dried Tomatoes

  You typically find sun-dried tomatoes packed in inexpensive oil; I try to pat off as much of this oil as I can. Packed with umami flavour, they can be puréed into dressings and sauces or chopped into salads, sautés, and pasta dishes.

- Whole and Diced Tomatoes

  Tomatoes are one of the few vegetables that I consider just as healthy canned as fresh; I always keep a few cans on hand for chili, pasta, and vegetables sautés.

## CONDIMENTS

My fridge door is filled with condiments; they are the flavour boosts that help plant foods sing. Some, like tomato paste or miso, come with their own health benefits.

- Dijon Mustard

  I love mustards and often have two or three types on hand at a time. However, Dijon holds a special place in my foodie heart. It is a salty, creamy, spunky ingredient that emulsifies salad dressings and adds zing to sauces.

- Gluten-Free Tamari

  Tamari is a richly flavoured, traditionally brewed soy sauce. Look for a gluten-free variety, as not all are gluten-free.

- Hot Sauces

  I usually have a few hot sauces on hand: Sriracha, a vinegar-based sauce (Valentina is my favourite), and Matouk's (a Caribbean scotch bonnet blend that is like a super-spicy, runny salsa).

- Miso

  Miso is fermented soybean paste; to enjoy its fermented benefits, eat it uncooked. I typically use either shiro (white) or aka (red) miso. Shiro miso is a blend of soybeans and rice, lightly fermented for a mild, sweet taste. It is wonderful for adding savoury depth to sauces, soups, and even baking. Aka miso has a longer ferment, for a saltier, funkier taste. It stands up well in sauces with other flavourful ingredients, like ginger or black beans. Use aka miso more sparingly than shiro. Note that not all miso is gluten-free; some, like mugi miso, contain barley.

- Tomato Paste

  Tomato paste is a concentrated form of tomato sauce that has the highest concentration of anti-inflammatory lycopene of any tomato product. It lends plenty of umami to any dish. I buy mine in handy tubes to bypass the common challenge of wasting what is left over when buying in it in the can.

- Vegan Mayonnaise

  Mayonnaise is a wonderful ingredient for adding creamy textures to plant-based recipes. Most vegan mayonnaise is made with soy oil; if you use it rarely, do not worry. However, if you use it frequently, it is better to make your own. It takes about three minutes to create homemade mayonnaise from monounsaturated avocado oil (see page 79) so you can indulge your love of the stuff in good health.

- Vinegars (apple cider, rice, wine)

  Getting the balance of acidity correct can really transform a dish. Unpasteurized apple cider vinegar has a pungent tang; as a fermented food, it also has small amounts of live cultures. Red wine vinegar has a bold, distinctive flavour; white wine vinegar is milder. Unseasoned rice vinegar has the lightest, freshest taste in comparison to apple cider or wine vinegars.

## FATS AND OILS

The quality and type of fats and oils you purchase are important when eating to fight inflammation; always select cold-pressed oils, as this preparation preserves the health benefits. Oils should be stored away from heat and light and purchased in a size that you can easily use within one to two months for freshness. I typically use about 1 quart (1 L) of olive oil per month!

- Avocado Oil

  A filtered avocado oil, free of solids, is a wonderful stand-in for olive oil for high-heat cooking: it has a smoke point of 500°F (260°C) degrees. It is also very mild in flavour, working in recipes where olive oil might not fit. Be forewarned: non-filtered varieties of avocado oil are available, and they are not appropriate for cooking. Save their rich avocado flavour for finishing a dish.

- Coconut Oil

  Virgin coconut oil has a lower smoke point than you might expect: usually below 300°F (150°C). For that reason, and for a more neutral flavour, I use naturally refined coconut oil, which has a smoke point in line with olive oil, for cooking.

- Extra-Virgin Olive Oil

  For cooking, you want an extra-virgin olive oil from the supermarket, as these are typically filtered to remove solids. It is the presence of solids that lowers the smoke point of the oil. You can easily cook with a standard oil up to medium-high on the stove, as the smoke point is typically around 375°F to 400°F (190°C to 200°C). I also bake and roast with olive oil most of the time. If you have the more expensive, cloudy varieties of olive oil, reserve these for dressings and drizzling only.

- Sesame Oil

  Dark toasted sesame oil has an unmistakable flavour; just a little goes a long way! Drizzle over stir-fries or fried rice dishes, and whisk it into sauces.

## SWEETENERS

On an anti-inflammatory diet, the total amount of sugars and the overall glycemic load of the meal matters in order to avoid inflammation-spiking blood sugar highs. I take the stance that real is always best and tend to avoid artificial sweeteners, preferring to use less of the good stuff than to increase sweetness with zero-calorie sweeteners that further stoke a sweet tooth.

- Cane Sugar

  Added sugars are definitely something to watch on an anti-inflammatory diet; however, in very small amounts, sometimes pure cane sugar is just the right fit for a recipe. It has a clean, neutral flavour and can be used to balance bitterness or acidity in a salad dressing or to sweeten baked goods without competing with a light flavour. Not all cane sugar is vegan, as it may be processed with animal products; look on the label for the vegan mark.

- Dates

  Dates add moisture to baked goods and provide natural sweetness; I look for plump, moist varieties like Medjool or Deglet Noor. If your dates are not moist, you can soak them in warm water for five minutes before using. Most dates are sold fresh; store them in the fridge.

- Pure Maple Syrup

  The sweetener I use most often, pure maple syrup is flavourful, allowing you to use less and still be satisfied. I usually purchase Grade B, which is lighter than Grade A. Maple syrup has trace amounts of minerals, but you would have to consume a lot (too much) to have a real impact on your nutrition status. While less processed, maple syrup is still a form of added sugar, and I always aim to use as little as possible. Store it in the fridge after opening.

## NUTS AND SEEDS

I try to incorporate nuts and seeds into meals throughout my day in smoothies, salads, snacks, or sauces. I always buy raw nuts, as roasting hastens the degradation of the healthy fats they contain as they sit on the shelf. Larger format packages are often more affordable; however, if buying more than you will use in a month, store in the freezer for optimal freshness. Store nut butters in the fridge.

- Almonds and Almond Butter

  I use raw, unsweetened almond butter; it has a natural sweetness on its own. I usually have whole and sliced almonds on hand to add to salads, nut cheeses, or baking. When soaked overnight, the skins of raw almonds slip off quite easily, so I do not often buy blanched varieties.

- Cashews

  Cashews are a staple in any plant-based kitchen. I soak raw cashews for four hours before use in creamy nut cheeses, sauces, and desserts. This step hydrates the flesh of the nuts for smoother blending and is essential if you are processing or blending in a standard blender. If you have a high-speed blender, you can skip this step!

- Chia Seeds

  Soaked chia absorbs water like a sponge because of its soluble fibre content. Chia makes a great egg substitute: soak 1 tablespoon (15 mL) chia seeds in 3 tablespoons (45 mL) hot water for each egg in a recipe. I use chia seeds to make chia puddings, instant fruit jams, and in baking.

- Ground Flaxseed

  Flaxseed needs to be ground, as its hard shell is almost impossible for the human gut to break down. When ground, all of the valuable omega-3 fatty acids, minerals, and lignans become bioavailable. You can use ground flaxseed to absorb liquid in a recipe, add fibre, and replace eggs using the same ratios as for chia seeds (see page 80).

- Hemp Seeds

  Hemp seed is one of my favourite plant-based proteins: 3 tablespoons (45 mL) of hemp seeds have 10 grams of protein, in addition to omega-3 fatty acids and minerals. I use hemp seeds in smoothies, dressings, and baking. You can also sprinkle them over salads, cereals, or any meal.

- Peanut Butter

  Richly savoury and smooth, peanut butter is a staple in my house. In smoothies, soups, and sauces or as a dip for fruit, this protein-rich legume is worth having on hand. I always buy natural, unsweetened varieties.

- Pumpkin Seeds

  Raw pumpkin seeds are a crunchy addition to trail mix, baking, and salads. When using fresh pumpkins at home, do not throw out the seeds! Although they are different than the pepita-style seed we typically buy in the store, you can rinse, season, and gently roast fresh pumpkin seeds for a delicious snack or salad topper.

- Tahini

  Tahini is sesame seed butter. It has become a staple in my kitchen for adding a creamy, savoury richness to sauces and dressings and even standing in for butter in baked goods. High in minerals like calcium, it is an essential ingredient in plant-based recipes.

- Walnuts

  Walnuts are richly flavoured and can be bitter if they are not fresh, which is why buying them at a store with high turnover is important. Walnuts are a nice addition to salads and make wonderful additions to desserts, where they help give depth to sweet notes.

## WHOLE GRAINS

It is so important to reiterate that grains and pseudo-grains absolutely have a place in an anti-inflammatory diet; while some people with advanced autoimmunity or digestive health issues may find relief in going grain-free for a while, whole grains provide nutrient density and tasty variety to an anti-inflammatory diet for the rest of us.

- Black Rice

  Chewy, dense, and richly flavoured, black rice is high in anti-inflammatory pigments. It makes a refreshing change from standard grains and is delicious as a coconut-based rice pudding.

- Brown Rice

  The glycemic impact of rice grains depends on variety and grain length. I always choose a long grain jasmine or basmati brown rice. If you eat a lot of rice and are concerned about arsenic content, consider buying rice grown in California, India, or Pakistan.

- Millet

  Less popular than quinoa, millet deserves a more regular place at the dinner table. Quick to cook with a mild, wheat-like flavour and a fluffy grain, millet works in almost any recipe that you would make with quinoa.

- Pasta

  Whole-grain pasta, cooked until just tender, can be enjoyed as part of an anti-inflammatory eating plan. I find that the nicest gluten-free varieties are often a blend of rice, which provides softness, and corn, giving the pasta a non-mushy structure. My new favourite for higher protein meals is chickpea flour–based pastas.

- Quinoa

  This classic Incan staple has an excellent amino acid profile, making it a great choice for plant-based diets. However, it is not actually high in protein, so do not use it as your sole protein source at a meal. It cooks up quickly and works well in a variety of dishes, from salads to casseroles.

## Meal Prep Your Way

I am, by nature, a bit of a food rebel. I have been known to roast vegetables with olive oil beyond its smoke point. Or eat dessert, like my Raspberry Cacao Slice (page 238), for breakfast. As a dietitian, I know that meal planning is the best way to save time and make eating well a breeze. However, I have a hard time following a set meal plan; my little rebel heart always wants to change its mind. So, traditional meal planning and prep is not something I come to naturally.

Of course, when eating a plant-based diet, a little prep makes things much easier. I find that doing a weekly prep of ingredients that take longer to prepare or cook makes week-day cooking super quick.

## 1. THE SUNDAY BATCH PREP

Some ingredients just take time to cook. I rarely make brown rice on a weeknight because it takes about forty-five minutes. However, if you magically have brown rice in the fridge or freezer, it feels like winning. So, I prep in advance.

If cooking for one or two, I suggest cooking one or two batches of grains and one or two batches of beans and legumes each week. If you do not want to cook beans from scratch, stock up on salt-free canned beans.

Grain prep is a great weekend activity because it takes very little active time, so you can do it while you are watching Netflix or folding the laundry. Just remember to set a timer! Reserve what you will use in a couple of days, then freeze the rest in 2-cup (500 mL) or 4-cup (1 L) portions, in resealable plastic freezer bags, for later. Be sure to label the bags with the variety and date. Each week, take inventory and prep some more as needed. Within a couple of weeks, you will have a nice rotation of grains and beans for effortless meals.

## 2. CHOP VEGETABLES A COUPLE TIMES A WEEK OR THE NIGHT BEFORE

The most intensive part of my recipes is chopping vegetables. If you are a more organized human than I am, you can chop the vegetables for your next three days of meals to dramatically reduce evening meal prep time. Alternatively, you can simply work one day in advance and chop vegetables for tomorrow's dinner before you go to bed. Most of the recipes in this book will come together in fifteen to twenty minutes if the vegetables are prepped in advance.

## 3. BATCH COOKING

My lunches are usually a combination of leftovers. When I make dinner, I often cook more for lunch the next day. For example, extra roasted vegetables can become a salad or wrap filling for lunch. Leftover rice can be fried with whatever vegetables you have in the fridge. Extra baked tofu can be added to a sandwich. If you are cooking for one, do not shy away from making a meal that serves four. You will have lunch the next day, and you can either freeze the rest for another meal next week or simply have dinner or lunch made for another day or two. Since you are already cooking, it takes little extra time to make a bit more.

## Cooking Grains, Beans, and Lentils

Cooking grains and beans is simple; all you need is water and time. A little pinch of salt in the cooking water will create a more flavourful grain.

### GRAINS

To cook most grains, bring them to a boil with the required amount of water, cover, and simmer until the water is absorbed and the grains are tender. Fluff with a fork and let sit covered for an additional ten minutes. I have noted any exceptions to the standard method.

| Grain | Dry Amount | Water Amount | Cooking Time (bring to a boil, then simmer) | Yield |
|---|---|---|---|---|
| Amaranth | 1 cup (250 mL) | 2½ cups (625 mL) | 20 minutes | 2½ cups (625 mL) |
| Black rice | 1 cup (250 mL) | 2 cups (500 mL) | 45 minutes | 3 cups (750 mL) |
| Brown rice | 1 cup (250 mL) | 2 cups (500 mL) | 35 to 45 minutes | 3 cups (750 mL) |
| Buckwheat | 1 cup (250 mL) | 2 cups (500 mL) | 10 to 15 minutes, uncovered | 3 cups (750 mL) |
| Millet | 1 cup (250 mL) | 2 cups (500 mL) | 15 to 20 minutes | 3½ cups (875 mL) |
| Quinoa | 1 cup (250 mL) | 2 cups (500 mL) | 15 minutes | 3 cups (750 mL) |

### BEANS AND LENTILS

Beans are easy and much more cost effective to cook from dried. Dried beans also have a nicer texture than most canned varieties. The only downside is that you have to plan ahead because they require overnight soaking, with the exception of lentils.

Before soaking, sort through the beans to ensure that there are no stones or other debris. Rinse the beans, place them in a pot, and fill to cover with at least 2 inches (5 cm) of water. Soak overnight or up to twenty-four hours.

When ready to cook, rinse again and fill the pot with fresh water to cover the beans with at least 2 inches (5 cm) of water. When you cook beans, do not salt them prior to cooking. The salt will hinder their softening during cooking. Instead, season at the end of cooking. If you want to add flavour, you can cook them with a bit of diced onion and garlic or some bay leaves.

Much quicker to cook than beans, red or yellow lentils will cook down to mush and add a thick texture to sauces, soups, and stews. Green and brown lentils hold their shape better but can also cook down very soft; these are the lentils often used in canning, and they may be delicate. I love using dried French green lentils, as they have a nicer, firmer texture.

Beluga, black, or du Puy lentils look like tiny black gems and have a wonderful firm and meaty texture when cooked that works very well in salads.

Your best guide to determining when beans are ready is your senses. Depending on how fresh, or what size, the beans are, cooking times vary, so check for tenderness with a fork or your teeth. Once cooked, drain and rinse the beans well.

If cooking beans *only* with the intention of making a dip or hummus, 1 teaspoon (5 mL) of baking soda will tenderize the beans, reduce cooking time, and make for the silkiest dip possible. Watch your beans carefully when cooking this way so that you do not end up with mush!

| Legume | Dry Amount | Water Amount | Cooking Time (bring to a boil, then simmer) | Yield |
|---|---|---|---|---|
| Black beans | 1 cup (250 mL) | Pot full | 45 to 60 minutes | 3 cups (750 mL) |
| Cannellini beans | 1 cup (250 mL) | Pot full | 60 to 90 minutes | 3 cups (750 mL) |
| Chickpeas | 1 cup (250 mL) | Pot full | 60 to 90 minutes | 3 cups (750 mL) |
| Lentils: green, brown, or black | 1 cup (250 mL) | 3 cups (750 mL) | 20 to 30 minutes | 3 cups (750 mL) |
| Lentils: red | 1 cup (250 mL) | 3 cups (750 mL) | 15 to 20 minutes | 3 cups (750 mL) |

## Save Money, Waste Less: Food Storage Hacks

One of the most common concerns I hear from clients is that they are worried about wasting produce if they overbuy. The more you commit to planning your meals, the less this will be a worry. However, sometimes vegetables go bad seemingly overnight, or that packet of herbs you bought for one recipe ends up forgotten at the back of the fridge.

First, there are separate fruit and veggie drawers for a reason. Many fruits, like avocado and apples, release ethylene gas as they ripen, which will wilt vegetables. Use those drawers! Here are a few other tips to help you make the most of your vegetable spend.

1. Treat herbs, such as parsley and cilantro, like plants: trim ends when you get them home, place upright in a cup of water, cover with a resealable plastic bag, and store in the fridge. A fresh bunch of herbs can last a couple of weeks if stored properly.

2. Wrap leafy greens tightly in plastic wrap and store them in the crisper of the refrigerator. Use within three to five days. You can also chop and freeze leafy greens such as kale, spinach, or Swiss chard for use in stews and smoothies. Use within a couple of weeks for best flavour.

3. With clamshells of salad greens and herbs, I find that placing a piece of paper towel in the bottom of the container helps absorb moisture that can lead to slime rot.

4. If bananas are getting past their prime, peel them, slice in coins, and freeze in a single layer on a rimmed cookie sheet. Once frozen, place in a resealable plastic freezer bag. The banana coins are yummy as a snack. You can add them to smoothies or blitz them for a few minutes in a food processor for banana "nice cream."

5. Plan your recipes based on storage: use leafy greens first, then transition to hardier vegetables like carrots and beets later in the week.

6. Purée unused herbs into a pesto. Pesto freezes beautifully, sealed in a glass container for up to a month for best flavour, and makes it super easy to whip up a weeknight pasta.

7. When using canned chickpeas, always pour off the soaking liquid (called aquafaba) into a jar and refrigerate for baking needs. It will keep for three to four days.

8. Use vegetable tops, like carrots and radishes, for pesto or adding to vegetable burgers.

# Plant Power to the People!

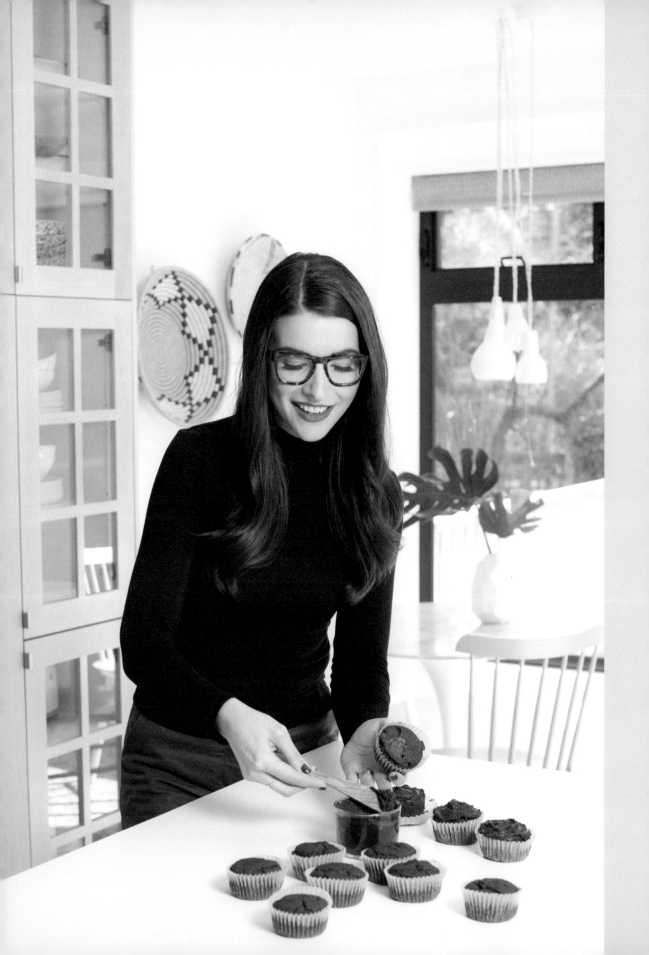

# 5

# Breakfasts Worth Waking Up For

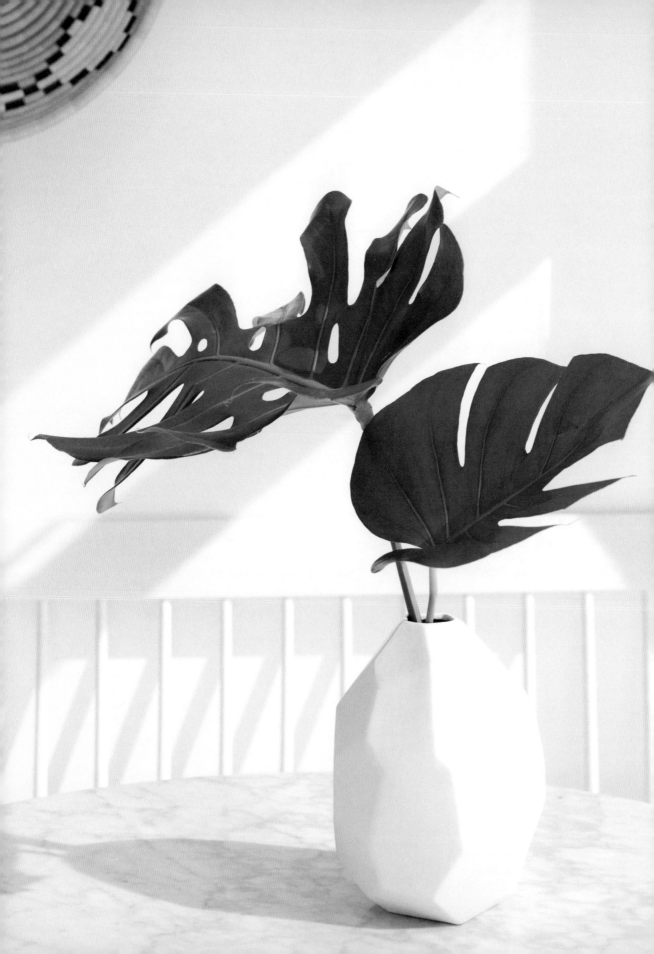

# Matcha Mango Chia Pudding

DAIRY-FREE | GLUTEN-FREE | NUT-FREE | PALEO-FRIENDLY | VEGAN | VEGETARIAN

SERVES 1

On a hectic morning, it is a relief to know you already have an energizing breakfast in the fridge. It is even better when it comes pre-caffeinated. Matcha, a powder ground from whole green tea leaves, provides a lift with fewer jitters than brewed coffee because of L-theanine, an amino acid that balances the effects of caffeine in the body. Prized for its high content of the polyphenol epigallocatechin gallate (EGCG), matcha is an anti-inflammatory all-star.

---

1. In a high-speed blender, combine the coconut milk, mango, maple syrup, and matcha. Blend until smooth and no visible chunks of mango remain. Pour into a mason jar or resealable container.

2. Add the chia seeds and coconut and stir vigorously with a fork for about 1 minute. Let sit for 2 minutes, and then stir again. This will ensure that the chia seeds do not clump together as they hydrate.

3. Store in the fridge overnight and you will have breakfast for the next morning.

Tip  If you taste the matcha mix before you add the chia seeds, you will notice that it tastes lovely and sweet. This sweetness will dissipate overnight, and the pudding will taste like an unsweetened matcha latte by morning. Stir in more maple syrup in the morning, if needed.

Make It Faster  If you have a wide-mouthed mason jar and a handheld immersion blender, you can blend the coconut milk, mango, maple syrup, and matcha directly in the jar and save a few dishes.

1 cup (250 mL) canned light coconut milk

½ cup (125 mL) fresh or partially thawed frozen mango chunks

1 teaspoon (5 mL) pure maple syrup

1 teaspoon (5 mL) matcha powder

3 tablespoons (45 mL) chia seeds

1 tablespoon (15 mL) unsweetened shredded coconut

# Golden Milk Porridge

DAIRY-FREE | GLUTEN-FREE | NUT-FREE | VEGAN | VEGETARIAN

SERVES 1

Turmeric is one of my favourite spices. Vibrant and earthy, turmeric is a powerful anti-inflammatory, and paired with millet it is an energizing way to start the day. Home-cooked porridge does not seem that doable on a busy morning, so I like to put everything in a pot and soak it overnight to reduce the cooking time in the morning.

1 cup (250 mL) unsweetened soy milk

¼ cup (60 mL) water

2 tablespoons (30 mL) freshly squeezed orange juice

2 tablespoons (30 mL) unsweetened coconut flakes

1 tablespoon (15 mL) pure maple syrup

1 teaspoon (5 mL) pure vanilla extract

½ teaspoon (2 mL) ground turmeric

¼ teaspoon (1 mL) ground cardamom

¼ teaspoon (1 mL) cinnamon

⅛ teaspoon (0.5 mL) ground ginger

5 whole fennel seeds

Salt

⅓ cup (75 mL) millet

For serving (optional)

Sliced banana

Sliced apple

Sliced persimmon

1. In a small saucepan, whisk together the soy milk, water, orange juice, coconut flakes, maple syrup, vanilla, turmeric, cardamom, cinnamon, ginger, fennel seeds, a pinch of salt, and millet. Cover and place in the fridge overnight. Be sure to use a stainless steel saucepan or the turmeric will permanently stain your precious enameled cookware.

2. In the morning, heat the porridge over medium-high heat and bring to a boil. Reduce to medium-low heat, partially covered, for about 12 minutes, stirring occasionally. The liquid will be mostly absorbed, but the mixture should not look dry.

3. Pour the porridge into a bowl, top with banana, apple, or persimmon (if using), and serve.

Tip  If you have a long, leisurely morning, you can make this in one go. Stir the golden milk mixture in a saucepan and then add the millet. Bring to a boil and lower to a simmer, partially covered, stirring occasionally for about 25 minutes.

Make It Faster  Bring a half-portion of the golden milk mixture to a boil, add a 1.7-ounce (50 g) packet of unsweetened instant gluten-free oats instead of millet, pack it in a Thermos, and you are out the door.

Make It Healthier  If you are a hard-core turmeric fan, add up to 1 teaspoon (5 mL). Any more than that and it will be too intense.

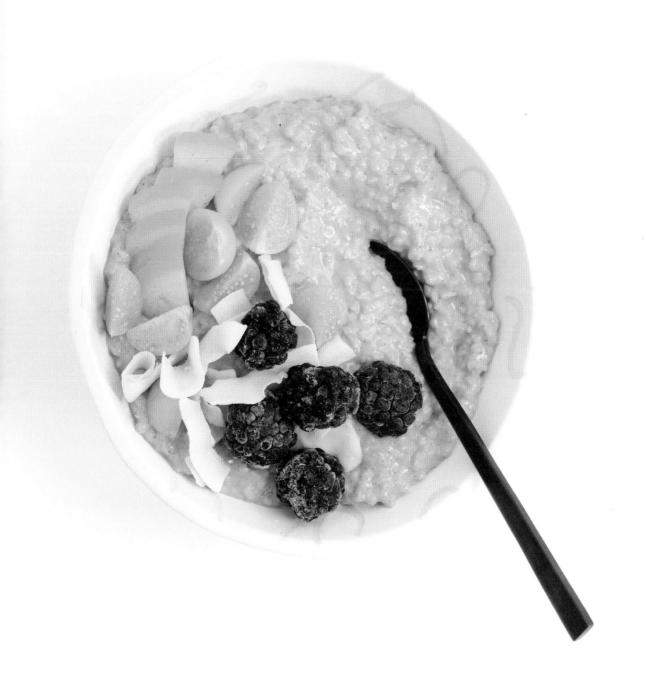

# Peaches and Cream Breakfast Parfait

DAIRY-FREE | GLUTEN-FREE | PALEO-FRIENDLY | VEGAN | VEGETARIAN

SERVES 2

Discovering cashew cream changed my dairy-free life. Soaked cashews make silky, dreamy creams that are full of healthful fats and energizing minerals. In fact, ¼ cup (60 mL) of cashews contains almost all of your copper needs for the day. Why is copper so special? This trace mineral is critical for not only energy production in the cell, but also immune function and production of one of the body's master antioxidant enzymes: superoxide dismutase, or SOD.

Sometimes, getting out of your breakfast rut is as simple as changing up how you serve it. Layers of rich cashew cream, ripe peaches, and crunchy granola feel far more decadent than they really are. If peaches are not in season, try berries or ripe pear.

---

½ cup (125 mL) raw cashews, soaked in water for at least 2 hours or overnight, drained, and rinsed

⅓ cup (75 mL) water

1 tablespoon (15 mL) pure maple syrup

1 teaspoon (5 mL) freshly squeezed lemon juice

¼ teaspoon (1 mL) grated peeled fresh ginger

¼ teaspoon (1 mL) pure vanilla extract

Salt

2 ripe medium peaches or 2 cups (500 mL) partially thawed frozen peach slices, diced

½ cup (125 mL) of your favourite gluten-free granola or chopped pecans

1. In a small blender, combine the cashews, water, maple syrup, lemon juice, ginger, vanilla, and a pinch of salt. Blend until smooth.

2. In two 1-cup (250 mL) mason jars, layer half the peaches, top with half the cashew cream, and add 2 tablespoons (30 mL) of granola to each jar. Repeat the layers, finishing with a layer of the remaining 2 tablespoons (30 mL) of granola in each jar.

Make It Faster  The parfait has a small amount of liquid, so it blends best in a large, wide-mouthed jar using an immersion blender or in a bullet blender. This means fewer dishes, too!

# Moroccan Mint Smoothie

DAIRY-FREE | GLUTEN-FREE | NUT-FREE | PALEO-FRIENDLY | VEGAN | VEGETARIAN

SERVES 1

This creamy, dreamy treat is a little vacation in a glass, inspired by Moroccan mint tea. Whole peppermint leaves are incredibly soothing to the digestive tract; peppermint is a carminative, meaning it eases muscular contractions of the gut. Not so good if you have acid reflux, but amazing for a bit of tummy upset. This is a delicious breakfast with an energy-boosting balance of healthy fats and protein. Plenty of greens and healthy omega-3 fats from hemp seeds make this smoothie an anti-inflammatory paradise.

1.  In a high-speed blender, combine the soy milk, avocado, kale, mint, banana, hemp seeds, lime juice, maple syrup, and ice. Blend on high until smooth. If using peppermint oil, start with 1 drop, stir and taste, and add more until you get a nice cooling sensation.

2.  Pour into a glass and serve.

Tip Culinary peppermint oil is made from the naturally occurring oils within the peppermint leaves, as opposed to extracts, which are made by steeping leaves in alcohol. Peppermint oil will give you a more intense mint flavour and that tingly, cool sensation that takes this smoothie to the next level. You can find peppermint oil at gourmet supply stores or online. In a pinch, feel free to substitute peppermint extract.

1¼ cups (300 mL) unsweetened soy milk

⅓ large avocado, pitted and peeled

1 cup (250 mL) lightly packed chopped kale leaves

⅓ cup (75 mL) lightly packed fresh mint leaves

1 small frozen ripe banana, roughly chopped

2 tablespoons (30 mL) hemp seeds

1 tablespoon (15 mL) freshly squeezed lime juice

1 teaspoon (5 mL) pure maple syrup

2 or 3 ice cubes

1 to 3 drops peppermint oil (optional)

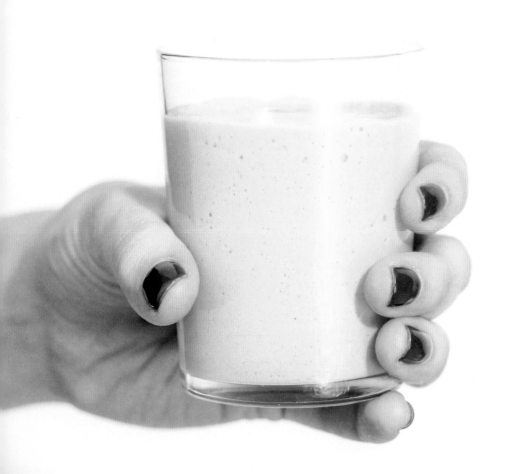

# Ginger Turmeric Smoothie

DAIRY-FREE | GLUTEN-FREE | PALEO-FRIENDLY | VEGAN | VEGETARIAN

SERVES 1

This spicy and sweet treat is the perfect way to bring your own anti-inflammatory sunshine to the breakfast table. Ginger is turmeric's botanical cousin and anti-inflammatory sidekick: compounds known as gingerols and shogaols in ginger have been shown to inhibit pro-inflammatory compounds and increase protection against oxidative damage. The crack of black pepper, while it may seem unusual, helps to improve the bioavailability of turmeric.

---

1. In a high-speed blender, combine the mango, ginger, cashew milk, cashews, turmeric, and a pinch each of salt and pepper. Blend until smooth.

2. Pour into a glass and serve immediately.

    Tip  1. If you have a high-speed blender, there is no need to soak the cashews for this smoothie. Otherwise, soak the cashews in water overnight in the fridge to be ready for breakfast the next day! 2. If you want a lighter texture, you can substitute coconut water for the cashew milk.

    Make It Healthier  If your taste buds are already attuned to the spicy, earthiness of turmeric, go ahead and use ½ to 1 teaspoon (2 to 5 mL) to pump up the plant power.

½ fresh mango, peeled and roughly chopped, or a heaping ½ cup (125 mL) frozen mango chunks

1-inch (2.5 cm) piece peeled fresh ginger, roughly chopped

1 cup (250 mL) unsweetened cashew milk or almond milk

¼ cup (60 mL) raw cashews

¼ teaspoon (1 mL) ground turmeric

Salt and freshly cracked pepper

# Blushing Beet Smoothie Bowl

DAIRY-FREE | GLUTEN-FREE | PALEO-FRIENDLY | VEGAN | VEGETARIAN

SERVES 2

Acai bowls are great, but berries that need to be flown across the globe are not the most eco-friendly choice when we have beets—an awesome homegrown superfood. I love beets because their intense jewel hue belies a bounty of anti-inflammatory benefits. They contain pigments called betalains, which help to fight inflammation, and if you tend to get a little hot under the collar, beets also help to lower blood pressure. The raspberries balance out the earthiness of the beets for a sweet-tart treat that will brighten your morning.

1½ cups (375 mL) frozen raspberries

½ cup (125 mL) peeled roughly chopped cooked red beets

½ frozen ripe banana, roughly chopped (about a 3-inch/8 cm piece)

1 tablespoon (15 mL) ground flaxseed

1 lemon slice (¼ inch/5 mm thick), skin on

½ cup (125 mL) unsweetened almond milk or soy milk

1 scoop vanilla protein (optional)

Toppings (optional)

Slivered raw almonds

Chia seeds

Unsweetened coconut flakes

Unsweetened granola

Pomegranate seeds

Lychee

1. In a high-speed blender, combine the raspberries, beets, banana, flaxseed, lemon, almond milk, and vanilla protein (if using). Blend until smooth. The mixture should be thick.

2. Pour into chilled bowls, add desired toppings, and serve immediately.

Tip Smoothie bowls are really just smoothies, heavy on the frozen fruit and light on the liquid. Cooking for one? Pour the remaining smoothie mixture into a freezer-safe container and store in the freezer for the next day. Remove from the freezer as soon as you wake up and it will be ready to eat in about 20 minutes.

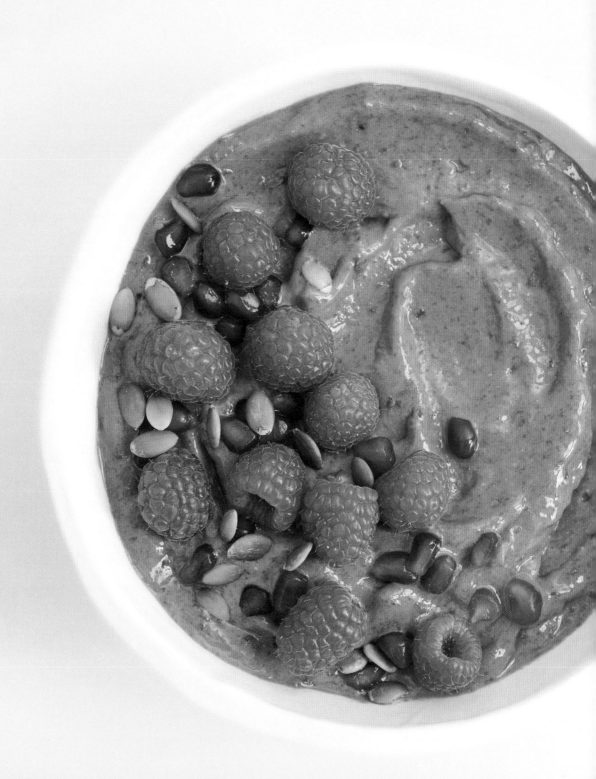

# Green Goddess Tofu Scramble

DAIRY-FREE | GLUTEN-FREE | NUT-FREE | VEGAN | VEGETARIAN

SERVES 2 TO 4

You might have had green juice for breakfast, but not like this. Instead of trying to mimic an eggy flavour, this high-protein tofu scramble gets its name from the savoury green herb juice that infuses the tofu. Piled high with kale, green peas, and parsley, it is filled with anti-inflammatory phytochemicals to help you take on the day. When it is served with cooked quinoa or millet, you can feed the family; otherwise, it is a great brunch for two when served with a slice of my Real Deal Gluten-Free Bread (page 267).

¾ cup (175 mL) low-sodium vegetable stock, divided

1 cup (250 mL) flat-leaf parsley leaves, divided

½ cup (125 mL) lightly packed fresh basil

1 tablespoon (15 mL) white miso

3 cloves garlic, roughly chopped, divided

2 tablespoons (30 mL) extra-virgin olive oil

1 cup (250 mL) finely chopped yellow onion (about ½ medium onion)

6 cups (1.5 L) lightly packed thinly sliced lacinato kale or baby spinach

1 package (12 ounces/350 g) firm tofu

1½ cups (375 mL) frozen peas

Salt

Red chili flakes

Freshly squeezed lemon juice

1.  In a small blender, combine ½ cup (125 mL) of the vegetable stock, ½ cup (125 mL) of the parsley, the basil, miso, and 1 clove of garlic. Set aside.

2.  In a large frying pan, heat the olive oil over medium heat. Add the onion and cook, stirring often, until soft and glossy, about 5 minutes.

3.  Add the kale and the remaining ¼ cup (60 mL) vegetable stock and cover the pan for 2 minutes to steam the kale. Stir in the remaining 2 cloves of garlic.

4.  Crumble the tofu into the pan, add the peas, and heat through, about 5 minutes.

5.  Pour the herb juice over the tofu scramble, stirring until the liquid is absorbed. Remove from the heat and season to taste with salt, chili flakes, and a squeeze of lemon juice. Mix in the remaining ½ cup (125 mL) parsley and serve.

Tip White (shiro) miso is lightly fermented rice and soybeans, and has a milder taste than yellow or red miso.

Make It Faster Whip up a batch of this scramble on the weekend and it makes a great filling for breakfast burritos all week long, wrapped in a brown rice tortilla. Store in an airtight container in the fridge for up to 5 days.

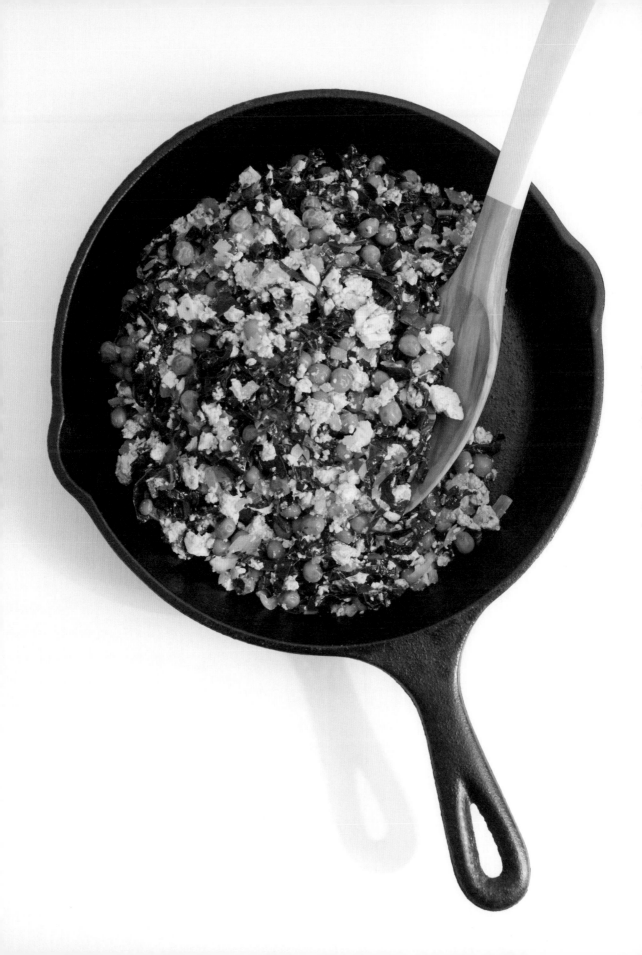

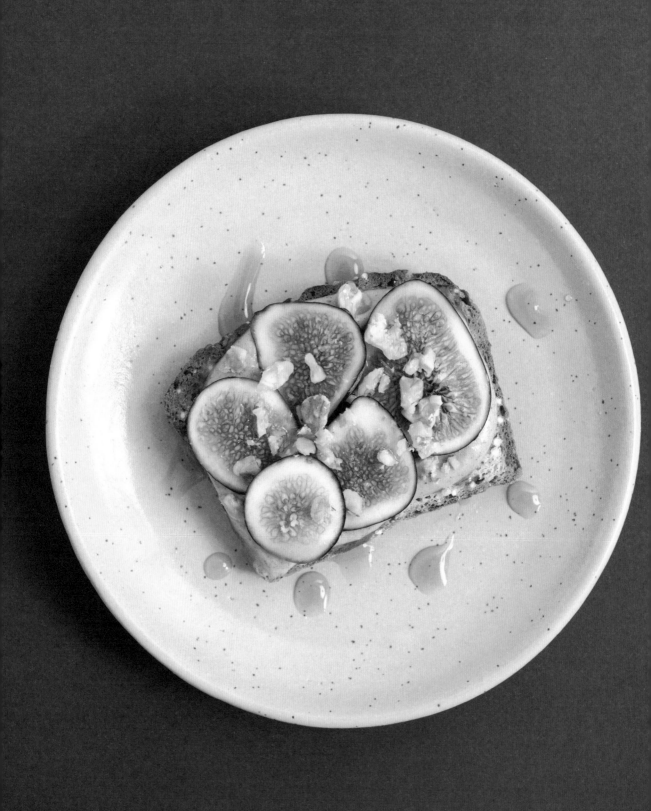

# Tahini Fig Toast

DAIRY-FREE | GLUTEN-FREE | NUT-FREE | VEGAN | VEGETARIAN

SERVES 2

You know that half-used jar of tahini in your fridge? This is how to make the most of it. I am not sure why it took me so long to realize that tahini—which is sesame butter—would make a delicious toast topper. I have favoured peanut butter for far too long! Tahini is rich in minerals, including zinc, which is critical for immune function and the production of cells involved in proper inflammatory response.

In just two minutes, you can take basic morning toast and turn it into a luscious, dessert-like masterpiece by whipping the tahini with banana and generously pouring it over your favourite bread. You might need to go buy some more tahini once you try this recipe.

---

1.  In a small blender, combine the tahini, banana, lemon juice, sugar, cinnamon, and a pinch of salt. Blend until smooth.

2.  Spread the tahini mixture over the toast, and then top with fig halves and a dusting of cinnamon.

Tip If fresh figs are not available and you like the chewy texture of dried figs, top the toast with sliced dried figs. Thinly sliced ripe pear is delicious, too!

¼ cup (60 mL) raw tahini

2 small very ripe bananas, roughly chopped

2 teaspoons (10 mL) freshly squeezed lemon juice

1 teaspoon (5 mL) cane sugar

½ teaspoon (2 mL) cinnamon, plus more for topping

Salt

4 slices of your favourite gluten-free bread, toasted (I use Little Northern Bakehouse Millet & Chia Loaf)

6 fresh figs, halved

# High-Protein Blueberry Almond Scones

DAIRY-FREE | GLUTEN-FREE | PALEO-FRIENDLY | VEGAN | VEGETARIAN

**MAKES 6 SCONES**

I do not have much of a sweet tooth, but I love baking. Making treats myself means using ingredients that I can feel good about eating. These scones are flavourful and satisfying and will not put you to sleep after eating them. Made from protein- and fibre-rich flours, without a lot of added sweetener, they help keep blood sugars balanced and are a far healthier choice than standard bakery fare. Consider your brunch game elevated.

---

2 tablespoons (30 mL) whole chia seeds

2½ cups (625 mL) almond flour

¼ cup (60 mL) coconut flour

2 teaspoons (10 mL) baking powder

¼ teaspoon (1 mL) cinnamon

⅛ teaspoon (0.5 mL) ground cardamom

Salt

⅓ cup (75 mL) coconut oil, chilled for 15 minutes

¼ cup (60 mL) pure maple syrup

1 teaspoon (5 mL) pure vanilla extract

½ cup (125 mL) fresh or frozen small wild blueberries or chopped dried cherries

1. Preheat the oven to 325°F (160°C). Line a baking sheet with parchment paper and set aside.

2. In a small bowl, combine the chia seeds with 6 tablespoons (90 mL) of warm water. Stir and set aside for 5 minutes, until thickened.

3. In a medium bowl, combine the almond flour, coconut flour, baking powder, cinnamon, cardamom, and a pinch of salt. Then, add the chilled coconut oil and combine with a pastry cutter or your fingers until the mixture has a crumbly texture.

4. Add the chia seed mixture, maple syrup, and vanilla to the flour mixture and mix into a soft, sticky dough. This really works best with your hands, so get in there!

5. Add the blueberries and gently work to distribute them evenly in the dough. Form the dough into a ball and flatten to a circle, about 1 inch (2.5 cm) thick. Cut into 6 wedges.

6. Place the scones on the prepared baking sheet and bake for 20 to 25 minutes, or until golden brown on the bottom (the scones will not brown much on top).

7. Remove from the oven and cool. The scones will be very delicate when first out of the oven but will firm up at room temperature. These scones are best eaten fresh but will keep, loosely covered on the counter, for 1 or 2 days.

Tip Large cultivated blueberries will not work in this recipe, as they break up the dough too much and you will end up with broken scones.

# Blackberry Ginger Muffins

DAIRY-FREE | GLUTEN-FREE | VEGAN | VEGETARIAN

MAKES 12 MUFFINS

There is something satisfying about freshly baked muffins; I love dreaming up ways of making baked goods that are nourishing to both body and soul. Nutrient-dense flours made from beans, nuts, and seeds replace the typical white, starchy stuff and keep inflammation-promoting blood sugar spikes at bay. Blackberry and ginger is a favourite combination of mine, but these muffins are a delicious way to savour any berry you have on hand. Freeze a batch for those mornings when all you have time for is coffee and a muffin to go. I also love to eat these muffins with a generous drizzle of my Masala Chai Almond Butter (page 261).

1½ cups (375 mL) almond flour

¾ cup (175 mL) gluten-free all-purpose flour

½ cup (125 mL) hemp hearts

3 tablespoons (45 mL) ground flaxseed

1 teaspoon (5 mL) baking powder

1 teaspoon (5 mL) baking soda

1 teaspoon (5 mL) ground cardamom

½ teaspoon (2 mL) cinnamon

¼ teaspoon (1 mL) salt

¾ cup (175 mL) unsweetened soy milk

¼ cup (60 mL) pure maple syrup

¼ cup (60 mL) extra-virgin olive oil

1 tablespoon (15 mL) liquid from canned chickpeas

2 teaspoons (10 mL) apple cider vinegar or freshly squeezed lemon juice

1 teaspoon (5 mL) pure vanilla extract

1 teaspoon (5 mL) grated peeled fresh ginger

¾ cup (175 mL) fresh or frozen blackberries, halved

2 tablespoons (30 mL) minced crystallized ginger

1. Preheat the oven to 350°F (180°C). Line a 12-cup muffin tin with paper liners or nonstick silicone muffin cups.

2. In a large bowl, whisk together the almond flour, all-purpose flour, hemp hearts, flaxseed, baking powder, baking soda, cardamom, cinnamon, and salt.

3. In a medium bowl, whisk together the soy milk, maple syrup, olive oil, chickpea liquid, apple cider vinegar, vanilla, and ginger.

4. Add the soy milk mixture to the flour mixture and stir to combine. Gently fold in the blackberries and crystallized ginger.

5. Scoop a heaping ¼ cup (60 mL) of batter into each muffin cup. Bake for 23 to 25 minutes, or until a toothpick inserted into the centre comes out clean. Let cool for 10 minutes, and then carefully transfer the muffins to a wire rack to cool completely. Muffins are delicate when warm but firm up when cool.

Tip  Cutting the blackberries in half and mincing the crystallized ginger ensures that the muffins hold together. If you are not a big ginger fan, you can omit the crystallized ginger.

Make It Healthier  The healthfulness of gluten-free flour mixes varies widely. I always use Bob's Red Mill All Purpose blend because it contains a large proportion of bean flours instead of white starches.

# Protein-Packed Savoury Tofu Muffins

DAIRY-FREE | GLUTEN-FREE | NUT-FREE | VEGAN | VEGETARIAN

MAKES 12 MUFFINS

¾ cup (175 mL) chickpea flour

½ cup (125 mL) water

¾ teaspoon (4 mL) salt

2 tablespoons (30 mL)
extra-virgin olive oil

1 cup (250 mL) finely
diced yellow onion
(about ½ medium onion)

¾ cup (175 mL) peeled
and finely diced carrots
(about 2 carrots)

3 cloves garlic, minced

Freshly cracked pepper

1 package (12 ounces/350 g)
medium-firm tofu

1 small zucchini, grated
(about 1 cup/250 mL)

½ cup (125 mL) roughly
chopped fresh herbs
(such as parsley, basil, dill)

¼ cup (60 mL) nutritional
yeast

1 teaspoon (5 mL)
baking powder

½ teaspoon (2 mL)
ground turmeric

½ teaspoon (2 mL)
ground cumin

¼ teaspoon (1 mL)
curry powder

Protein is critical in keeping blood sugars balanced and supporting immune function. In my practice, I commonly see clients omit protein from their meals, leading to increased hunger and decreased energy. On a plant-based diet, it is easy to eat protein with foods like these protein-packed muffins.

I love these savoury little muffins because they are the perfect grab-and-go breakfast or snack. Essentially a mini tofu frittata, they are high in fibre and pack in plenty of veggies, too. Make a batch on the weekend for brunch, or to prep for busy weekday mornings. These muffins would be delicious served with the Ginger Turmeric Smoothie (page 97) as a satisfying meal on the go.

---

1. Preheat the oven to 375°F (190°C). Line a 12-cup muffin tin with paper liners or nonstick silicone muffin cups.

2. In a medium bowl, whisk together the chickpea flour, water, and salt. Let sit for 10 minutes so the flour can hydrate while you cook the vegetables.

3. In a medium frying pan, heat the olive oil over medium-high heat. Add the onion and sauté for 3 minutes, stirring occasionally, until it begins to soften. Add the carrots and sauté for another 3 minutes until softened, then add the garlic and sauté for another 1 minute. Remove from the heat and season to taste with salt and pepper.

4. In a food processor, purée the tofu until smooth. Add the chickpea flour mixture and purée until combined. Add the sautéed vegetables, zucchini, herbs, nutritional yeast, baking powder, turmeric, cumin, and curry powder. Blend until combined.

5. Divide the mixture evenly among the muffin cups.

6. Bake for 30 to 35 minutes, or until a toothpick inserted into the centre comes out clean and the muffins are just starting to turn golden at the edges. Carefully remove the muffins from the tin and let cool for 5 minutes before serving.

7. The muffins will keep in a resealable container in the fridge for 3 to 4 days.

Tip 1. It is important to finely dice the onions and carrots. If the vegetable chunks are too big, the muffins will not hold together as well. 2. I like to use a balance of strongly aromatic herbs such as dill, thyme, or basil and more neutral-flavoured herbs such as parsley. However, feel free to experiment with a mix of your favourite herbs. I use ¼ cup (60 mL) freshly chopped flat-leaf parsley, 2 tablespoons (30 mL) freshly chopped basil, and 2 tablespoons (30 mL) freshly chopped dill. If you prefer, you could substitute finely chopped baby spinach for some or all of the herbs for a milder flavour.

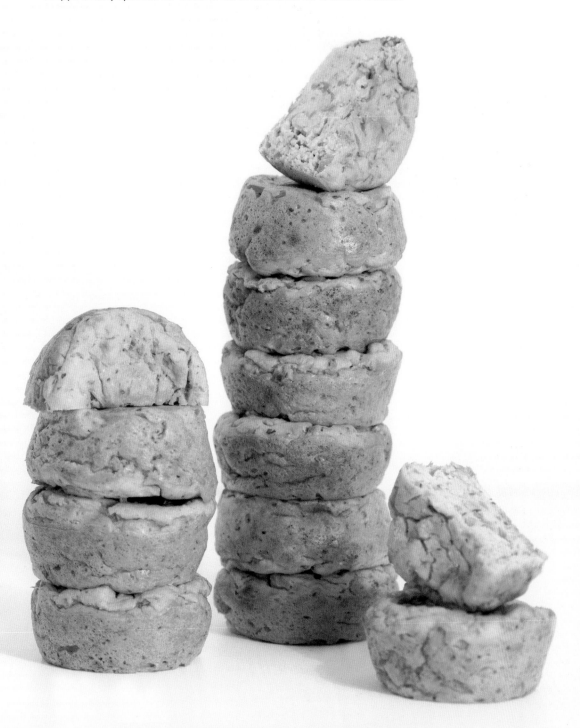

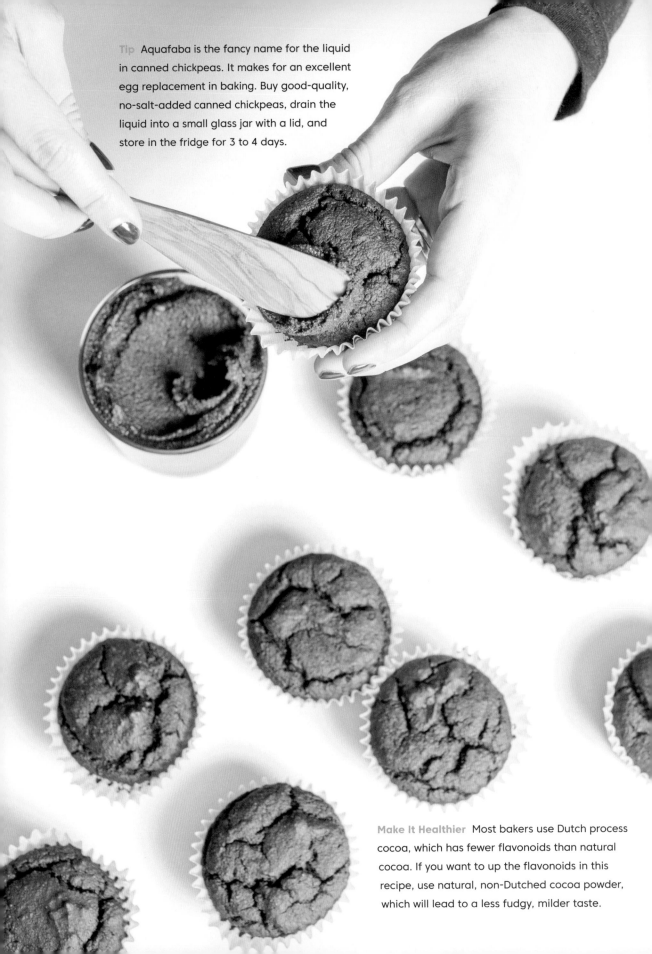

**Tip** Aquafaba is the fancy name for the liquid in canned chickpeas. It makes for an excellent egg replacement in baking. Buy good-quality, no-salt-added canned chickpeas, drain the liquid into a small glass jar with a lid, and store in the fridge for 3 to 4 days.

**Make It Healthier** Most bakers use Dutch process cocoa, which has fewer flavonoids than natural cocoa. If you want to up the flavonoids in this recipe, use natural, non-Dutched cocoa powder, which will lead to a less fudgy, milder taste.

# Healthy Breakfast Cupcakes with Salted Chocolate Frosting

DAIRY-FREE | GLUTEN-FREE | VEGAN | VEGETARIAN

SERVES 12

Most café muffins are really just sugary cupcakes, so I figured I might as well create a luscious chocolate cupcake that is really a healthy muffin in disguise! Cocoa is an anti-inflammatory, after all. With flavonoid-rich cocoa and high-protein almond flour forming the base of this cupcake, it's safe to say that this might be the first cupcake this dietitian has ever advocated eating on a daily basis. Tahini is the perfect substitute for buttercream; it is rich, thick, and luscious—you will want to eat this fudge-like frosting with a spoon! That is okay, because tahini is rich in minerals such as anti-inflammatory magnesium, calcium, and iron.

---

1. Preheat the oven to 350°F (180°C). Line a 12-cup muffin tin with paper liners or nonstick silicone muffin cups.

2. **Make the Healthy Breakfast Cupcakes** In a large bowl, whisk together the almond flour, all-purpose flour, cocoa, flaxseed, baking powder, cardamom, cinnamon, and salt to combine.

3. In a small bowl, whisk together the soy milk, olive oil, maple syrup, lemon juice, chickpea liquid, and vanilla.

4. Add the soy milk mixture to the flour mixture and mix until well blended.

5. Scoop ¼ cup (60 mL) of batter into each muffin cup. Bake for 35 to 38 minutes, or until a toothpick inserted into the centre comes out clean.

6. Let the muffins cool in the tin for 5 minutes before carefully transferring to a rack to cool fully. The muffins will firm up as they cool.

7. **Make the Salted Chocolate Frosting** In a small bowl, whisk together the tahini, maple syrup, cocoa, salt, and cinnamon until well blended. Spread on cooled cupcakes and serve immediately or refrigerate until ready to serve.

8. The cupcakes will keep in a resealable container in the fridge for 2 to 3 days. Bring iced cupcakes to room temperature before enjoying for best flavour.

## Healthy Breakfast Cupcakes

- 1½ cups (375 mL) almond flour
- ½ cup (125 mL) gluten-free all-purpose flour
- ½ cup (125 mL) cocoa powder
- 1 tablespoon (15 mL) ground flaxseed
- 2 teaspoons (10 mL) baking powder
- ½ teaspoon (2 mL) ground cardamom
- ½ teaspoon (2 mL) cinnamon
- ½ teaspoon (2 mL) salt
- ¾ cup (175 mL) unsweetened soy milk
- ¼ cup (60 mL) extra-virgin olive oil
- ⅓ cup (75 mL) pure maple syrup
- 1 tablespoon (15 mL) freshly squeezed lemon juice
- 1 tablespoon (15 mL) liquid from canned chickpeas (see Tip)
- 1 teaspoon (5 mL) pure vanilla extract

## Salted Chocolate Frosting

- ½ cup (125 mL) raw tahini, room temperature
- ¼ cup (60 mL) pure maple syrup
- ¼ cup (60 mL) cocoa powder
- ¼ teaspoon (1 mL) salt
- ⅛ teaspoon (0.5 mL) cinnamon

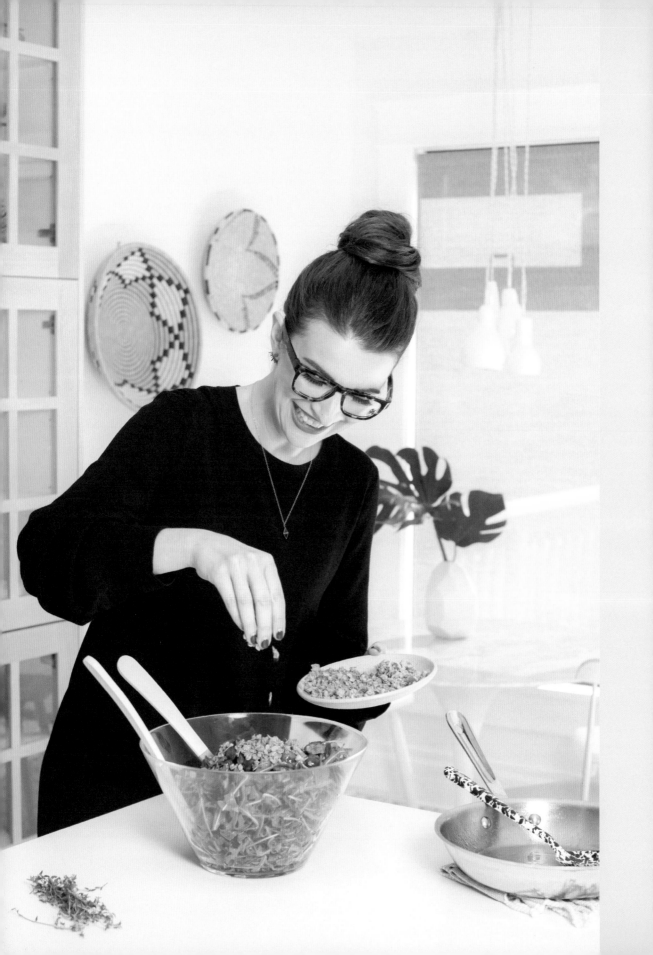

# 6

# Salads That Go Beyond Lettuce

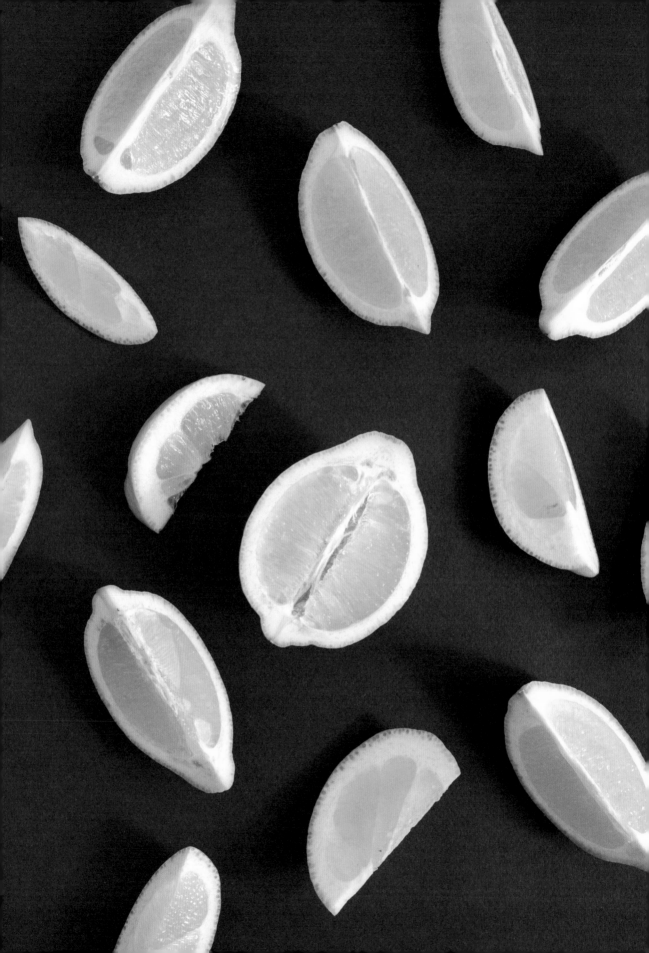

# Roasted Asparagus, Almond, and Lemony Millet Salad

DAIRY-FREE | GLUTEN-FREE | VEGAN | VEGETARIAN

SERVES 4 AS A SIDE

Nothing is a surer sign of spring than the arrival of the first bunches of asparagus at the grocery store. In addition to being delicious, you might be surprised at the anti-inflammatory benefits of asparagus: high in prebiotic fructans, asparagus is also rich in vitamin K and glutathione, a powerful antioxidant substance. A garlicky lemon tahini dressing makes this salad so tasty you might want a big bowl all to yourself. If you add 1 cup (250 mL) of roasted chickpeas to the mix, this recipe will make a satisfying meal for two.

---

1. Preheat the oven to 425°F (220°C). Line a baking sheet with parchment paper.

2. **Make the Asparagus, Almond, and Lemony Millet Salad** Toss the asparagus spears with olive oil, ⅛ teaspoon (0.5 mL) of the salt, and pepper and place on the prepared baking sheet. Roast until the edges turn golden, 11 to 14 minutes. Chop into bite-sized pieces and set aside.

3. In a small saucepan, add the millet, water, lemon peel, and the remaining ¼ teaspoon (1 mL) salt and bring to a boil over high heat. Reduce the heat to medium-low and simmer, partially covered, until the water is absorbed, 10 to 12 minutes. Remove from the heat, discard the lemon peel, and let cool.

4. **Make the Lemon Tahini Dressing** In a small food processor or using a large, wide-mouthed jar with a handheld immersion blender, add the tahini, lemon zest and juice, water, garlic, and salt and blend until smooth.

5. In a large bowl, add the asparagus, cooked millet, parsley, almonds, and hemp seeds. Toss with the dressing and serve.

**Make It Faster** You can prepare the millet, asparagus, and dressing up to 1 day in advance. I recommend not assembling the salad until just before serving, as the millet tends to absorb the dressing.

## Asparagus, Almond, and Lemony Millet Salad

1 pound (450 g) asparagus, trimmed

1 tablespoon (15 mL) extra-virgin olive oil

⅛ teaspoon (0.5 mL) + ¼ (1 mL) salt, divided

Freshly cracked pepper

½ cup (125 mL) uncooked millet

1 cup (250 mL) water

1 piece (2 inches/5 cm long) lemon peel

1 cup (250 mL) lightly packed chopped fresh curly parsley

⅓ cup (75 mL) raw slivered almonds

¼ cup (60 mL) hemp seeds

## Lemon Tahini Dressing

¼ cup (60 mL) raw tahini

Zest of ¼ lemon

¼ cup (60 mL) freshly squeezed lemon juice

2 tablespoons (30 mL) water

1 clove garlic, crushed or grated on a microplane

⅛ teaspoon (0.5 mL) salt

# Zucchini Zoodles with Sungold Cherry Tomato Sauce

DAIRY-FREE | GLUTEN-FREE | PALEO-FRIENDLY | VEGAN | VEGETARIAN

SERVES 4 AS A MAIN, 8 AS A SIDE

When I first started gardening, my tomato plant got out of hand! If you want to test the limits of your devotion to a single vegetable, try to eat five pounds of it in a single week. That is how I came up with this delicious zucchini noodle dish. Tomatoes are packed with anti-inflammatory lycopene—a fat-soluble compound—so they pair beautifully with flavourful extra-virgin olive oil.

This is the kind of recipe where ingredients are everything. In the middle of winter, this is a nice, simple dish for a busy night. In the middle of summer, particularly when picking perfectly ripe produce from your garden or the farmers' market, it is a transcendent experience. The sweet acidity of Sungold cherry tomatoes makes it borderline addictive.

---

2 pints (1 L) ripe Sungold cherry tomatoes or other cherry tomatoes, halved

½ cup (125 mL) tightly packed fresh basil leaves, thinly sliced into ribbons

¼ cup (60 mL) extra-virgin olive oil

3 tablespoons (45 mL) chopped drained capers or pitted and chopped Kalamata olives

1 clove garlic, minced or finely grated on a microplane

Salt and pepper

Freshly squeezed lemon juice

4 to 6 firm, small zucchini, spiralized (about 2 pounds/900 g)

1 cup Almond Ricotta Cheese (page 260) or 1 can (14 ounces/398 mL) white cannellini beans

1. In a large bowl, add the tomatoes, basil, olive oil, capers, and garlic and crush together with your fingers to release the juices and blend ingredients into a sauce. Taste and season with salt and pepper and with lemon juice for more acidity, if required. If tomatoes are not in season or naturally sweet, add ½ teaspoon (2 mL) of sugar to boost the flavour. Let sit while you spiralize the zucchini, so the flavours can blend.

2. Toss the spiralized zucchini noodles with the tomato sauce. Divide among 4 bowls and top each with ¼ cup (60 mL) Almond Ricotta Cheese.

Tip 1. If you are looking for a heartier meal, instead of zucchini use 1 package (12 ounces/340 g) of gluten-free spaghetti, cooked according to package directions, and a couple of handfuls of baby arugula for extra greens. 2. No spiralizer? Use a sharp vegetable peeler to peel the zucchini lengthwise into ribbons.

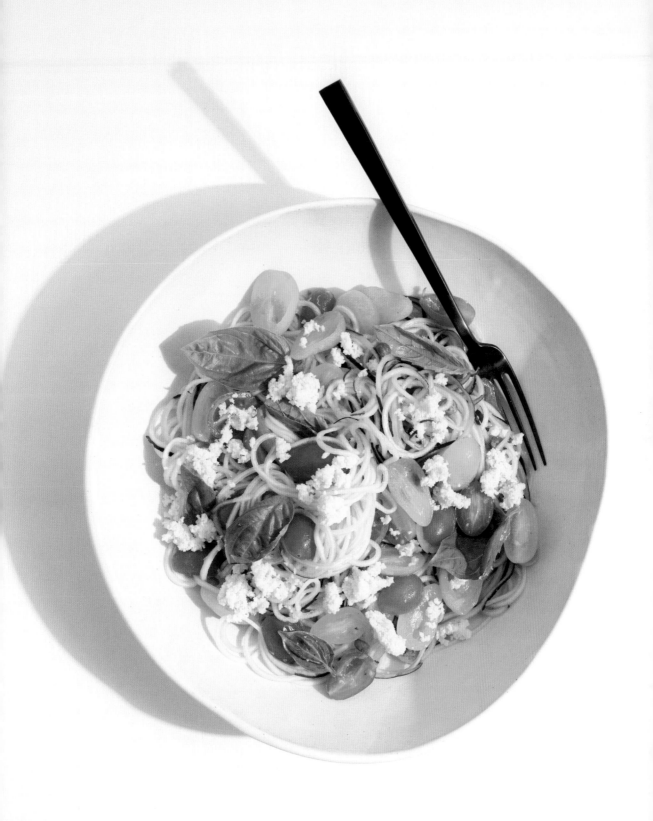

# Pink Grapefruit, Fennel, and Watermelon Radish Salad

DAIRY-FREE | GLUTEN-FREE | NUT-FREE | PALEO-FRIENDLY | VEGAN | VEGETARIAN

SERVES 4 AS A SIDE

Assembled lovingly on a platter and lavished with olive oil, this dish is a showstopper for guests. Beautiful slices of pink grapefruit pay homage to Italian crudo, which is essentially Italian-style sashimi. This salad is all juicy, vibrant flavour with plenty of crunch from the fennel and radish. Flavonoids in the grapefruit, along with vitamin C, make them a natural anti-inflammatory choice. If you have one, slice the radish and fennel using a mandolin for a finer texture that is more pleasant to chew.

## Dressing

2 tablespoons (30 mL) extra-virgin olive oil

1 teaspoon (5 mL) white wine vinegar

1 teaspoon (5 mL) Dijon mustard

¼ teaspoon (1 mL) cane sugar

⅛ teaspoon (0.5 mL) salt

Freshly cracked pepper

## Salad

2 pink grapefruits, peel and pith removed, thinly sliced into rounds

2 watermelon radishes, thinly sliced

1 cup (250 mL) thinly sliced fennel bulb

1 cup (250 mL) pea shoots or sunflower sprouts

1 tablespoon (15 mL) capers, drained and roughly chopped

1 tablespoon (15 mL) shallot

1. **Make the Dressing** In a small bowl, whisk together the olive oil, white wine vinegar, mustard, sugar, salt, and pepper.

2. **Assemble the Salad** Arrange slices of grapefruit on a serving platter or individual plates. Layer the radish slices on top. Sprinkle the fennel slices over the radish and top with pea shoots, capers, and shallot.

3. Drizzle the dressing over the salad and serve.

Tip A watermelon radish is larger than standard red radishes; it has a lime green skin that, when cut, reveals a gorgeous pink flesh. If not available, absolutely go for red egg or breakfast radishes.

# Roasted Cauliflower Salad with Creamy Caper-Raisin Dressing

DAIRY-FREE | GLUTEN-FREE | PALEO-FRIENDLY | VEGAN | VEGETARIAN

**SERVES 4 AS A SIDE**

Cauliflower is one of my kitchen staple ingredients, for not only its versatility but also its anti-inflammatory power. Just like its emerald-hued cousins, cauliflower is a member of the cruciferous veggie family. What makes the crucifers unique is the presence of sulphur-based molecules known as glucosinolates. These compounds are thought to protect against DNA damage, lower the production of pro-inflammatory mediators, and support phase II detoxification enzymes in the liver. This salad is delicious, creamy, sweet, salty, and so flavourful. I love serving it alongside my Celeriac Lentil Fritters with Date Jam (page 197) for a filling and satisfying meal. To save time, in a small bowl, soak the raisins in hot water while you bake the cauliflower.

---

1. Preheat the oven to 450°F (230°C). Line a baking sheet with parchment paper.

2. **Make the Roasted Cauliflower Salad** Place the cauliflower florets in a large bowl. Drizzle with the olive oil, season with salt and pepper, and toss to coat. Place on the prepared baking sheet and roast until golden brown, 15 to 20 minutes.

3. **Make the Creamy Caper-Raisin Dressing** Meanwhile, drain the raisins and place half in a small food processor, or use an immersion blender and a wide-mouthed jar. Add the water, red wine vinegar, tahini, garlic, thyme, olive oil, and salt and pepper. Blend until smooth. Stir in the capers and the remaining raisins.

4. In a large salad bowl, add the parsley, almonds, and roasted cauliflower and toss with the Creamy Caper-Raisin Dressing. Serve warm or cold.

**Make It Faster** The secret to a faster roasting time is to cut your florets small! More surface area means more caramelization in less time.

## Roasted Cauliflower Salad

1 medium head cauliflower, cut into small florets (7 to 8 cups/1.75 to 2 L)

2 tablespoons (30 mL) extra-virgin olive oil

Salt and freshly cracked pepper

1 cup (250 mL) packed chopped fresh curly parsley

¼ cup (60 mL) sliced raw almonds

## Creamy Caper-Raisin Dressing

⅓ cup (75 mL) Thompson raisins, soaked in hot water, divided

2 tablespoons (30 mL) water

1 tablespoon (15 mL) red wine vinegar

1 tablespoon (15 mL) raw tahini

½ clove garlic, chopped

1 teaspoon (5 mL) fresh thyme leaves or ½ teaspoon (2 mL) dried thyme

2 tablespoons (30 mL) extra-virgin olive oil

Salt and freshly cracked pepper

2 tablespoons (30 mL) capers, drained

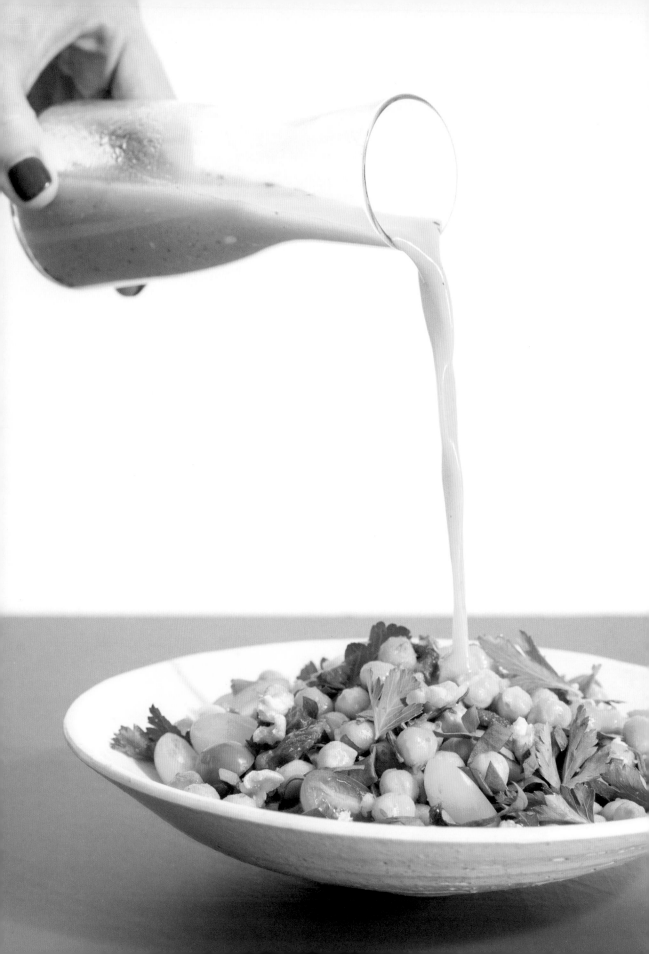

# Spiced Chickpea, Sundried Tomato, and Spinach Salad

DAIRY-FREE | GLUTEN-FREE | PALEO-FRIENDLY | VEGAN | VEGETARIAN

SERVES 3 AS A MAIN, 6 AS A SIDE

Creating a truly satisfying salad is all about a balance of flavour and textures. Here, creamy chickpeas are spiked with earthy spices and accented with sweet and umami flavours from the tomatoes. Chewy, fresh, crunchy, and satisfying. This salad makes use of one of my favourite salad greens, parsley. Long neglected as mere garnish, parsley is packed with vitamins K and C in addition to anti-inflammatory flavonoids.

1. **Make the Dressing** In a small bowl, whisk together the olive oil, lemon juice, red wine vinegar, mustard, maple syrup, salt, and pepper to taste. Set aside.

2. **Make the Salad** Heat the olive oil in a medium skillet over medium heat. Add the garlic and stir for 1 minute.

3. Add the chickpeas, stirring occasionally until they appear to absorb the oil in the skillet, 3 to 4 minutes. Add the cumin, turmeric, and coriander and stir to coat, about 30 seconds. Remove from the heat and stir in the sundried tomatoes and salt.

4. To serve, in a large bowl, toss together the parsley, spinach, tomatoes, and walnuts with the roasted chickpeas and dressing. Taste and adjust seasoning, if necessary. Serve warm or chilled.

   **Make It Healthier** I always cook with unsalted chickpeas. If you have salted chickpeas on hand, season with ¼ teaspoon (1 mL) of salt instead of ½ teaspoon (2 mL).

   **Make It Faster** You can make the chickpea mixture 1 day in advance and refrigerate until needed.

## Dressing

- 2 tablespoons (30 mL) extra-virgin olive oil
- 2 tablespoons (30 mL) freshly squeezed lemon juice
- 1 tablespoon (15 mL) red wine vinegar
- 1 teaspoon (5 mL) Dijon mustard
- ½ teaspoon (2 mL) pure maple syrup
- ¼ teaspoon (1 mL) salt
- Freshly cracked pepper

## Salad

- 3 tablespoons (45 mL) extra-virgin olive oil
- 2 cloves garlic, minced
- 2 cans (14 ounces/398 mL each) chickpeas, drained and rinsed
- 1 teaspoon (5 mL) ground cumin
- ¼ teaspoon (1 mL) ground turmeric
- ¼ teaspoon (1 mL) ground coriander
- ¼ cup (60 mL) chopped sundried tomatoes, packed in oil and patted dry
- ½ teaspoon (2 mL) salt
- 2 cups (500 mL) lightly packed fresh flat-leaf parsley
- 2 cups (500 mL) tightly packed baby spinach, sliced into thin ribbons
- 1 cup (250 mL) yellow or red cherry tomatoes, halved
- ⅓ cup (75 mL) raw walnut pieces

# Roasted Sunchoke, Fennel, and Pistachio Salad

DAIRY-FREE | GLUTEN-FREE | PALEO-FRIENDLY | VEGAN | VEGETARIAN

**SERVES 2 AS A MAIN, 4 AS A SIDE**

Anti-inflammatory living is heavily inspired by Mediterranean cuisine—one of the healthiest ways of eating on the planet. Fennel is a Mediterranean ingredient that deserves a larger place in your kitchen. In addition to its vitamin C content, fennel contains a volatile oil known as anethole that is thought to moderate anti-inflammatory pathways. Here, both pickled and fresh fennel complement creamy roasted sunchokes for a salad that is totally addictive.

1 cup (250 mL) white wine vinegar

1 cup (250 mL) water

3½ teaspoons (17 mL) salt, divided

1 tablespoon (15 mL) cane sugar

2 small fennel bulbs, thinly sliced on a mandolin, divided (4 cups/1 L sliced)

1 pound (450 g) sunchokes, scrubbed and sliced ¼ inch (5 mm) thick

3 tablespoons (45 mL) extra-virgin olive oil, divided

Freshly cracked pepper

Zest of ½ lemon

2 tablespoons (30 mL) freshly squeezed lemon juice

½ cup (125 mL) shelled raw pistachios

1. Preheat the oven to 425°F (220°C). Line a baking sheet with parchment paper.

2. In a small saucepan, bring the white wine vinegar, water, 1 tablespoon (15 mL) of the salt, and sugar to a boil and stir until the sugar and salt dissolve.

3. Place half of the fennel in a 1-quart (1 L) mason jar or bowl and pour the vinegar mixture over the fennel. Let sit uncovered as you prepare the rest of the salad, at least 15 minutes.

4. In a medium bowl, toss the sunchokes with 1 tablespoon (15 mL) of the olive oil, ¼ teaspoon (1 mL) of the salt, and pepper and place on the prepared baking sheet. Roast for 12 to 15 minutes, until fork-tender.

5. In a small bowl, whisk together the remaining 2 tablespoons (30 mL) olive oil, lemon zest and juice, the remaining ¼ teaspoon (1 mL) salt, and pepper.

6. Drain the pickled fennel, gently squeezing out excess liquid. In a medium serving dish, combine the remaining fresh fennel, pickled fennel, roasted sunchokes, and pistachios and toss with the dressing. Serve warm or chilled.

Tip This salad keeps very well in the fridge for 3 or 4 days but is at its flavourful best when fresh.

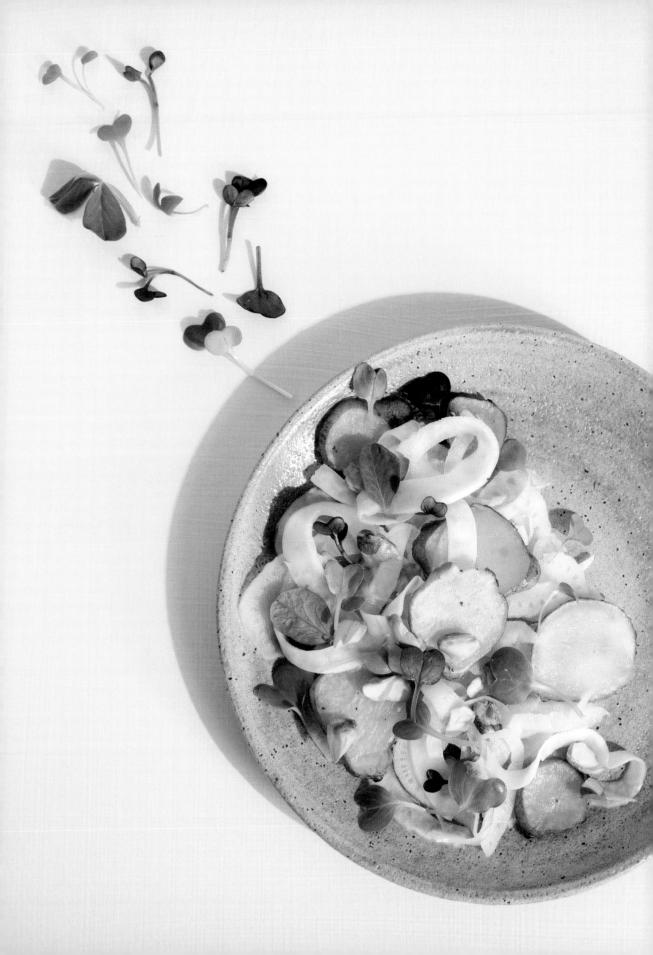

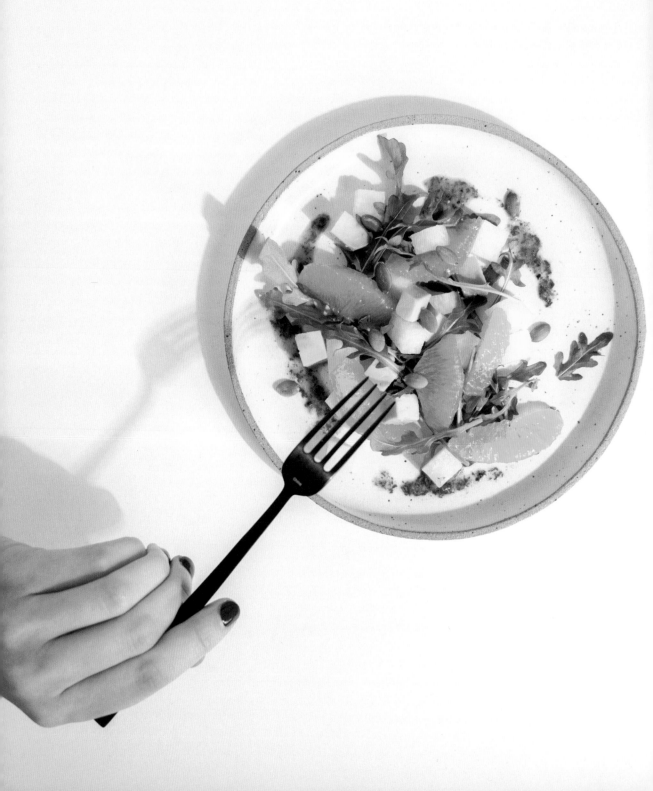

# Jicama, Orange, and Pumpkin Seed Salad

DAIRY-FREE | GLUTEN-FREE | NUT-FREE | PALEO-FRIENDLY | VEGAN | VEGETARIAN

SERVES 2 AS A MAIN, 4 AS A SIDE

Juicy, sweet, and crunchy, this salad is incredibly refreshing. Jicama is a tuber common in Mexican cuisine that lends a satisfying, fresh crispness to the dish. Oranges and avocado are rich in soluble fibre, which is soothing to irritable digestive tracts and helps slow the rise of blood sugars after a meal, keeping energy levels on an even keel and inflammation at bay. Pumpkin seeds and hemp oil provide a boost of anti-inflammatory omega-3 fatty acids. Paired with a zesty cilantro-lime dressing, this is the perfect meal for lazy days on the patio or when you want to transport yourself there in spirit!

1. **Make the Cilantro and Lime Dressing** In a small food processor or using a large, wide-mouthed jar with a handheld immersion blender, combine the cilantro, lime juice, olive oil, hemp oil, jalapeño, cumin, salt, and pepper. Process until well blended.

2. **Make the Jicama, Orange, and Pumpkin Seed Salad** In a serving bowl, toss the jicama, orange sections, arugula, and pumpkin seeds with the Cilantro and Lime Dressing. Top with avocado and serve.

Tip For the nicest texture and presentation, section the orange so no membrane or pith remains. To do this, slice off the top and bottom of the orange to reveal the flesh. Next, cut away the peel and pith completely from the sides, taking care not to cut away too much of the actual fruit. Run a paring knife in between the flesh and the membrane of one section to release it from the fruit. You will end up with a beautiful, juicy orange section, free of any membrane.

## Cilantro and Lime Dressing

¼ cup (60 mL) lightly packed fresh cilantro leaves

3 tablespoons (45 mL) freshly squeezed lime juice

1 tablespoon (15 mL) extra-virgin olive oil

1 tablespoon (15 mL) hemp oil or extra-virgin olive oil

2 teaspoons (10 mL) chopped pickled jalapeño pepper

¼ teaspoon (1 mL) ground cumin

¼ teaspoon (1 mL) salt

Freshly cracked pepper

## Jicama, Orange, and Pumpkin Seed Salad

1½ cups (375 mL) diced jicama (half of a 4-inch/ 10 cm wide jicama)

1 orange, peel and pith removed, sections halved (see Tip)

4 cups (1 L) lightly packed baby arugula

⅓ cup (75 mL) raw pumpkin seeds

1 avocado, pitted, peeled and chopped

# Quinoa, Beet, and Kale Salad with Pistachio Butter Dressing

DAIRY-FREE | GLUTEN-FREE | VEGAN | VEGETARIAN

SERVES 2 AS A MAIN, 4 AS A SIDE

## Pistachio Butter Dressing

1 cup (250 mL) shelled raw pistachios

2 tablespoons (30 mL) extra-virgin olive oil

2 tablespoons (30 mL) freshly squeezed lemon juice

¼ cup (60 mL) water

1 clove garlic, roughly chopped

½ teaspoon (2 mL) fresh thyme leaves

¼ teaspoon (1 mL) salt

Red chili flakes

## Quinoa, Beet, and Kale Salad

1 large bunch curly or black kale, torn into bite-sized pieces

1 tablespoon (15 mL) extra-virgin olive oil, plus more for frying

1 tablespoon (15 mL) freshly squeezed lemon juice

Salt and pepper

1 medium peeled cooked red beet, finely diced

1 cup (250 mL) cooked white quinoa

¼ cup (60 mL) drained capers, patted dry with a paper towel

This salad is inspired by my first meal at Ava Gene's in Portland, Oregon—it nearly brought tears to my eyes because it was the first time I had experienced a restaurant that created salads with the same complexity of flavour traditionally reserved for more serious dishes. Still one of my favourite greens, kale, rich in anti-inflammatory sulphur-based glucosinolates, is massaged with a lemon and olive oil mixture to make it tender. Then it is paired with sweet, earthy beets and laid on a bed of creamy, buttery, almost hummus-like pistachio dressing. Pistachios boast more antioxidants, including lutein, zeaxanthin, and polyphenols, than most nuts.

1. **Make the Pistachio Butter Dressing** In a small blender or using a large, wide-mouthed jar with a handheld immersion blender, purée the pistachios with the olive oil, lemon juice, water, garlic, thyme, salt, and a pinch of chili flakes. Add up to ⅓ cup (75 mL) more water slowly, as needed, to aid blending and thin to a creamy texture similar to a loose hummus.

2. **Make the Quinoa, Beet, and Kale Salad** In a large bowl, combine the kale with the olive oil, lemon juice, salt and pepper, to taste, and massage with your hands until the kale begins to soften and wilt. Add the diced beet and quinoa and toss to combine.

3. In a small skillet, heat a thin layer of olive oil over medium-high heat. Add the capers and let sizzle until they begin to crisp, brown, and bloom, watching carefully and stirring occasionally, 1 to 2 minutes. Remove from the heat and drain on a paper towel.

4. To serve, spread a dollop of Pistachio Butter Dressing on the bottom of a plate. Place the salad mixture on top and sprinkle with fried capers.

Make It Faster You can find pre-cooked beets in most supermarkets to save on time and mess!

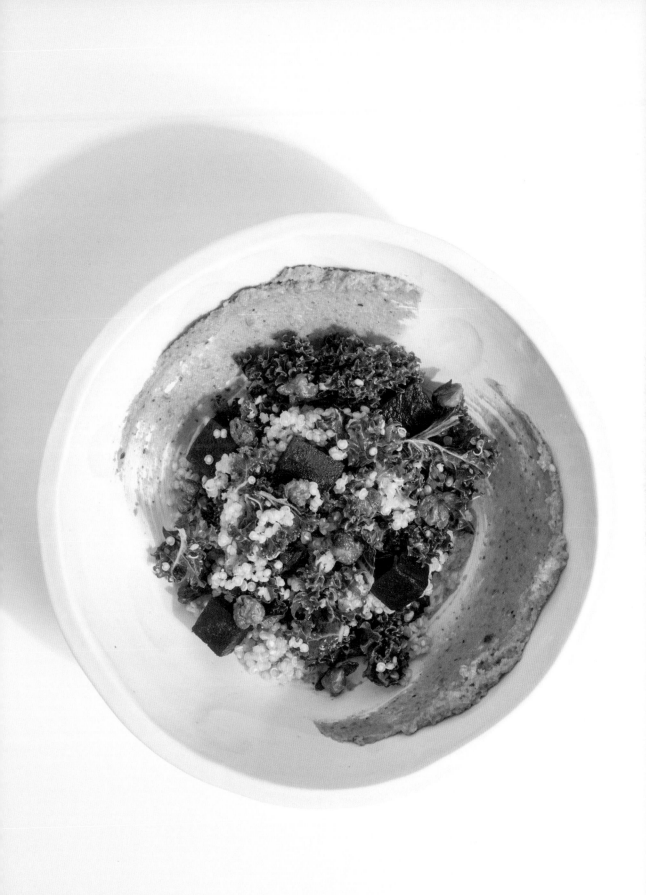

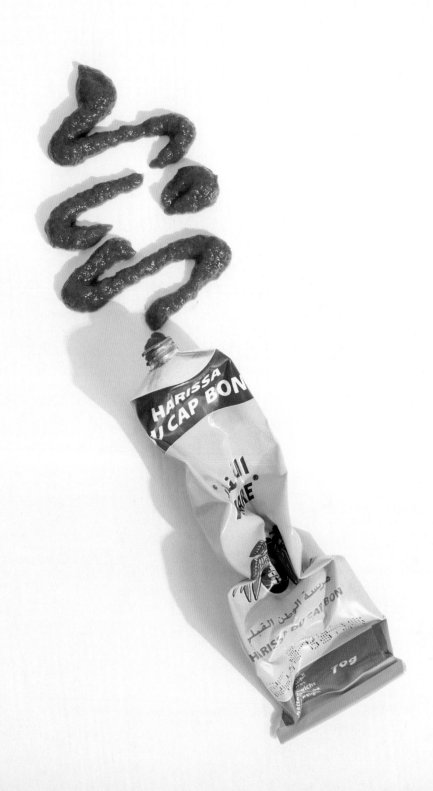

# Harissa-Spiked Carrot and White Bean Salad

DAIRY-FREE | GLUTEN-FREE | NUT-FREE | VEGAN | VEGETARIAN

SERVES 4 AS A SIDE

Soft, buttery white beans are my secret nutritional weapon because they do not taste like the health food they are. Packed with plant protein, indigestible fibres in beans feed beneficial bacteria in the gut, promoting a healthy community of bacteria that helps to ease inflammation. Combined with sweet, caramelized carrots and fiery, earthy harissa paste, this salad is an almost addictive and deeply satisfying dish. This salad makes a wonderful accompaniment to my Mujadara Neat-Balls in Spiced Tomato Sauce (page 177).

1. In a medium skillet, heat 2 tablespoons (30 mL) of the olive oil over medium-high heat. Add the carrots and cook until softened and beginning to caramelize, stirring occasionally, 10 to 12 minutes. Remove from the heat.

2. In a medium serving bowl, whisk together the remaining 2 tablespoons (30 mL) olive oil, lemon juice, shallots, harissa, tomato paste, cumin, and salt. Add the carrots, beans, parsley, and pumpkin seeds and toss well to coat with dressing.

3. Serve warm or cold.

Tip  Harissa is a spice paste common in North African and Middle Eastern cuisines; you can find it at Middle Eastern markets and gourmet stores. Note that some, often European, harissa pastes are very mild. Be sure to taste your harissa the first time you use it! Mild harissa varieties will result in a bland salad.

Make It Faster  This salad keeps very well covered in the fridge and can be made 2 to 3 days in advance.

4 tablespoons (60 mL) extra-virgin olive oil, divided

¾ pound (340 g) carrots, thinly sliced on a mandolin (about 4 large carrots)

3 tablespoons (45 mL) freshly squeezed lemon juice

1 tablespoon (15 mL) finely diced shallots

2 teaspoons (10 mL) hot harissa paste

1 teaspoon (5 mL) tomato paste

½ teaspoon (2 mL) ground cumin

¼ teaspoon (1 mL) salt

1 can (14 ounces/398 mL) butter or cannellini beans, drained and rinsed

½ cup (125 mL) packed fresh curly parsley

¼ cup (60 mL) raw pumpkin seeds

# Vietnamese Cucumber Salad with Ginger and Mint

DAIRY-FREE | GLUTEN-FREE | NUT-FREE | PALEO-FRIENDLY | VEGAN | VEGETARIAN

SERVES 4 AS A SIDE

Cool as a cucumber? What if you heat things up with chili flakes and ginger? Inspired by traditional Vietnamese cucumber salad, this dish has a trio of gut-friendly ingredients: ginger, mint, and chili. Capsaicin, the compound that gives chilies their heat, may help ease digestive distress by improving motility, as does ginger. Mint is known to be anti-spasmodic, meaning that it eases the contractions of the smooth muscle of the gut. So, perhaps this spicy salad will really keep you as cool as the cucumber it is made from!

10 mini cucumbers or 2 small English cucumbers

1 tablespoon (15 mL) salt

1 tablespoon (15 mL) finely diced shallot

1 tablespoon + 2 teaspoons (25 mL) freshly squeezed lime juice

1½ teaspoons (7 mL) cane sugar

½ teaspoon (2 mL) freshly grated peeled ginger

½ teaspoon (2 mL) toasted sesame oil

⅛ teaspoon (0.5 mL) red chili flakes or a few thin slices of red chili pepper

½ cup (125 mL) fresh mint leaves, thinly sliced into ribbons

1. Cut half of the cucumber into small ½-inch (1 cm) chunks and thinly slice the other half with a knife or on a mandolin. You are aiming for 5 cups (1.25 L) of cucumbers.

2. In a medium bowl, combine the cucumber and salt, tossing well with your fingers. Transfer the cucumber to a colander and set it over the bowl so the cucumber can drain for 10 minutes.

3. Rinse off excess salt from the cucumber and pat dry with paper towel. Rinse and dry the bowl.

4. In the same bowl, whisk together the shallot, lime juice, sugar, ginger, sesame oil, and chili flakes.

5. Add the cucumber to the dressing mixture, toss, and let sit for 5 minutes. Toss with the mint, taste, and add more salt or lime juice, if needed, and serve.

Make It Faster  This salad can be made up to 1 day in advance, but add the mint just before serving, as the mint will lose flavour and taste a bit muddy over time. Do not skip the salting step; otherwise, the salad will be swimming in water.

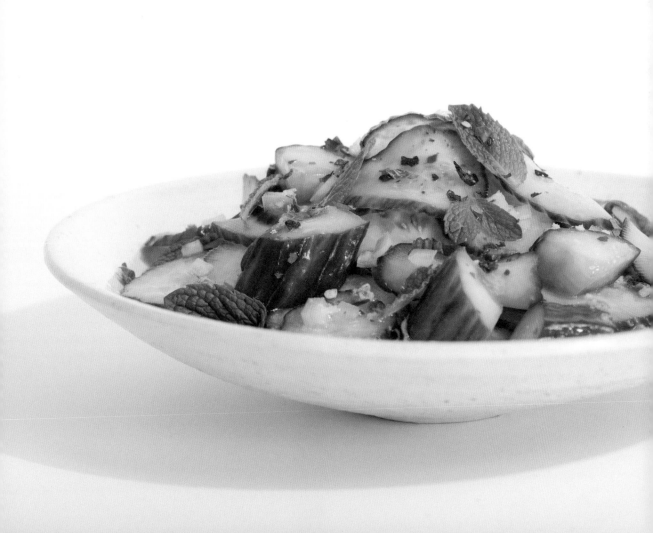

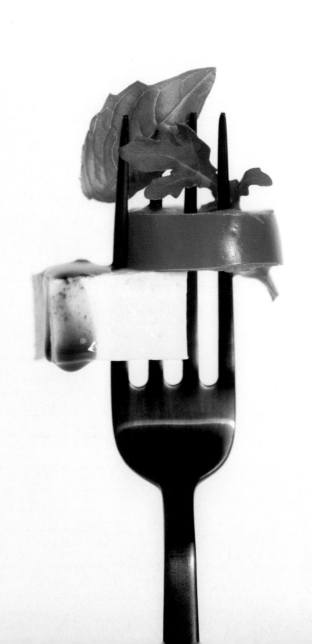

# Grilled Tofu Caprese Salad

DAIRY-FREE | GLUTEN-FREE | NUT-FREE | PALEO-FRIENDLY | VEGAN | VEGETARIAN

**SERVES 2 AS A MAIN, 4 AS A SIDE**

There are few things in life as effortlessly perfect as a caprese salad. When I learned that you could cure tofu with lemon juice to impart a cheese-like freshness, I knew I had to create a plant-based version of one of my longtime favourites. Despite the misconceptions about nightshade vegetables being pro-inflammatory, tomatoes are packed with anti-inflammatory compounds like vitamin C and lycopene. Paired with a potent basil-infused oil, this is a beautiful salad.

---

1. Cut the tofu into sixteen ½-inch (1 cm) slices. In a medium resealable container, marinate the tofu in lemon juice, 1 tablespoon (15 mL) of the olive oil, and salt for at least 20 minutes or up to 12 hours in the fridge. The longer the tofu marinates, the more it will have a tangy, fresh mozzarella–like flavour. Reserve 1 teaspoon (5 mL) of the marinade for the dressing.

2. In a small blender or using a wide-mouthed jar with a handheld immersion blender, purée the basil, reserved marinade, and the remaining ¼ cup (60 mL) olive oil. Adjust seasoning with salt and set aside.

3. Prepare a grill for direct cooking over high heat. Or, preheat a cast iron grill pan over medium-high heat. Place the tofu directly on the grill and cook until grill marks appear, 3 to 4 minutes. Flip and grill for another 3 to 4 minutes. You are not trying to cook the tofu, just to enhance the flavour by grilling it.

4. Drizzle the basil mixture onto a serving platter or individual plates. Top with a few handfuls of baby arugula (if using). Layer on the tofu and tomato slices. Drizzle with the balsamic glaze and finish with a pinch each of sea salt and pepper.

   **Make It Faster** If you do not have a grill, you can assemble the salad and skip the grilling. You will lose that nuance of flavour, but the salad is still delicious.

1 package (12 ounces/350 g) extra-firm or pressed tofu, drained and patted dry

3 tablespoons (45 mL) freshly squeezed lemon juice

⅓ cup (75 mL) extra-virgin olive oil, divided

½ teaspoon (2 mL) salt

½ cup (125 mL) lightly packed fresh basil leaves

2 cups (500 mL) baby arugula (optional)

2 large ripe tomatoes, sliced

Balsamic glaze, for garnish

Flaky sea salt (I use Maldon)

Freshly cracked pepper

**Tip** You want to use a thick balsamic glaze to keep the balsamic and the basil oil distinct and not looking muddy. Balsamic glaze also has a more intense flavour, with a syrupy instead of acidic finish.

# Green Pea, Radish, and Date Salad with Apple Miso Dressing

DAIRY-FREE | GLUTEN-FREE | VEGAN | VEGETARIAN

SERVES 4 AS A SIDE

### Apple Miso Dressing

2 tablespoons (30 mL) raw apple cider vinegar

1 tablespoon (15 mL) extra-virgin olive oil

1 tablespoon (15 mL) white miso

1 teaspoon (5 mL) pure maple syrup

1½ teaspoons (7 mL) minced shallot

⅛ teaspoon (0.5 mL) red chili flakes

Salt

### Green Pea, Radish, and Date Salad

2 cups (500 mL) freshly shelled peas or thawed frozen peas

1 bunch radishes, trimmed and thinly sliced (6 to 8 radishes)

1 cup (250 mL) diced cucumbers

4 Medjool dates, pitted and sliced

¼ cup (60 mL) blanched slivered almonds

¼ cup (60 mL) lightly packed fresh mint leaves, sliced

Green peas are easy to underestimate; many of us grew up eating them straight out of the can. Of course, their green colour should be a hint that they contain anti-inflammatory riches. In addition to flavonols, green peas contain high amounts of anti-inflammatory vitamin K and energizing minerals. As a legume, they also contain 9 grams of protein per cup, putting them on par with quinoa. This salad has a delicate sweetness and a dressing that is downright delicious.

1. **Make the Apple Miso Dressing** In a small bowl, whisk together the apple cider vinegar, olive oil, miso, maple syrup, shallot, chili flakes, and a tiny pinch of salt. Taste and adjust seasoning if needed.

2. **Make the Green Pea, Radish, and Date Salad** If using fresh peas, bring a medium pot of water to a boil over high heat. Blanch the peas for 1 minute, drain in a colander, and rinse with cold water.

3. Add the peas to a medium serving bowl with the radish, cucumber, dates, almonds, and mint. Pour the Apple Miso Dressing over the salad, toss to combine, and serve.

Tip Medjool dates and Deglet Noor dates are two varietals that are larger, very soft, and moist. If the dates you have on hand seem dry, soak them in hot water for 5 minutes before using.

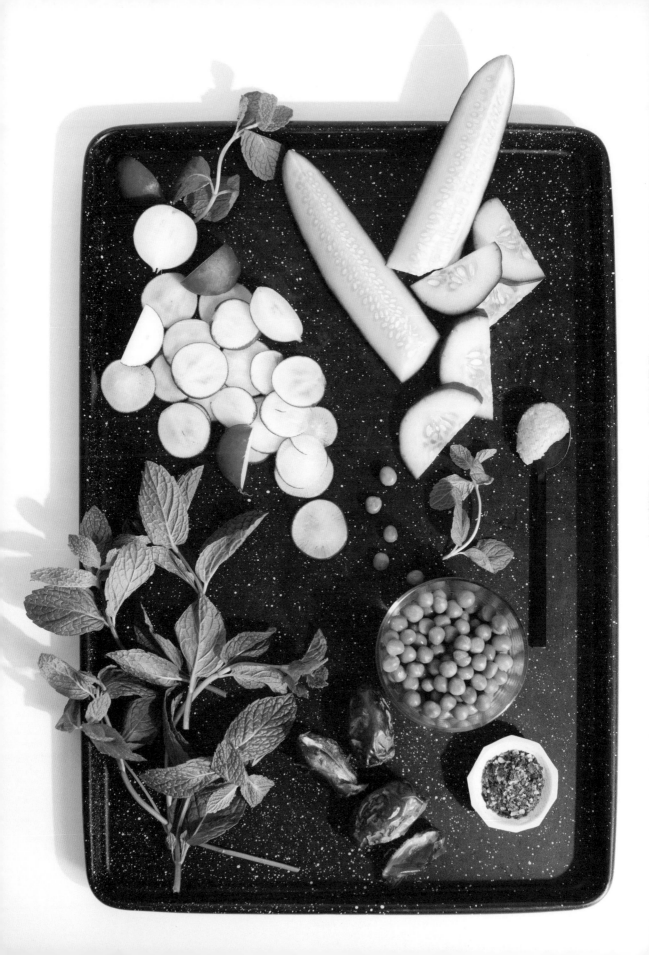

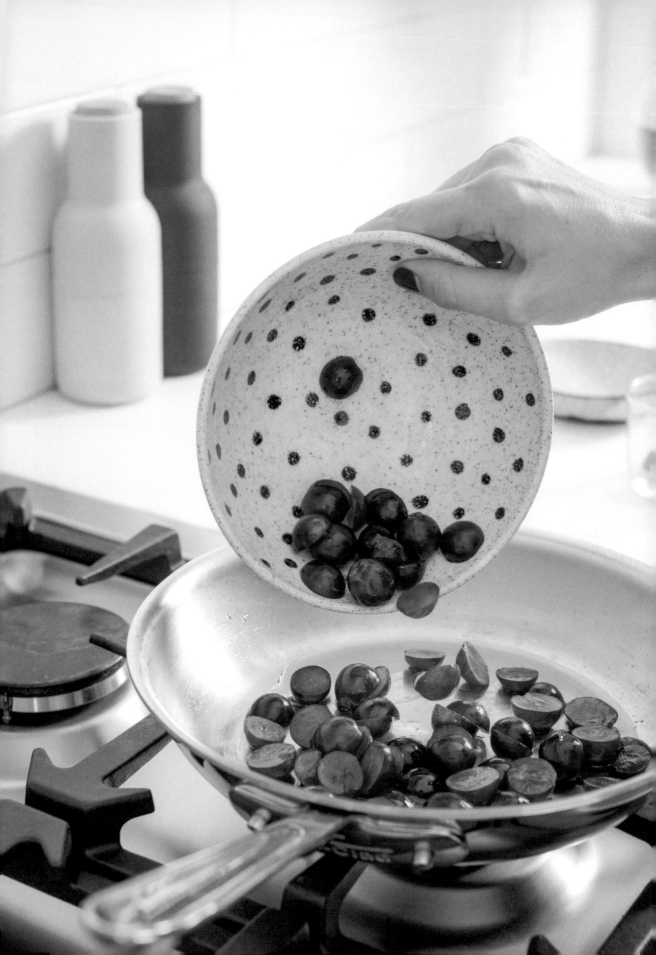

# Pan-Roasted Grape and Arugula Salad with Oat and Walnut Crumble

DAIRY-FREE | GLUTEN-FREE | VEGAN | VEGETARIAN

SERVES 4 AS A SIDE

As much as my family claims to love grapes, I always seem to be looking for ways to use up the much-unloved bag sitting in the fridge. This salad is an unexpected combination of warm, sweet grapes and a brooding, savoury walnut crumble. It turns the notion of comfort food on its leafy head. Red grapes contain powerful polyphenols in their skin that, when paired with omega-3-rich walnuts, are an anti-inflammatory match made in heaven.

---

1.  **Make the Oat and Walnut Crumble**  In a small bowl, combine the rolled oats, walnuts, oat flour, brown sugar, salt, and thyme.

2.  In a medium skillet, heat the olive oil over medium heat and then add the crumble mixture, stirring constantly as the mixture begins to clump and toast. Watch carefully so it does not burn. Cook until it becomes golden brown, 3 to 4 minutes. Remove from the heat and transfer the mixture to a small bowl to cool. Wipe the skillet clean.

3.  **Make the Lemon Thyme Dressing**  In another small bowl, whisk together the olive oil, lemon zest and juice, shallot, thyme, and salt and set aside.

4.  **Prepare the Pan-Roasted Grape and Arugula Salad**  In the clean skillet, heat the olive oil over medium heat. Add the grapes, and cook until they begin to soften, 4 to 5 minutes. Remove from the heat.

5.  To assemble, add the arugula and grapes to a medium serving bowl. Add the dressing and toss to combine. Add the crumble, toss again, and serve warm.

Tip  Not all oat products are gluten-free due to cross-contamination in agriculture and food processing. If you have celiac disease or diagnosed gluten intolerance, be sure to look for the gluten-free symbol on your oat products.

Make It Faster  You can make the crumble and dressing 1 day in advance. Refrigerate in separate resealable containers until ready to use.

## Oat and Walnut Crumble

½ cup (125 mL) gluten-free quick rolled oats

½ cup (125 mL) finely chopped raw walnuts

2 tablespoons (30 mL) gluten-free oat flour

1 tablespoon (15 mL) brown cane sugar

¼ teaspoon (1 mL) salt

¼ teaspoon (1 mL) fresh thyme leaves

2 tablespoons (30 mL) extra-virgin olive oil

## Lemon Thyme Dressing

2 tablespoons (30 mL) extra-virgin olive oil

Zest of ⅓ lemon

2 tablespoons (30 mL) freshly squeezed lemon juice

1 teaspoon (5 mL) minced shallot

⅛ teaspoon (0.5 mL) fresh thyme leaves

⅛ teaspoon (0.5 mL) salt

## Pan-Roasted Grape and Arugula Salad

1 tablespoon (15 mL) extra-virgin olive oil

2 cups (500 mL) red skinned grapes, halved

4 cups (1 L) lightly packed baby arugula

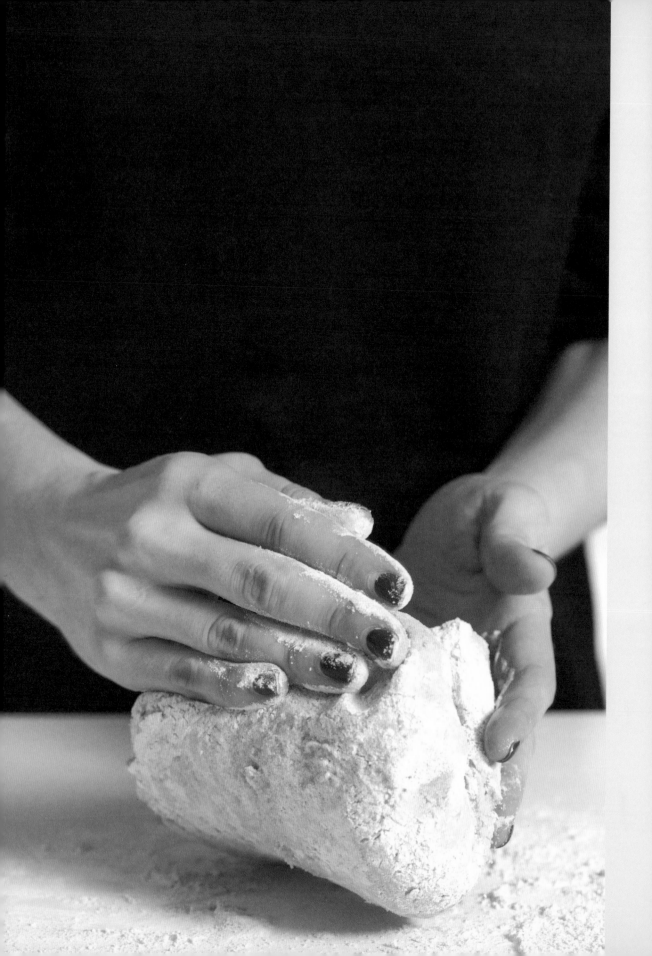

# 7

# Soul-Satisfying Plant-Based Meals

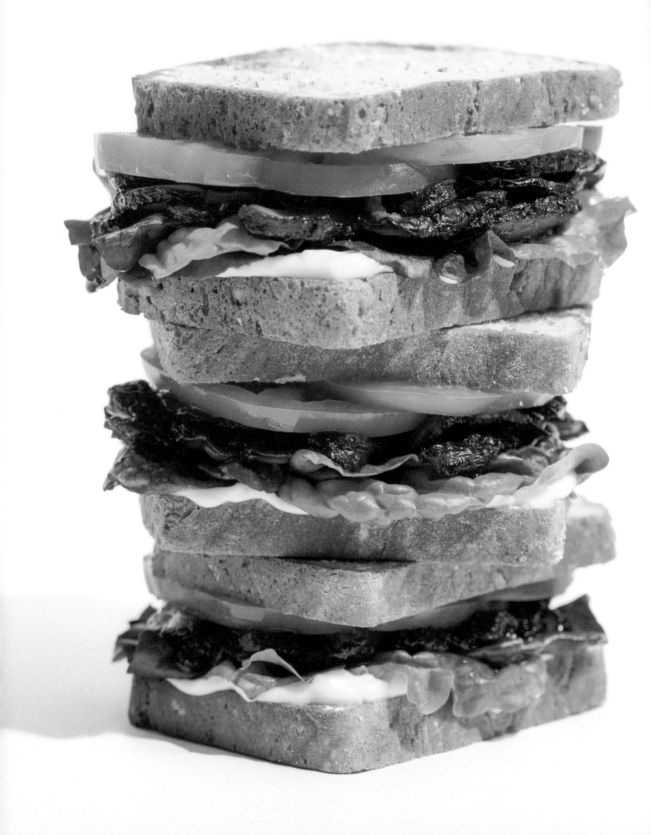

# Shiitake BLT Sandwich

DAIRY-FREE | GLUTEN-FREE | NUT-FREE | VEGAN | VEGETARIAN

SERVES 2

When trying to eat well, sometimes it is the classic comforts you miss the most. BLT sandwiches were a childhood favourite of mine, but I had given them up long ago, until some genius figured out that shiitake mushrooms, with their chewy, meaty texture, make a great whole food substitute for bacon. In addition, isn't it comforting to know that one of your favourite treats can be anti-inflammatory, too? Long overlooked in a sea of prettier, more colourful veggies, shiitake mushrooms contain a unique vitamin D precursor and plant polysaccharides that help to support immune function and fight inflammation. As well, they contain anti-inflammatory copper and selenium. After trying this recipe, you will not overlook shiitakes again.

---

1. In a small bowl, whisk together 2 tablespoons (30 mL) of the avocado oil with the tamari, maple syrup, garlic, a pinch of paprika (if using), and a pinch of salt.

2. In a large skillet, heat the remaining 2 tablespoons (30 mL) avocado oil over medium heat. Add the mushrooms and let sizzle for 2 minutes until they start to brown. Then flip them over and let sizzle for 1 more minute.

3. Pour the avocado oil and tamari mixture over the mushrooms and cook until the liquid reduces, about 1 minute. Remove from heat.

4. Toast the bread. Spread each slice with a bit of mayonnaise. Then layer the lettuce and tomato on one of the slices. Top with the mushroom mixture and a slice of toast. Repeat to assemble the second sandwich.

Tip Ensure that you use a large enough skillet so you do not crowd the mushrooms as they sizzle away for best texture. You want them to brown, not to steam!

¼ cup (60 mL) avocado oil, divided

2 tablespoons (30 mL) gluten-free tamari

2 teaspoons (10 mL) pure maple syrup

2 cloves garlic, minced or finely grated on a microplane

Smoked paprika (optional)

Salt

2 cups (500 mL) shiitake mushrooms, sliced

4 slices gluten-free bread

2 tablespoons (30 mL) vegan mayonnaise

Small handful of romaine lettuce or red leaf lettuce

1 tomato, sliced

# Green Machine Burgers

DAIRY-FREE | GLUTEN-FREE | NUT-FREE | VEGAN | VEGETARIAN

**MAKES 4 BURGERS**

2 cups (500 mL) frozen shelled edamame

2 cups (500 mL) finely sliced kale

1 cup (250 mL) grated zucchini

½ cup (125 mL) gluten-free rolled or instant oats

2 cloves garlic, minced

3 tablespoons (45 mL) ground flaxseed

3 tablespoons (45 mL) hemp seeds

½ teaspoon (2 mL) ground cumin

1 tablespoon (15 mL) gluten-free tamari

1 tablespoon (15 mL) freshly squeezed lemon juice

1 tablespoon (15 mL) unseasoned rice vinegar

¼ teaspoon (1 mL) salt

½ to 1 teaspoon (2 to 5 mL) Sriracha

3 tablespoons (45 mL) water

3 tablespoons (45 mL) extra-virgin olive oil

4 gluten-free hamburger buns

### Garnish

Turmeric Mayonnaise (page 259)

Avocado slices

Shredded cabbage

Fresh pineapple, thinly sliced

We all love a good burger, and these Asian-inspired gems are full of omega-3-rich seeds and greens; they are practically an anti-inflammatory salad. I love serving these burgers bun-less, with a dollop of Turmeric Mayonnaise (page 259) and slices of avocado, but they are delicious with all the traditional fixings, too. These burgers hold together very well while remaining soft and moist. They are delicious served with the Vietnamese Cucumber Salad with Ginger and Mint (page 128) and Chili Garlic Brussels Sprouts (page 214).

1. Cook the edamame according to package directions. Place the kale in a colander in the sink. When the edamame is cooked, slowly pour it out over the kale to wilt the greens.

2. In a food processor, combine the edamame, kale, zucchini, rolled oats, garlic, flaxseed, hemp seeds, cumin, tamari, lemon juice, rice vinegar, salt, Sriracha, and water. Process until the ingredients form a uniform mixture but are still visible and the mixture starts to come together as a dough. Form into 4 patties, each about 1 inch (2 cm) thick.

3. In a large skillet, heat the olive oil over medium heat. Add the burger patties and cook, resisting the urge to fuss with them so they can form a crust, 4 to 6 minutes. Flip the burgers carefully, as they will be soft, and cook for another 4 to 6 minutes. The burgers are soft while still warm and firm up as they cool.

4. To serve, spread the Turmeric Mayonnaise on the buns and top with the burgers. Layer on avocado, cabbage, and pineapple.

**Make It Faster** These burgers freeze beautifully, wrapped between sheets of parchment paper and stored in a resealable plastic bag, for up to 1 month. Make a double batch and have them at the ready! Thaw in the refrigerator prior to cooking, and then reheat in a skillet with 2 tablespoons (30 mL) olive oil, cooking for 6 to 8 minutes per side.

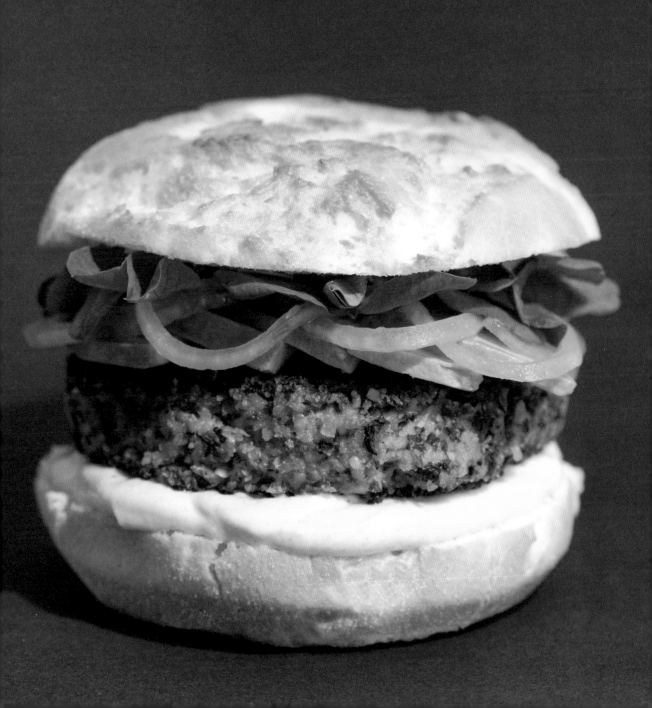

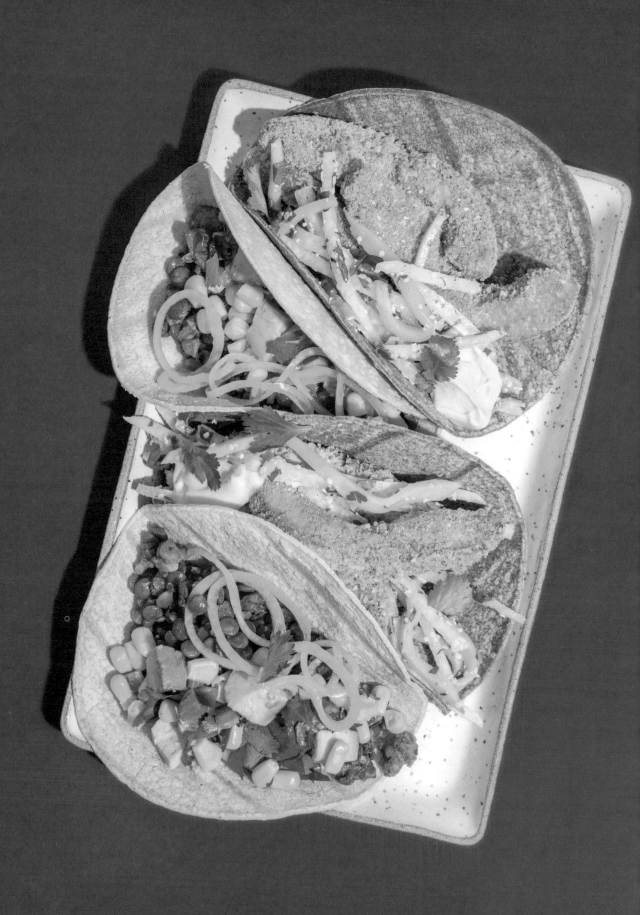

# Lentil and Walnut Tacos with Turmeric Pickled Onions and Corn and Avocado Salsa

DAIRY-FREE | GLUTEN-FREE | VEGAN | VEGETARIAN

SERVES 4

Every once in a while, you happen on a seemingly simple arrangement of ingredients that turns into a mind-blowing meal. High in fibre and healthy fats, these tacos are insanely flavourful and quick to prepare. They come together in 15 minutes if you have already made the pickled onions and lentils or in 40 minutes if you want to do it all on the fly. Trust me, you want to make the pickled onions! These onions, with their prebiotic fibres and anti-inflammatory sulphur-based compounds, become almost delicate in flavour and very addictive. You will never have a reason to skip taco Tuesday again.

---

1. **Make the Turmeric Pickled Onions**  Add the onion, lemon juice, salt, sugar, and turmeric to a 1-quart (1 L) mason jar. Place the lid on tightly and shake. Let sit at room temperature for 30 minutes to 1 hour. You can store the pickled onions in the fridge for up to 1 week.

2. **Make the Corn and Avocado Salsa**  In a medium bowl, add the corn, avocado, cilantro, lime juice, jalapeño, and salt and stir to combine.

3. **Make the Lentil and Walnut Filling**  In a large skillet, heat the olive oil over medium heat. Add the garlic and cook, stirring often, for 1 minute. Add the oregano, cumin, chili powder, and paprika and stir until fragrant, about 30 seconds. Add the lentils, walnuts, water, tomato paste, and salt (if using) and simmer for 5 minutes.

4. To serve, fill the tortillas with the Lentil and Walnut Filling, then top with Turmeric Pickled Onions and Corn and Avocado Salsa.

**Make It Faster**  Need to make this a 10-minute meal? Serve the Lentil and Walnut Filling with pre-shredded cabbage and store-bought salsa.

**Make It Healthier**  If you want to add a dose of fermented foods to this fibre-rich meal, substitute the Lacto-Fermented Turmeric Onions (page 274) for the Turmeric Pickled Onions.

## Turmeric Pickled Onions

1 sweet yellow onion, thinly sliced on a mandolin

½ cup (125 mL) freshly squeezed lemon juice (about 3 juicy lemons)

1½ teaspoons (7 mL) salt

1 teaspoon (5 mL) cane sugar

½ teaspoon (2 mL) ground turmeric

## Corn and Avocado Salsa

2 cups (500 mL) fresh or thawed frozen corn kernels

2 avocados, pitted, peeled, and diced

1 cup (250 mL) lightly packed chopped fresh cilantro

¼ cup (60 mL) freshly squeezed lime juice

½ jalapeño pepper, seeded and diced

¼ teaspoon (1 mL) salt

## Lentil and Walnut Filling

2 tablespoons (30 mL) extra-virgin olive oil

2 cloves garlic, minced

1 teaspoon (5 mL) dried oregano

1 teaspoon (5 mL) dried cumin

1 teaspoon (5 mL) chili powder

½ teaspoon (2 mL) sweet paprika

2 cups (500 mL) cooked French lentils

1 cup (250 mL) finely chopped raw walnuts

½ cup (125 mL) water

1 tablespoon (15 mL) tomato paste

½ teaspoon (2 mL) salt (omit if using salted canned lentils)

## For serving

8 small corn tortillas (or Bibb lettuce or large collard leaves)

# Jicama Avocado Tacos

DAIRY-FREE | GLUTEN-FREE | NUT-FREE | VEGAN | VEGETARIAN

**SERVES 4**

## Crispy Avocado Fries

½ cup (125 mL) brown rice flour

½ teaspoon (2 mL) salt, divided

½ cup (125 mL) unsweetened cashew milk or soy milk

Hot sauce

¼ cup (60 mL) gluten-free bread crumbs

¼ cup (60 mL) nutritional yeast

2 large ripe avocados, pitted, peeled, and each cut into 8 slices

Olive oil cooking spray (optional)

## Jicama-Mango Slaw

1½ cups (375 mL) jicama, cut into matchsticks (about half of a 4-inch/ 10 cm diameter jicama)

½ cup (125 mL) peeled and thinly sliced ripe Ataulfo mango

½ cup (125 mL) lightly packed chopped fresh cilantro

1 tablespoon (15 mL) freshly squeezed lime juice

1 tablespoon (15 mL) hemp seeds

Salt

## Sriracha Mayonnaise

⅓ cup (75 mL) vegan mayonnaise

1 tablespoon (15 mL) Sriracha

## For serving

8 small corn tortillas

I do not think you can ever have too many tacos. These tacos are filled with avocado fries, rich in omega-9 oleic acid. Jicama is a root veggie with a flesh that is slightly starchy, moist, and crisp. It is lower in carbohydrates than other root vegetables, great for snacking, and perfect for making slaw paired with sweet-tart mango, which is high in anti-inflammatory beta-carotene and vitamin C. These tacos are perfect served with a side of refried black beans for extra protein.

1. Preheat the oven to 425°F (220°C). Line a baking sheet with parchment paper.

2. **Make the Crispy Avocado Fries** Set up 3 small bowls on the kitchen counter for breading the avocado. In the first bowl, combine the brown rice flour and ¼ teaspoon (1 mL) of the salt; in the second bowl, combine the cashew milk and a dash of hot sauce; and in the third bowl, combine the bread crumbs, nutritional yeast, and the remaining ¼ teaspoon (1 mL) salt.

3. Dredge each avocado slice in the brown rice flour mixture, then in the cashew milk, and finally in the bread crumb mixture and place on the prepared baking sheet. Try not to handle the avocado too much. I like to use a spoon to coat the avocado once it is in the dredging mixtures instead of risking squishing the slices.

4. For extra crispness, give the avocado fries a light spray of olive oil (if using) and then bake until light golden brown, about 8 minutes. Carefully flip the fries, spray with more olive oil (if using), and bake for another 8 minutes. Remove from the oven.

5. **Make the Jicama-Mango Slaw** In a medium bowl, combine the jicama, mango, cilantro, lime juice, hemp seeds, and a pinch of salt. Let sit until the Crispy Avocado Fries are ready.

6. **Make the Sriracha Mayonnaise** In a small bowl, mix together the mayonnaise and Sriracha.

7. To serve, spread each corn tortilla with a smear of Sriracha Mayonnaise. Add 2 Crispy Avocado Fries and a bit of Jicama-Mango Slaw.

# Smoky Peanut Corn Chowder

DAIRY-FREE | GLUTEN-FREE | VEGAN | VEGETARIAN

SERVES 4

Although so many of my food memories come from my grandmother, corn chowder is a meal that I strongly associate with my mother's cooking. Sweet, creamy, and smoky, it was always one of my favourite comfort dishes. I have taken this childhood favourite and given it a little plant sass. Cauliflower rice replaces potatoes for a more nutrient-dense, less starchy soup. Peanut butter is a flavourful, healthy replacement for full cream. Crunchy smoked tofu croutons up the protein and make this a complete meal.

2½ cups (625 mL) cauliflower florets

¼ cup (60 mL) extra-virgin olive oil, divided

1 package (7 ounces/210 g) smoked tofu, cut into ½-inch (1 cm) cubes

½ medium yellow onion, diced

2 stalks celery, diced

2 cups (500 mL) fresh or thawed frozen corn kernels

2 cloves garlic, minced

1¼ teaspoons (6 mL) salt, divided

1 teaspoon (5 mL) ground cumin

¾ teaspoon (4 mL) dried thyme

½ teaspoon (2 mL) hot smoked paprika, plus more for garnish

4 cups (1 L) water

¼ cup (60 mL) natural peanut butter

1. Place the cauliflower florets in a food processor and pulse until it resembles rice. Set aside.

2. In a large pot over medium heat, heat 2 tablespoons (30 mL) of the olive oil. Add the tofu and cook until the edges start to crisp, 4 to 5 minutes, stirring often so they do not stick. Remove from the heat and transfer to a plate. Set aside.

3. Heat the remaining 2 tablespoons (30 mL) olive oil in the same pot over medium heat. Add the onion and celery and cook, stirring often, until soft and glossy, 5 to 7 minutes. Do not worry if it is browning on the bottom of the pot. That is the good stuff.

4. Add the cauliflower, corn, and garlic and cook for 3 minutes until the cauliflower begins to soften. Add ½ teaspoon (2 mL) of the salt, cumin, thyme, and paprika and stir for 1 minute.

5. Pour in the water and bring to a boil for 5 minutes, until the vegetables are fork-tender. Scrape all that good stuff off the bottom of the pot as you add the water.

6. Add the peanut butter and the remaining ¾ teaspoon (4 mL) salt. Let simmer on low for 10 minutes, stirring occasionally, so the flavours can blend. Remove from the heat.

7. Using a handheld immersion blender, purée the soup until smooth, adding a bit of extra water if the mixture looks too thick.

8. Ladle into large soup bowls and garnish each serving with tofu cubes and a sprinkle of paprika.

Make It Faster You can often find pre-made cauliflower rice in the produce section of the grocery store. Substitute 2 cups (500 mL) of pre-made cauliflower rice for the cauliflower florets.

# Winter Sunchoke Soup with Cilantro Pesto

DAIRY-FREE | GLUTEN-FREE | PALEO-FRIENDLY | VEGAN | VEGETARIAN

SERVES 4 TO 6

### Winter Sunchoke Soup

2 cups (500 mL) peeled and chopped sunchokes (about 1 pound/450 g)

1 cup (250 mL) small cauliflower florets

3 cloves garlic, unpeeled

2 tablespoons (30 mL) extra-virgin olive oil

Salt and freshly cracked pepper

½ cup (125 mL) raw cashews, soaked in water for at least 4 hours, drained, and rinsed

4 cups (1 L) low-sodium vegetable stock, divided

1 tablespoon (15 mL) white miso

½ teaspoon (2 mL) ground cumin

½ teaspoon (2 mL) dried thyme

### Cilantro Pesto

1 cup (250 mL) lightly packed fresh cilantro leaves

¼ cup (60 mL) raw almonds

¼ cup (60 mL) olive oil

½ jalapeño pepper, seeded and chopped

⅛ teaspoon (0.5 mL) salt

Zest of ½ lemon

1 tablespoon (15 mL) freshly squeezed lemon juice

Sunchokes would not win any beauty contests, unless you believe that true beauty comes from within (and you should). This brown and knobby root vegetable, also known as a Jerusalem artichoke, is packed with prebiotic inulin to feed the trillions of beneficial bacteria living in your gut. That prebiotic fibre also makes for a smooth soup that is warm, comforting, and decadently healthy. Roasting the sunchokes takes a little extra time, but it is worth it.

1. Preheat the oven to 400°F (200°C).

2. **Make the Winter Sunchoke Soup** On a baking sheet lined with parchment paper, toss the sunchokes, cauliflower, and garlic with the olive oil, a generous pinch of salt, and a few cracks of pepper. Roast for 25 to 30 minutes, until the cauliflower is golden brown at the edges. Watch carefully after 15 minutes so that the garlic does not overcook. Remove the garlic if done before the other vegetables.

3. **Make the Cilantro Pesto** Meanwhile, in a high-speed blender, add the cilantro, almonds, olive oil, jalapeño, salt, lemon zest and juice and purée. Scrape the pesto into a small bowl and set aside. Rinse the blender.

4. Remove the vegetables from the oven. Carefully remove the skin from the roasted garlic and discard. Add the roasted vegetables, garlic, and cashews to the high-speed blender, then add enough vegetable stock to cover and purée until smooth.

5. Pour the soup into a medium pot and heat over medium-low heat. Stir in the remaining vegetable stock, miso, cumin, and thyme and season to taste with salt and pepper.

6. Once heated, ladle the soup into bowls, swirl a spoonful of Cilantro Pesto on top, and serve.

**Make It Faster** This soup takes about 45 minutes to make but comes together faster if the Cilantro Pesto is made ahead and the vegetables are roasted the night before. Then you will have this soup ready in about 15 minutes! Store remaining pesto in a resealable container in the fridge for 3 to 4 days.

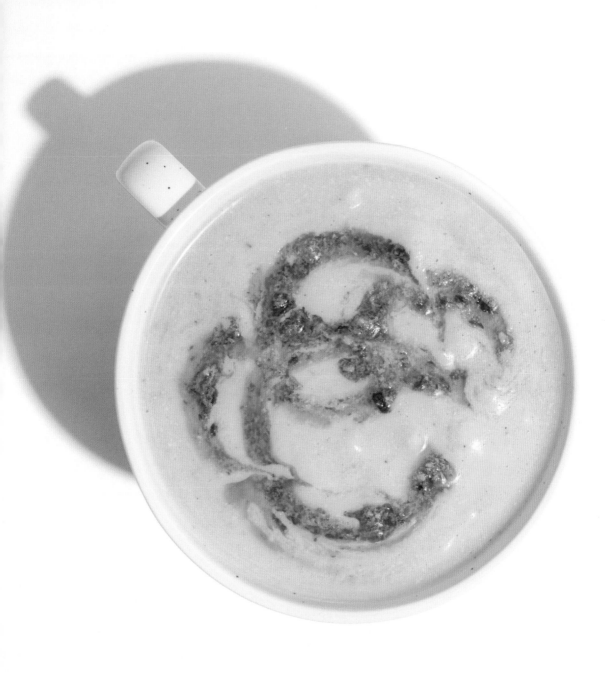

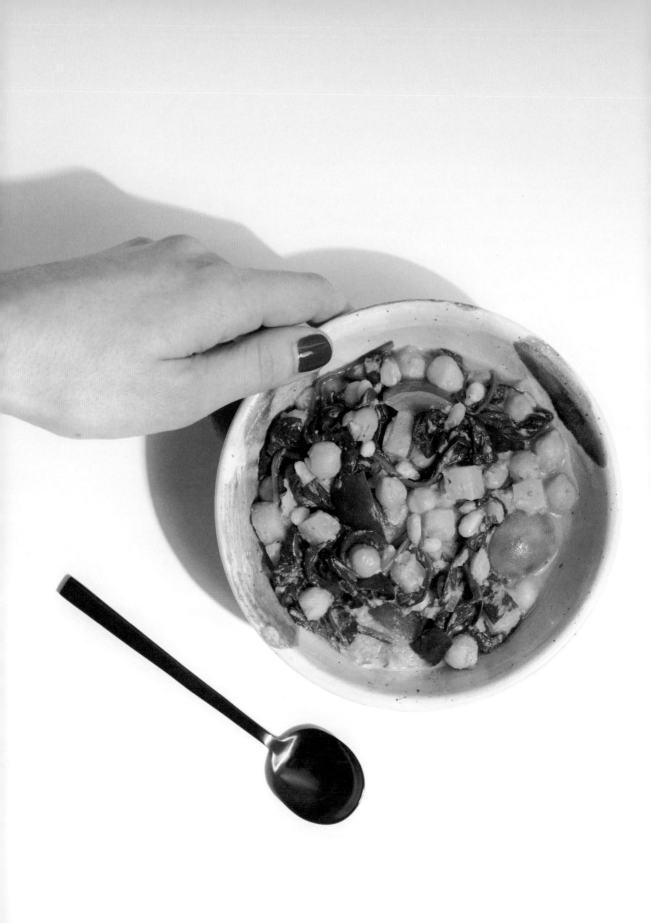

# Red Grape, Chickpea, and Pine Nut Stew

DAIRY-FREE | GLUTEN-FREE | VEGAN | VEGETARIAN

SERVES 4

One-pot meals are my favourite. I love combining a variety of flavours and textures into one hearty bowl of goodness. One of my secrets for making a truly satisfying meal is keeping it high in fibre; chickpeas contain a whopping 8 grams of fibre per cup (250 mL). All that fibre helps to feed beneficial bacteria in the gut and keep inflammation at bay. Garlic and shallot, with their anti-inflammatory sulphur-based compounds, also keep gut bacteria happy with their prebiotic fructans. This is a wonderful weeknight meal that comes together quickly without too much chopping!

1. In a large pot, heat the olive oil over medium heat. Add the shallot, cumin, thyme, sumac, and garlic and cook for 2 minutes, stirring often, until the shallot begins to soften and the spices become aromatic.

2. Add the zucchini and cook until it turns golden, stirring occasionally, 3 to 5 minutes. Add the chickpeas, red grapes, and salt and let it all sizzle away for 5 minutes, stirring occasionally.

3. Stir in the vegetable stock and tahini, let simmer for 5 minutes, and then remove from the heat. Stir in the spinach, pine nuts, and lemon juice until the spinach wilts, and serve.

Tip Sumac is a spice made from the dried red berries of the sumac bush. It has a tart, lemony flavour that adds a special touch to the dish. In a pinch, add lemon zest instead.

⅓ cup (75 mL) extra-virgin olive oil

½ cup (125 mL) diced shallot (about 1 medium shallot)

1½ teaspoons (7 mL) ground cumin

1 teaspoon (5 mL) dried thyme

½ teaspoon (2 mL) ground sumac

3 cloves garlic, minced

1½ cups (375 mL) diced zucchini

2 cans (14 ounces/398 mL each) chickpeas, drained and rinsed

1 cup (250 mL) red grapes, halved

¾ teaspoon (4 mL) salt

2 cups (500 mL) low-sodium vegetable stock

2 tablespoons (30 mL) raw tahini

4 cups (1 L) packed baby spinach

½ cup (125 mL) raw pine nuts

1 tablespoon (15 mL) freshly squeezed lemon juice

# Portuguese Green Bean Stew

DAIRY-FREE | GLUTEN-FREE | NUT-FREE | PALEO-FRIENDLY | VEGAN | VEGETARIAN

SERVES 4

My grandmother is not a cook; she is a culinary magician. She makes all of her soups without broth and can turn a handful of ingredients into an insanely flavourful meal. I still remember all the childhood summers I spent shelling peas and trimming beans alongside my grandmother. More accurately, eating all the peas and beans my grandmother shelled! Tomatoes, with their abundance of the carotenoid lycopene, are an important part of an anti-inflammatory diet because of their lycopene, with well-researched benefits. A fat-soluble nutrient, the bioavailability of lycopene actually improves when you cook it in a healthy fat. Serve this simple stew with millet or quinoa.

---

2 pounds (900 g) fresh green beans, trimmed and cut into bite-sized pieces

⅓ cup (75 mL) extra-virgin olive oil

1 cup (250 mL) diced yellow onion

2 cloves garlic, minced

1 teaspoon (5 mL) ground cumin

1 can (28 ounces/796 mL) no-salt-added crushed tomatoes

¾ teaspoon (4 mL) salt

1. Bring a large pot of water to a boil over high heat. Add the green beans and boil for 7 to 8 minutes until they start to soften. Remove from the heat and drain.

2. In a large skillet, heat the olive oil over medium heat. Add the onion, garlic, and cumin and cook until the onion begins to soften, about 5 minutes.

3. Add the tomatoes, salt, and cooked green beans and let boil gently, partially covered, for 15 minutes, or until beans are fork-tender. Serve warm or at room temperature with millet or quinoa.

Make It Faster  The only thing that takes time in this recipe is trimming the beans. You can either do this ahead of time or buy fine green beans, which are often sold pre-trimmed. You can skip the parboiling step for these more delicate beans, but it is absolutely needed for thick, woodier beans.

# Stir-Fried Black Rice with Kimchi and Asian Greens

DAIRY-FREE | GLUTEN-FREE | NUT-FREE | VEGAN | VEGETARIAN

SERVES 4

The first time I tried kimchi, it was breakfast. I was jet-lagged and not sure I could fall in love with this pungent, garlicky, spicy stuff called kimchi. It took about three days and then I looked forward to it at every meal.

One of my favourite rules for eating well is to make half of your plate fruits or vegetables. I love this rule for its flexibility: you can add more vegetables to almost any meal and make it healthier, which is what I have done here. By using many nutrient-dense greens, along with fermented cabbage in kimchi, you are getting plenty of anti-inflammatory plant power. Black rice is also a bit of an upgrade because it is rich in flavonoid compounds that, while they do degrade in cooking somewhat, are still very different from the relative nothingness that white rice offers. To preserve the fermented benefits of kimchi, add it at the very end so it does not reach steaming temperatures.

---

1. In a large skillet or wok, heat the coconut oil over medium-high heat. Add the garlic and greens and fry, stirring constantly, until the greens wilt, 2 to 4 minutes depending on variety.

2. Reduce the heat to medium, then add the crumbled tofu, sesame oil, tamari and heat through, stirring constantly to avoid it sticking to the bottom of the skillet, about 2 minutes.

3. Add the rice and stir to thoroughly combine and heat through, 3 to 4 minutes. Remove from the heat, stir in the kimchi, taste, and adjust seasoning with tamari if necessary.

Tip Cooked and cooled rice has the best texture for fried rice. If you can, make the rice up to 3 days in advance and this meal will come together in 20 minutes.

3 tablespoons (45 mL) refined coconut oil or avocado oil

1 clove garlic, minced

6 cups (1.5 L) chopped Asian greens (gailan, bok choy, yu choy, amaranth greens)

Half of a 12-ounce (350 g) package extra-firm tofu, crumbled

1 tablespoon (15 mL) toasted sesame oil

1 tablespoon (15 mL) gluten-free tamari

2½ cups (625 mL) cooked and cooled long-grain black rice

1 cup (250 mL) vegan kimchi, chopped

# Plant-Style Teppanyaki Noodles

*DAIRY-FREE | GLUTEN-FREE | NUT-FREE | VEGAN | VEGETARIAN*

**SERVES 4**

⅓ cup (75 mL) gluten-free tamari

2 tablespoons (30 mL) black sesame seeds

2 teaspoons (10 mL) hot sauce

1 teaspoon (5 mL) cane sugar

1 teaspoon (5 mL) toasted sesame oil

2 tablespoons (30 mL) coconut oil or avocado oil

1 small yellow onion, thinly sliced into half-moons

4 stalks celery, finely sliced

1 tablespoon (15 mL) minced peeled fresh ginger

2 cloves garlic, minced

2 medium sweet potatoes, spiralized (about 6 cups/ 1.5 L spiralized)

¼ cup (60 mL) water

1 sweet red pepper, thinly sliced

1 small package (about 4 cups/1 L) coleslaw mix

1 can (19 ounces/540 mL) black beans, drained and rinsed

1 cup (250 mL) bean sprouts

As a teenager, one of my favourite treats was getting teppanyaki noodles at the food court. They seemed so healthy at the time, even covered in a sweet and salty sauce that is anything but healthy. I thought it was high time to reimagine this nostalgic dish and pack it full of vegetables. With the anti-inflammatory trio of garlic, ginger, and onion as the flavour base and sweet potato standing in for doughy noodles, this super-quick meal will help you feel energized and comforted at the same time.

---

1.  In a small bowl, whisk together the tamari, sesame seeds, hot sauce, sugar, and sesame oil. Set aside.

2.  In a wok or large skillet, heat the coconut oil over medium-high heat. Add the onion, celery, ginger, and garlic and sauté for 3 to 4 minutes until softened.

3.  Add the spiralized sweet potato and water and cover with a lid to let steam for 3 minutes. Remove the lid, add the red pepper and coleslaw, and cook, stirring often, for 2 minutes.

4.  Stir in the tamari mixture and black beans and heat for 1 to 2 minutes. Divide among 4 plates, top with the bean sprouts and serve.

**Tip** If you have a mandolin, use it to slice the onion, celery, and red pepper for a perfect, light, and silky texture when cooked. Be sure to use the hand guard!

**Make It Faster** Buy spiralized sweet potatoes to save time! In addition, you can slice all the veggies the night before and store them in the fridge.

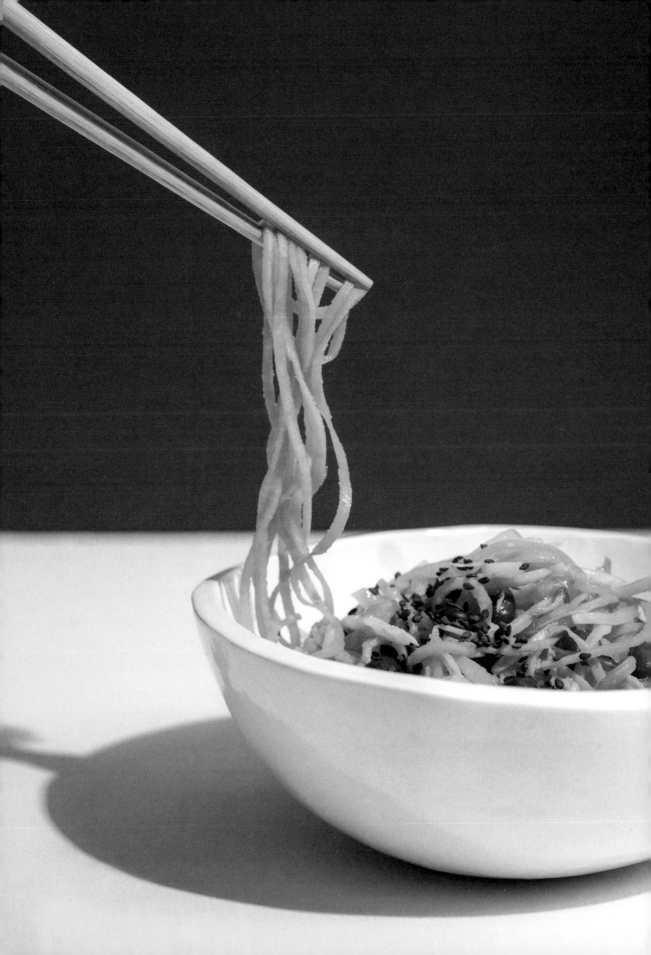

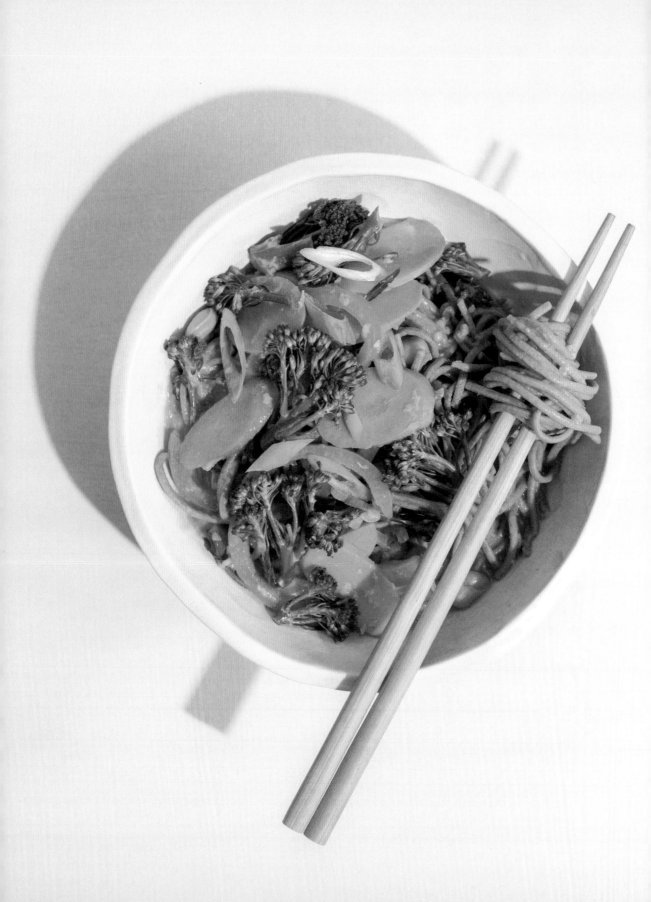

# Spicy Miso Soba Bowl

DAIRY-FREE | GLUTEN-FREE | NUT-FREE | VEGAN | VEGETARIAN

SERVES 4

On a cold day, a hot bowl of noodles always does the trick, fortifying both body and soul. I love using miso to create an almost instant broth that is still rich and flavourful. Miso is a wonderful fermented food; preserve its benefits by not boiling it! Use whatever veggies you have on hand; this recipe is a great way to use up whatever is languishing in the veggie drawer. Just be sure to keep the anti-inflammatory fire-power: garlic, ginger, and onion. Pure buckwheat soba noodles can be a bit hard to find; if your local market does not carry them, gluten-free ramen or Thai rice noodles would be delicious, too.

1 package (9 ounces/250 g) buckwheat soba noodles

2 cups (500 mL) frozen shelled edamame

⅓ cup (75 mL) red miso

1 teaspoon (5 mL) Sriracha, plus more for serving

2 tablespoons (30 mL) unseasoned rice vinegar

1 tablespoon (15 mL) gluten-free tamari

1 teaspoon (5 mL) toasted sesame oil

2 tablespoons (30 mL) coconut oil

2 tablespoons (30 mL) minced peeled fresh ginger

4 cloves garlic, minced

½ yellow onion, thinly sliced into half-moons

1 small bunch broccolini, cut into bite-sized pieces

4 large carrots, thinly sliced

1 large sweet red pepper, thinly sliced

Salt

For serving

Sliced green onions

Sesame seeds

1. Bring a medium pot of water to a boil. Cook the soba noodles according to package directions, adding the edamame when there is 5 minutes left on the cook time. Reserve 2 cups (500 mL) of cooking water. Drain, rinse the soba noodles and edamame, and set aside.

2. In a large bowl, whisk together the reserved cooking liquid, miso, Sriracha, rice vinegar, tamari, and sesame oil until well blended. Set aside.

3. In a large skillet or wok, heat the coconut oil over medium-high heat. Stir-fry the ginger, garlic, and onion for 2 minutes to soften. Add the broccolini and carrots and cook, stirring often, for 3 to 4 minutes. Add the red pepper and cook for 1 minute. Remove from the heat and season with a pinch of salt.

4. To serve, divide the noodle and edamame mixture among 4 large bowls. Top with vegetables and pour about ½ cup (125 mL) miso broth over each noodle bowl. Top with green onions and sesame seeds and more hot sauce, if desired.

# Carrot Tofu Hippie Scramble

DAIRY-FREE | GLUTEN-FREE | NUT-FREE | VEGAN | VEGETARIAN

SERVES 4

When I was a teenager, one of the first vegetarian dishes I cooked was a carrot tofu scramble from the *Vegetarian Times Cookbook*. This variation is so easy to make, and kids and grownups like it in equal measure. Rich in anti-inflammatory carotenoids, naturally sweet carrots and umami-filled tamari transform humble tofu into craveable comfort food. I have added a couple of tweaks of my own, like omega-3-rich hemp seeds, and it is still a firm favourite in my home.

---

2 tablespoons (30 mL) extra-virgin olive oil

1 tablespoon (15 mL) minced fresh ginger

2 cloves garlic, minced

1 package (12 ounces/350 g) extra-firm or pressed tofu, crumbled

¼ cup (60 mL) gluten-free tamari, divided

1 pound (450 g) carrots, grated

2 teaspoons (10 mL) toasted sesame oil

¼ cup (60 mL) hemp seeds

Hot sauce

1.  In a large skillet, heat the olive oil over medium heat. Add the ginger and garlic and cook for 2 minutes, stirring occasionally.

2.  Add the crumbled tofu and 1 tablespoon (15 mL) of the tamari. Cook for 5 minutes, stirring occasionally.

3.  Add the carrots, stirring to distribute them through the tofu, and heat through, about 2 minutes. Remove from the heat and stir in the remaining 3 tablespoons (45 mL) tamari, sesame oil, hemp seeds, and a dash of hot sauce. Divide among 4 bowls and serve.

Make It Faster  Grating carrots in your food processor (or buying pre-grated carrots!) will turn a 15-minute task into a 1-minute task, and then this dinner will come together in less than 20 minutes.

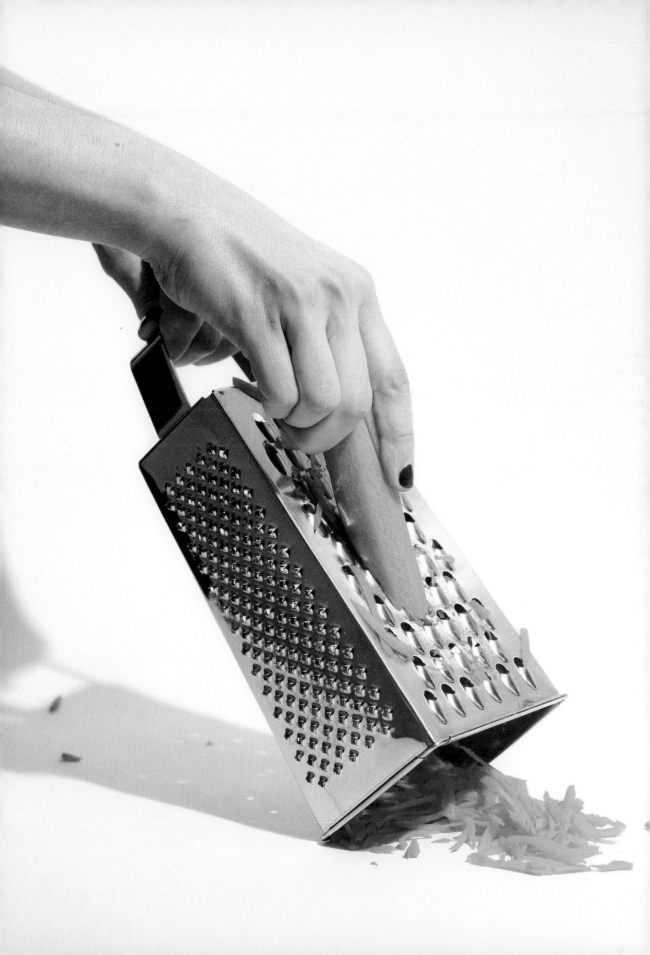

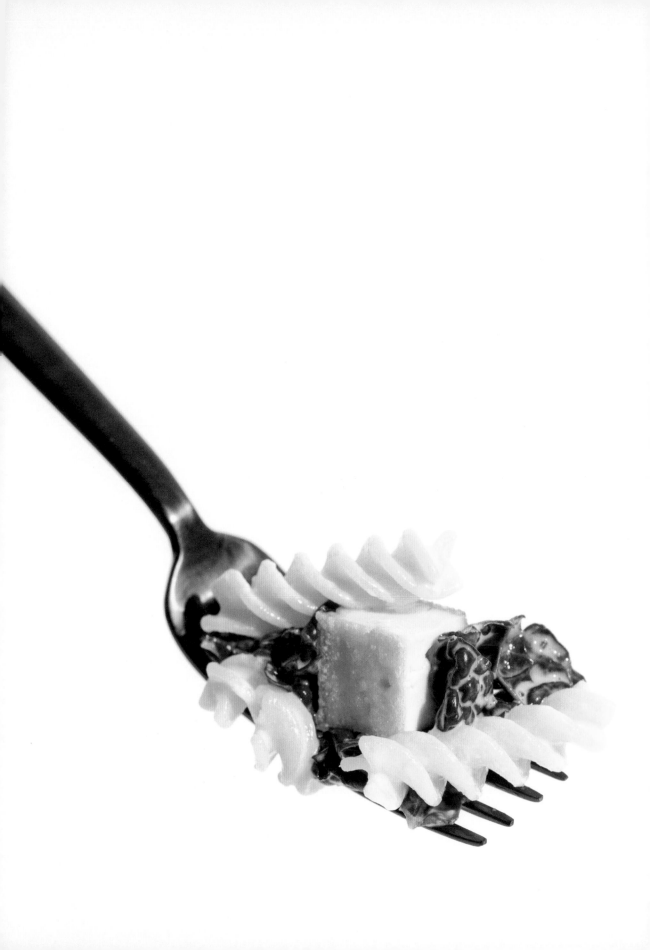

# Creamy Pasta with Smoked Tofu and Kale

DAIRY-FREE | GLUTEN-FREE | NUT-FREE | VEGAN | VEGETARIAN

SERVES 4

After a good salad, pretty much anything in a cream sauce is a favourite for me. As much as I love a cashew cream, soy milk makes a wonderfully creamy alternative. For additional protein, I add smoked tofu, an ingredient that does not get enough attention. It is essentially marinated and pre-cooked tofu. If cooking tofu still intimidates you, smoked tofu is the perfect way to enjoy this mineral-rich ingredient. Soybeans contain peptides and isoflavones that are associated with lower inflammation; my preference is always for foods made from organic whole soybeans as opposed to supplementing with isolated or extracted soy proteins, which I do not recommend. This savoury, creamy main dish packs plenty of protein and fibre-rich greens for a truly nourishing dinner.

1. In a large pot, cook the pasta according to package directions. Drain, reserving 2 tablespoons (30 mL) of the cooking liquid. Do not rinse pasta.

2. In a large skillet, heat 3 tablespoons (45 mL) of the olive oil over medium heat. Add the garlic and shallots and cook, stirring often, until soft and glossy, 2 to 3 minutes.

3. Add the tofu and thyme, stirring occasionally until the edges of the tofu begin to turn golden brown, 3 to 5 minutes. Add the kale and stir until wilted, about 2 minutes. Season with salt and pepper and then scrape the mixture into a large bowl.

4. Return the skillet to medium heat and add the remaining 1 tablespoon (15 mL) olive oil. Whisk in the flour for 1 minute to hydrate it, then slowly whisk in the soy milk and tamari. Bring to a gentle boil and reduce the heat to medium-low, whisking often, until the sauce thickens, about 5 minutes. Remove from the heat, add the tofu and kale mixture, pasta, and reserved pasta cooking liquid, and toss to combine. Season with salt and pepper to taste. Divide among 4 bowls and serve.

3 cups (750 mL) dried gluten-free pasta (about three-quarters of a 12-ounce/ 340 g package)

¼ cup (60 mL) extra-virgin olive oil, divided

2 cloves garlic, minced

½ large shallot, diced

1 package (7 ounces/210 g) smoked tofu, cut into ½-inch (1 cm) cubes

1 teaspoon (5 mL) dried thyme

2 large bunches black kale, stems removed and thinly sliced in ribbons

¼ teaspoon (1 mL) salt

Freshly cracked pepper

1 tablespoon (15 mL) gluten-free all-purpose flour or arrowroot starch

2 cups (500 mL) unsweetened soy milk

1 tablespoon + 1 teaspoon (20 mL) gluten-free tamari

# Chipotle Tofu Mole

DAIRY-FREE | GLUTEN-FREE | VEGAN | VEGETARIAN

SERVES 4 TO 6

2 packages (12 ounces/350 g each) extra-firm tofu, cut into ½-inch (1 cm) cubes

2 tablespoons (30 mL) avocado oil

1 small yellow onion, diced

1 cup (250 mL) cherry tomatoes, halved, or Roma tomatoes, cubed

4 chipotle peppers canned in adobo sauce, chopped

¼ cup (60 mL) Thompson raisins

2 cloves garlic, minced

3 cups (750 mL) low-sodium vegetable stock, divided

⅓ cup (75 mL) raw almond butter

2 tablespoons (30 mL) cocoa powder

1 teaspoon (5 mL) ground cumin

¾ teaspoon (4 mL) salt

½ teaspoon (2 mL) cinnamon

½ teaspoon (2 mL) dried oregano

¼ teaspoon (1 mL) allspice

Freshly squeezed lime juice

For serving

Cooked whole grain (brown rice, quinoa, millet, buckwheat)

Fresh cilantro leaves

Lime wedges

Mole is an insanely complex chili-cocoa sauce that can have upward of thirty ingredients and requires soaking dried chilies, but these days I do not have time for that!

I propose a simpler but no less delicious option: a savoury mole-inspired sauce that uses cocoa powder and chipotle peppers and comes together in thirty minutes, including roasting the tofu. Cocoa powder, particularly the non–Dutched processed variety, is high in anti-inflammatory flavonoid compounds. Savory, earthy, and smooth, I love serving this sauce over cauliflower rice and my Jicama, Orange, and Pumpkin Seed Salad (page 123) to up the veggie count. It also makes a great protein sauce combination for Mexican-inspired grain bowls.

1.  Preheat the oven to 425°F (220°C). Line a baking sheet with parchment paper.

2.  Place the tofu on the baking sheet, without any oil or seasoning, and bake for 15 minutes.

3.  Meanwhile, in a large skillet, heat the avocado oil over medium heat. Add the onion and cook, stirring occasionally, until soft and glossy, 5 to 7 minutes.

4.  Add the tomatoes, chipotle peppers, raisins, garlic, and 1 cup (250 mL) of the vegetable stock and let it bubble away, stirring occasionally, for 5 minutes to soften the tomatoes.

5.  Add the remaining 2 cups (500 mL) vegetable stock and stir in the almond butter, cocoa, cumin, salt, cinnamon, oregano, and allspice. Bring to a boil and then reduce the heat to low for 5 minutes.

6.  Remove the sauce from the heat and purée using a handheld immersion blender. If the mixture seems too thick, thin it with up to ¼ cup (60 mL) water so it has the texture of a thick gravy. Return to low heat, add the tofu, and let sit for 2 minutes so the tofu can soak up the sauce a bit. Taste and adjust the seasoning with a generous squeeze of lime juice and salt.

7.  Serve the tofu mole over your favourite whole grain, top with fresh cilantro, and serve with a lime wedge.

# Lemon Millet Risotto with Roasted Radicchio

DAIRY-FREE | GLUTEN-FREE | NUT-FREE | VEGAN | VEGETARIAN

SERVES 4

This is a true anti-inflammatory risotto but made from millet. Millet makes a creamier risotto than quinoa because of its starchier texture. Rich in lutein and zeaxanthin, millet also boasts plenty of fibre and immune-supporting zinc and magnesium. A bit of calcium-rich tahini enhances the creaminess of the dish. Roasting the radicchio softens the intense bitterness and even reveals a bit of sweetness. If you are not a fan of radicchio, I suggest serving this risotto with some roasted Brussels sprouts or broccolini instead.

---

1. Preheat the oven to 425°F (220°C). Place the oven rack close to the heat source. Line a baking sheet with parchment paper.

2. **Make the Lemon Millet Risotto**  In a large skillet, heat the olive oil over medium heat. Add the shallots and cook, stirring often, until soft, 2 to 3 minutes. Add the garlic and stir for 1 minute.

3. Add the millet and stir to coat with the olive oil. Pour in 3 cups (750 mL) of the vegetable stock, increase the heat to high, and bring to a boil. Cover with a lid slightly vented, reduce the heat to medium-low, and cook until the millet is just a little chewy and has absorbed most of the stock, 14 to 16 minutes.

4. **Make the Roasted Radicchio**  Meanwhile, generously coat the radicchio with olive oil, massaging it with your fingers to ensure an even coating. Place on the prepared baking sheet, season with salt and pepper, and roast for 4 to 5 minutes, until the top looks wilted and loses its bright red colour. Gently turn it over and roast for another 4 to 5 minutes. Set aside.

5. To finish the risotto, add the tahini and the remaining 1 cup (250 mL) vegetable stock to the risotto, stirring until mostly absorbed but still moist, 1 to 2 minutes. Remove from the heat and add the lemon zest and juice, stirring to incorporate. Taste and adjust the seasoning with salt and pepper.

6. To serve, divide the risotto among 4 plates or shallow bowls and top with a radicchio half.

## Lemon Millet Risotto

2 tablespoons (30 mL) extra-virgin olive oil

1 large shallot, minced

1 clove garlic, minced

1 cup (250 mL) dried millet

4 cups (1 L) low-sodium vegetable stock, divided

¼ cup (60 mL) raw tahini

Zest of 1 lemon

3 tablespoons (45 mL) freshly squeezed lemon juice

## Roasted Radicchio

2 small radicchio, halved

¼ cup (60 mL) extra-virgin olive oil

¼ teaspoon (1 mL) salt

Freshly cracked pepper

# Carrot White Bean Risotto

DAIRY-FREE | GLUTEN-FREE | NUT-FREE | PALEO-FRIENDLY | VEGAN | VEGETARIAN

SERVES 4

Cooking risotto is much easier than you think! Although white rice is not an anti-inflammatory ingredient, the carrot juice packs high levels of carotenoids that are anti-inflammatory, and the white beans increase fibre and protein to help lower the glycemic impact of this recipe while still staying in the creamy, buttery flavour zone. This recipe is a perfect example of how anti-inflammatory living is a lifestyle that leaves room for a few exceptions to the rules every now and again.

4 cups (1 L) low-sodium vegetable stock

2 cups (500 mL) fresh carrot juice

¼ cup (60 mL) extra-virgin olive oil

½ large yellow onion, diced

4 carrots, diced

2 cloves garlic, minced

½ teaspoon (2 mL) ground cumin

¼ teaspoon (1 mL) cinnamon

¼ teaspoon (1 mL) ground ginger

¼ teaspoon (1 mL) ground turmeric

1½ cups (375 mL) Arborio rice or Carnaroli rice

2 cans (14 ounces/398 mL each) cannellini beans or navy beans

Salt and pepper

1. In a medium saucepan, add the vegetable stock and carrot juice and bring to a simmer over medium heat. Reduce the heat to medium-low to keep warm.

2. In a large skillet, heat the olive oil over medium-high heat. Add the onion and sauté for 3 minutes until it begins to soften. Add the carrots, garlic, cumin, cinnamon, ginger, and turmeric, stirring constantly for 2 minutes.

3. Add the rice to the vegetables, stirring for 1 minute so that the grains are coated in oil.

4. Add 1 cup (250 mL) of the vegetable stock and carrot juice mixture, stirring constantly until absorbed. Add the remaining stock, 1 cup (250 mL) at a time, and repeat the stirring process until you have used up all of the stock and the grains are just tender. With the remaining 1 cup (250 mL) of stock, add the beans to heat through.

5. Taste and adjust seasoning with salt and pepper, divide among 4 bowls, and serve.

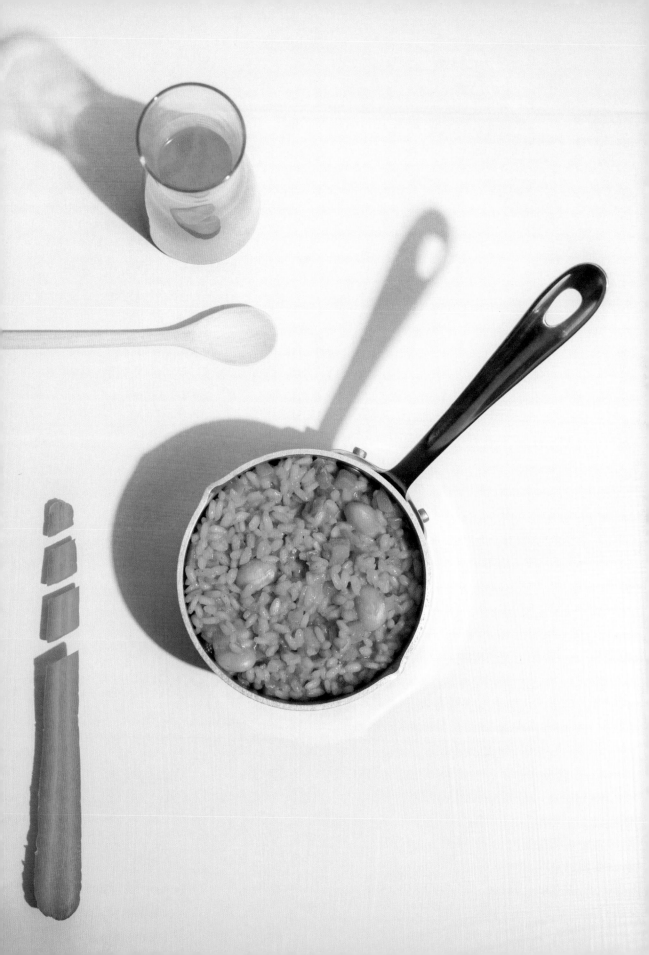

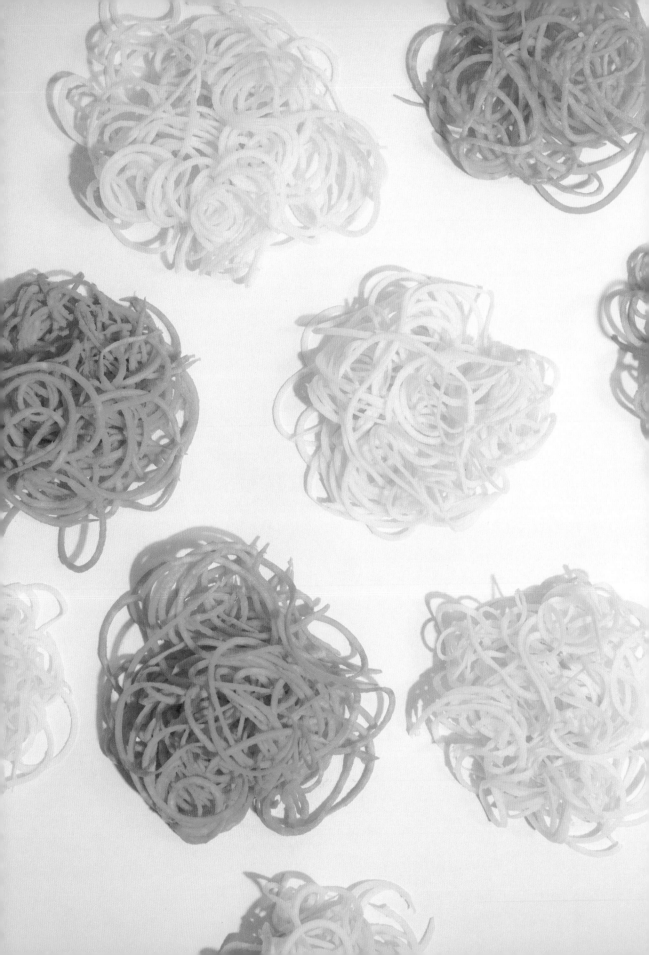

# Sweet Potato Pasta with Mushrooms and Walnut Cream

DAIRY-FREE | GLUTEN-FREE | PALEO-FRIENDLY | VEGAN | VEGETARIAN

SERVES 4

I love swapping in vegetables for traditional starches wherever I can, because any excuse to eat more vegetables is a good one! Spiralized sweet potatoes are a great substitute for pasta, offering more anti-inflammatory vitamin C and beta-carotene. I love yellow-fleshed sweet potatoes here, as they are less sweet; however, for a serious boost of beta-carotene, feel free to use orange-fleshed varieties.

Mushrooms, walnuts, and leeks are an anti-inflammatory trifecta, providing omega-3 fats, prebiotic fibres, and polysaccharides that support immune function.

- ⅓ cup (75 mL) extra-virgin olive oil, divided
- 1 small leek, thinly sliced (white and light green parts only)
- 1 pound (450 g) cremini mushrooms, sliced
- 1 clove garlic, chopped
- 1 teaspoon (5 mL) gluten-free tamari
- 1 cup (250 mL) raw walnuts, soaked in water for at least 2 hours, drained, and rinsed
- 1 cup (250 mL) water
- 2 teaspoons (10 mL) white miso
- 1 teaspoon (5 mL) minced fresh rosemary or ¼ teaspoon (1 mL) dried rosemary
- 1 teaspoon (5 mL) freshly squeezed lemon juice
- 1 teaspoon (5 mL) pure maple syrup
- ¼ teaspoon (1 mL) salt
- 2 large yellow sweet potatoes, skin on and spiralized (about 8 cups/2 L spiralized)

1. In a large nonstick skillet, heat 1 tablespoon (15 mL) of the olive oil over medium heat. Add the leek and cook, stirring occasionally, for 1 minute.

2. Increase the heat to medium-high. Add the mushrooms and sauté for 5 to 7 minutes until they release their moisture, stirring constantly so the leeks do not burn. Add the garlic and stir for 1 minute. Remove from the heat and season with the tamari.

3. In a high-speed blender, add one-third of the mushroom-leek mixture along with the walnuts, water, miso, rosemary, lemon juice, maple syrup, and salt. Purée until smooth, 1 to 2 minutes. Set aside while you cook the sweet potatoes.

4. Transfer the remaining mushroom-leek mixture to a large bowl and add 2 tablespoons (30 mL) olive oil to the skillet over medium heat. Add half of the spiralized sweet potatoes, stirring constantly so they do not stick to the bottom of the skillet for about 5 minutes, or until they are fork-tender. Transfer the cooked sweet potatoes to the bowl with the mushroom-leek mixture and cook the remaining spiralized sweet potatoes in the remaining 2 tablespoons (30 mL) olive oil until fork-tender.

5. Reduce the heat to low and return the reserved sweet potatoes and mushroom-leek mixture to the skillet. Add the puréed mushroom-leek mixture, stir to combine and cook for 1 minute to warm through. Divide the pasta among 4 plates and serve.

Tip Soaking the walnuts helps to reduce any natural bitterness, but I find they do not hold up to soaking as well as cashews, so try to avoid overdoing it. Soaking them in the morning, so you can get cooking right after work, is fine, but ideally do not let them soak overnight.

Make It Faster You can often find prepared sweet potato spirals in the produce section of the grocery store.

# Chickpea Gnocchi with Olive Tomato Sauce

DAIRY-FREE | GLUTEN-FREE | NUT-FREE | VEGAN | VEGETARIAN

SERVES 4

## Chickpea Gnocchi

3 cups (750 mL) cooked or canned chickpeas (reserve ¼ cup/60 mL chickpea liquid)

1 cup (250 mL) chickpea flour

3 tablespoons (45 mL) extra-virgin olive oil

1 clove garlic, minced or grated on a microplane

½ teaspoon (2 mL) ground cumin

Zest of 1 lemon

½ teaspoon (2 mL) salt

## Olive Tomato Sauce

¼ cup (60 mL) extra-virgin olive oil

2 pints (1 L) cherry tomatoes, halved

3 cloves garlic, minced or grated on a microplane

½ cup (125 mL) pitted Kalamata olives, halved

Salt and pepper

## Garnish

1 cup (250 mL) lightly packed fresh flat-leaf parsley

Freshly squeezed lemon juice (optional)

Gnocchi are delightful little pillows of awesomeness but given that they are usually made from mashed potatoes, they do not offer a whole lot of nutritional benefits. When made with my secret weapon—chickpeas—they achieve a whole other level of awesome. Fibre and protein help keep you feeling full and satisfied and your blood sugars balanced. This recipe contains chickpeas in three ways: cooked, ground into flour, and aquafaba, which is really just a fancy way of saying "chickpea cooking water." Whoever figured out that chickpea liquid can be used as an egg substitute is a genius.

If it seems overly ambitious to make your own gnocchi on a week-night, never fear. It is ridiculously easy. By the time your pasta pot has come to a boil, you will be ready.

1.  Bring a large pot of salted water to a boil over high heat.

2.  **Make the Chickpea Gnocchi** In a food processor, add the chickpeas, reserved chickpea liquid, chickpea flour, olive oil, garlic, cumin, lemon zest, and salt. Blend until combined. Divide the chickpea dough into 4 portions. Roll each portion on a lightly floured work surface until it forms a log about ¾ inch (2 cm) thick. With a knife or pizza cutter, cut the gnocchi into ½-inch (1 cm) pieces. You will have little rectangular pillows, which you can leave as is or fancy up by smoothing the edges or gently pressing with a fork.

3.  **Make the Olive Tomato Sauce** Heat the olive oil in a large frying pan over medium-high heat. Add the cherry tomatoes and cook for 3 to 5 minutes, stirring occasionally so they start to release their juices. Add the garlic and olives and cook for 2 to 3 minutes. Remove from the heat and season well with salt and pepper.

4.  In 2 batches, cook the gnocchi in the boiling water for 2 to 4 minutes, until they rise to the surface. Do not cook longer than 4 minutes or they will start to disintegrate at the edges and look sloppy. Remove with a slotted spoon and place onto plates. Top with the Olive Tomato Sauce, fresh parsley, and a squeeze of lemon juice (if using) and serve.

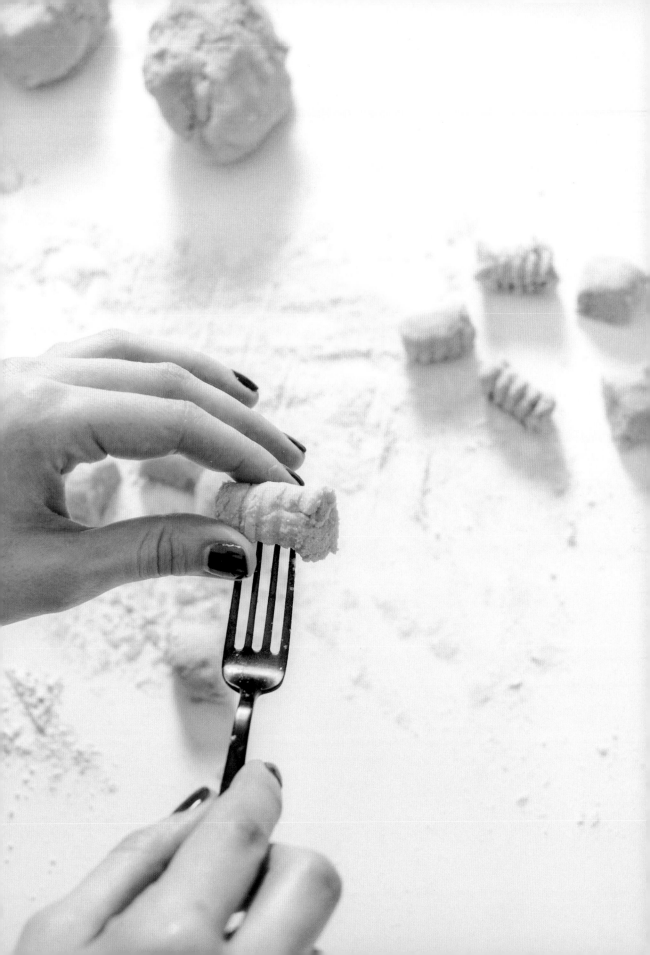

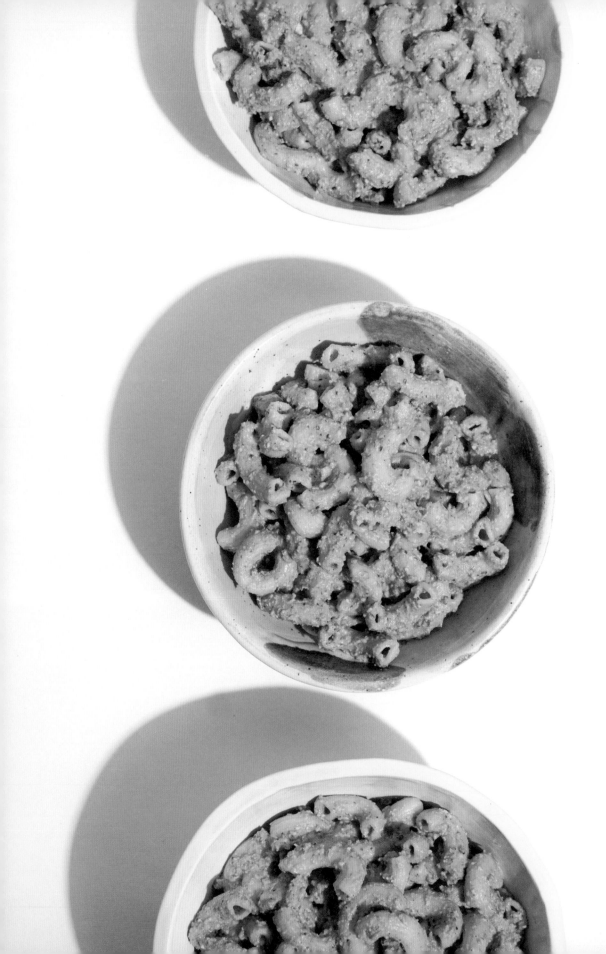

# Martian Macaroni

DAIRY-FREE | GLUTEN-FREE | VEGAN | VEGETARIAN

SERVES 4

This is my grown-up version of one of my standard mom meals. My kids love macaroni, but I cannot leave well enough alone and always add a bunch of peas for a hit of green. That is how Martian Macaroni was born! Healthier than you might think, green peas contain almost 5 grams of protein per ½ cup (125 mL), along with admirable amounts of zinc, iron, and magnesium.

I have created a vibrant green pesto sauce with a light, fresh flavour to make eating your greens new again. This is a super-quick meal that will keep you energized.

---

1. In a large pot of boiling water, cook the pasta according to package directions. Drain the pasta in a colander.

2. In a large skillet, heat the olive oil over medium heat. Add the celery and cook, stirring occasionally, until soft and glossy, about 5 minutes. Add the garlic, peas, and greens and cook until the greens are wilted, 1 to 2 minutes. Remove from the heat and season with the salt.

3. In a high-speed blender, combine the vegetable mixture with the almond milk, pistachios, and mint. Blend until smooth.

4. In the skillet, add the cooked pasta and green pesto sauce and toss to coat. Divide among 4 bowls and serve.

1 package (12 ounces/340 g) gluten-free pasta

¼ cup (60 mL) extra-virgin olive oil

2 stalks celery, diced

3 cloves garlic, sliced

2 cups (500 mL) frozen peas

4 cups (1 L) packed baby greens (spinach, kale, or a mixture)

½ teaspoon (2 mL) salt

½ cup (125 mL) unsweetened almond milk or cashew milk

⅓ cup (75 mL) shelled raw pistachios

¼ cup (60 mL) lightly packed fresh mint leaves

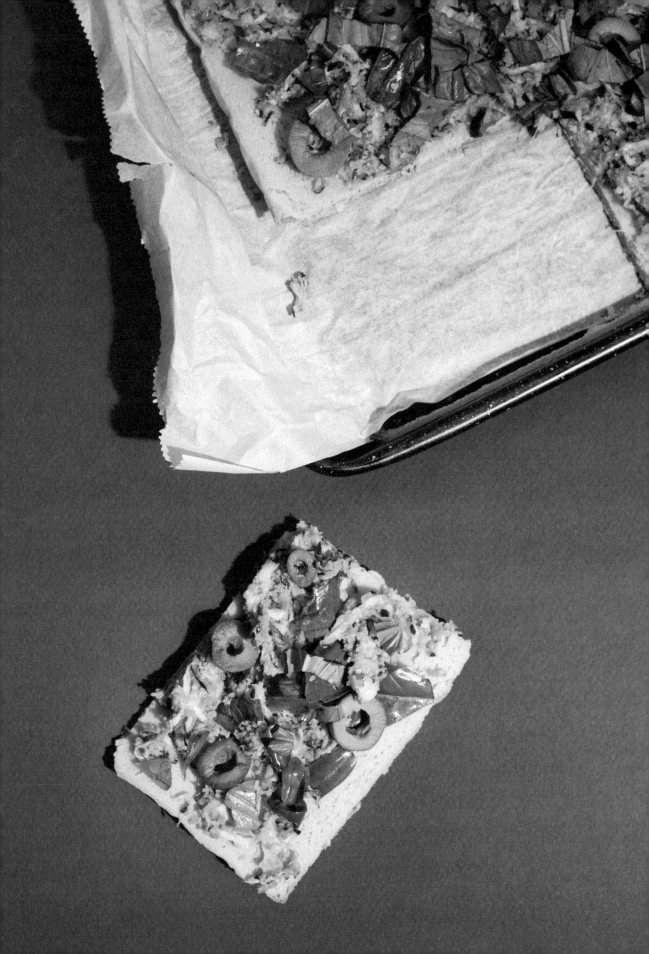

# Socca Pizza with Zucchini, Olives, and Basil

DAIRY-FREE | GLUTEN-FREE | NUT-FREE | VEGAN | VEGETARIAN

**SERVES 2 AS A MAIN, 4 AS A SIDE**

I used to make my own pizza dough, but then I had kids. Since then, I have been on the hunt for a pizza base that comes together in minutes, and this is it. This just might be the easiest pizza you will ever make. It looks like a lot of steps, but this whole recipe comes together in about 45 minutes. In addition, because you are using chickpea flour, the pizza base will be savoury, high in fibre, and high in protein. You can top it with whatever you want. Just in case you need inspiration, I have a way of making zucchini that wows even the zucchini-haters in my family. I love serving this with either my Roasted Sunchoke, Fennel, and Pistachio Salad (page 120) or my Grilled Tofu Caprese Salad (page 131).

---

1. Preheat the oven to 450°F (230°C). Place a baking sheet in the oven to heat. Cut a piece of parchment paper to the size of the baking sheet, with extra paper to hang over the edges, and set aside.

2. In a medium bowl, combine the chickpea flour, water, olive oil, 1 teaspoon (5 mL) of the salt, and pepper. Stir thoroughly and let sit for 10 minutes. This allows the chickpea flour to hydrate, which will give the crust better texture and digestibility.

3. In a separate medium bowl, combine the grated zucchini and the remaining 1 teaspoon (5 mL) salt. Move the zucchini to a colander, place the colander over the bowl, and let sit for 10 minutes so that the zucchini starts to release its water. Do not skip this step or the pizza will be a mushy mess.

4. Once the oven is preheated, remove the baking sheet and carefully place the parchment paper on it. Brush the paper with olive oil and pour the chickpea flour mixture onto it. Give it a little jiggle to spread the dough and bake for 5 to 7 minutes, until firm and starting to become golden, but not brown.

5. Meanwhile, in small handfuls, squeeze the zucchini to remove all of the water. You should easily get about ½ cup (125 mL) of liquid, which you can discard. Mix the zucchini with the panko, nutritional yeast, and garlic.

*recipe continues*

1½ cups (375 mL) chickpea flour

1¼ cups (300 mL) warm water

2 tablespoons (30 mL) extra-virgin olive oil, plus extra for greasing the pan

2 teaspoons (10 mL) salt, divided

Freshly cracked pepper

3½ cups (875 mL) grated zucchini (about 2 medium zucchini)

¼ cup (60 mL) gluten-free panko crumbs

¼ cup (60 mL) nutritional yeast

1 clove garlic, grated on a microplane

½ cup (125 mL) fresh basil leaves, torn or thinly sliced

½ cup (125 mL) Kalamata olives, pitted and halved

6.   When done, remove the chickpea flour crust from the oven, brush with a little more olive oil, and spread the zucchini mixture on top. Return to the oven and bake for 10 to 12 minutes, until the edges turn golden brown.

7.   Remove from the oven and, holding the edges of the parchment paper, carefully place the pizza on a cutting board. Top with basil and olives, cut into 8 slices, and serve. The crust will not be rigid and crisp, but it holds together beautifully.

Tip   Depending on where you live, you will find either pure chickpea flour or a chickpea fava blend, such as Bob's Red Mill Garbanzo and Fava Flour. Both are delicious and will work beautifully.

# Channna Masala

DAIRY-FREE | GLUTEN-FREE | VEGAN | VEGETARIAN

**SERVES 4 TO 6**

One fine day in Kauai, my friend Pardeep made her channa masala. I had yet to make a version I enjoyed as much as hers, so replicating her magic became a bit of an obsession. After a couple of not-quite-there attempts, Pardeep made it for me and wrote down the ingredients because food friends are the best friends.

I have added a couple of my own touches, and the result is a high-fibre, high-protein meal that is packed with anti-inflammatory spices without being too spicy. Chickpeas are a phenomenal, mineral-rich food that is easily one of my favourite plant-based staples.

¼ cup (60 mL) coconut oil

1 small yellow onion, diced

⅛ teaspoon (0.5 mL) baking soda

4 cloves garlic, minced

1-inch (2.5 cm) piece peeled fresh ginger, minced

1 tablespoon (15 mL) garam masala

1 teaspoon (5 mL) ground cumin

½ teaspoon (2 mL) ground turmeric

¼ teaspoon (1 mL) hot curry powder

¼ teaspoon (1 mL) ground cardamom

3 cans (14 ounces/398 mL each) chickpeas, drained and rinsed

2 tablespoons (30 mL) tomato paste

1¼ teaspoons (6 mL) salt

2 tablespoons (30 mL) freshly squeezed lemon juice

1. In a large skillet, heat the coconut oil over medium heat. Add the onion and baking soda and cook, stirring occasionally, until the onions begin to caramelize and break down, 5 to 7 minutes.

2. Add the garlic, ginger, garam masala, cumin, turmeric, curry powder, and cardamom and stir for 30 seconds until the spices become fragrant.

3. Add the chickpeas, tomato paste, and salt and stir to mix well. Reduce the heat to medium-low and simmer for 10 to 15 minutes to allow the flavours to blend.

4. Remove from the heat, stir in the lemon juice, and serve with your favourite whole grain.

**For serving**

Cooked whole grain (brown rice, quinoa, millet, buckwheat)

**Tip** Adding a pinch of baking soda helps the onions break down and caramelize more quickly so they dissolve into the chickpeas.

**Make It Healthier** Wilt 6 cups (1.5 L) of baby spinach or baby kale into the chickpeas during the last 5 minutes of cooking to add more vegetables.

# Chickpea Panisse with Edamame and Lemon

DAIRY-FREE | GLUTEN-FREE | NUT-FREE | VEGAN | VEGETARIAN

SERVES 4

Panisse is essentially a creamy polenta cake made from chickpea flour instead of corn. Chickpea flour is one of my favourite ingredients because it offers plenty of protein that supports the immune system and minerals to keep you feeling energized. Served with garlicky lemon spinach, it is a lovely and hearty main dish that will bust the myth that plant-based eating is not filling. For smaller appetites, or those still new to high-fibre diets, I recommend making and serving a half batch of the panisse.

4½ cups (1.125 L) water, divided

¼ cup (60 mL) + 2 tablespoons (30 mL) extra-virgin olive oil, divided, plus more for frying

1 teaspoon (5 mL) salt

2 cups (500 mL) chickpea flour

2 cloves garlic, sliced

⅛ teaspoon (0.5 mL) red chili flakes

2 cups (500 mL) frozen shelled edamame

4 cups (1 L) packed baby spinach

1 tablespoon (15 mL) freshly squeezed lemon juice

1 teaspoon (5 mL) Dijon mustard

Turmeric Mayonnaise (page 259), for serving (optional)

1. Preheat the oven to 200°F (100°C). Lightly oil a 9-inch (2.5 L) square baking dish.

2. In a medium pot, add 4 cups (1 L) of the water, ¼ cup (60 mL) of the olive oil, and salt and bring to just shy of a boil over high heat. Reduce the heat to medium and add the chickpea flour, whisking constantly for 5 minutes until hydrated and thickened. Pour the mixture into the prepared baking dish and let sit at room temperature for 15 minutes while you cook the vegetables.

3. In a medium skillet, heat the remaining 2 tablespoons (30 mL) olive oil over medium heat. Add the garlic and chili flakes and cook, stirring occasionally, until softened, about 2 minutes. Add the edamame and the remaining ½ cup (125 mL) water and cook until the water is mostly evaporated, about 3 minutes.

4. Stir in the spinach to warm, not fully wilt, about 1 minute. Remove from the heat, stir in the lemon juice and mustard, and season with salt. Transfer to a medium bowl. Wipe the skillet clean.

5. Place a plate in the preheated oven to keep the chickpea panisse warm once fried.

6.	Slice the chickpea panisse into 4 equal squares. In the skillet over medium heat, add a thin layer of olive oil to coat the pan. Cook 2 squares of chickpea panisse at a time until brown and crispy, 4 to 5 minutes, resisting the urge to fuss with them. Carefully flip the squares using a silicone flipper and cook until brown and crispy on the other side, about 3 minutes. Transfer to the plate in the oven to keep warm while you cook the remaining squares.

7.	To serve, place a square of chickpea panisse on a plate, smear with a bit of Turmeric Mayonnaise (if using), and top with one-quarter of the lemony vegetable mixture.

Tip  If you can find green chickpeas, they make a great change from edamame.

Make It Faster  You can prepare the chickpea panisse the night before, and then this meal will come together in 20 minutes. If you pre-cook the chickpea panisse squares, you can warm them in a 200°F (100°C) oven; then it will take less than 15 minutes to prepare the vegetables and assemble.

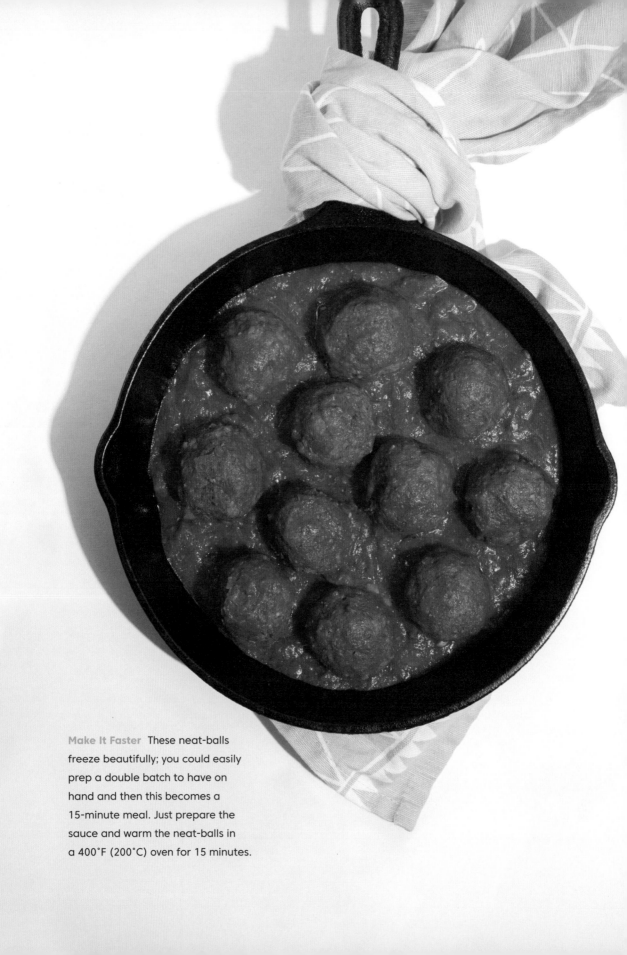

**Make It Faster** These neat-balls freeze beautifully; you could easily prep a double batch to have on hand and then this becomes a 15-minute meal. Just prepare the sauce and warm the neat-balls in a 400°F (200°C) oven for 15 minutes.

# Mujadara Neat-Balls in Spiced Tomato Sauce

DAIRY-FREE | GLUTEN-FREE | NUT-FREE | VEGAN | VEGETARIAN

SERVES 4

Mujadara is a traditional Lebanese dish of lentils, rice, and caramelized onions that I have transformed into a new take on a classic Italian comfort food! Lentils are packed with plant power: high in protein, fibre, and minerals, they keep your blood sugars balanced and your gut healthy. These sweetly aromatic neat-balls are a nutrient-dense yet light main course; any leftovers make a great neat-ball sub for lunch the next day. If you already have the rice and lentils prepared, the whole dish comes together in about 40 minutes. For a heartier meal, serve with brown rice or buckwheat.

1. Preheat the oven to 400°F (200°C). Line a baking sheet with parchment paper and lightly grease with olive oil.

2. **Make the Mujadara Neat-Balls** In a food processor, blend the lentils, rice, onion, garlic, dates, flaxseed, bread crumbs, cumin, turmeric, salt, thyme, and pepper, scraping the sides occasionally, until about two-thirds puréed. You want the ingredients to be uniform and sticky, but not a paste.

3. Scoop out the lentil-rice mixture by the heaping tablespoon (18 mL), form into balls, and place on the prepared baking sheet ½ inch (1 cm) apart. You should get about 24 balls. If the mixture starts sticking to your hands, just rinse your hands well with water.

4. Bake for 12 minutes until a crust forms on the bottom. Turn the balls carefully, as they will be soft, and bake for another 12 minutes. Let cool for a few minutes to allow them to firm up.

5. **Make the Spiced Tomato Sauce** Meanwhile, in a medium skillet heat the olive oil over medium heat. Add the garlic and cook, stirring often, about 1 minute.

6. Add the cumin, cinnamon, allspice, and coriander and stir for 30 seconds until the spices become fragrant. Then add the tomatoes and simmer over medium-low heat for 15 minutes. To finish, stir in the lemon juice and salt.

7. To serve, ladle the Spiced Tomato Sauce into shallow bowls and arrange 6 Mujadara Neat-Balls in each bowl.

## Mujadara Neat-Balls

2 cans (14 ounces/398 mL each) lentils, or 3½ cups (875 mL) cooked green or brown lentils

1 cup (250 mL) cooked brown rice

½ small yellow onion, diced

1 clove garlic, minced

5 Medjool dates, pitted and diced

¼ cup (60 mL) ground flaxseed

¼ cup (60 mL) gluten-free bread crumbs

2 teaspoons (10 mL) ground cumin

1 teaspoon (5 mL) ground turmeric

¾ teaspoon (4 mL) salt

½ teaspoon (2 mL) dried thyme

Freshly cracked pepper

## Spiced Tomato Sauce

1 clove garlic, minced

2 tablespoons (30 mL) extra-virgin olive oil

1 teaspoon (5 mL) ground cumin

½ teaspoon (2 mL) cinnamon

¼ teaspoon (1 mL) allspice

¼ teaspoon (1 mL) ground coriander

1 can (28 ounces/798 mL) no-salt-added diced tomatoes

2 teaspoons (10 mL) freshly squeezed lemon juice

½ teaspoon (2 mL) salt

# Cauliflower Peperonata Sauté

DAIRY-FREE | GLUTEN-FREE | NUT-FREE | VEGAN | VEGETARIAN

SERVES 4

¼ cup (60 mL) extra-virgin olive oil

½ yellow onion, thinly sliced into half moons

2 sweet red peppers, thinly sliced

2 tomatoes, quartered, seeded, and flesh cut into slices

¼ teaspoon (1 mL) salt, divided

Freshly cracked pepper

6 cups (1.5 L) cauliflower florets (1 small cauliflower)

¼ cup (60 mL) + 2 tablespoons (30 mL) water, divided

3 cloves garlic, minced

1 tablespoon (15 mL) tomato paste

2 cans (14 ounces/398 mL each) cannellini beans or chickpeas, drained and rinsed

½ cup (125 mL) packed curly parsley, chopped

⅓ cup (75 mL) sliced Kalamata olives

Zest of 1 lemon

Juice of ½ lemon

2 tablespoons (30 mL) gluten-free bread crumbs

Cooked millet or brown rice, for serving (optional)

Cauliflower is by far one of my favourite kitchen chameleons; in an anti-inflammatory eating plan, it helps you reduce your intake of high glycemic starch while boosting your intake of phytochemicals. This colourful sauté was inspired by the Roman bell pepper stew of the same name; it has a great balance of saltiness and sweetness with a nice little crunch. Enjoy this as a satisfying main dish when you add legumes or as a side dish without.

1. In a large skillet, heat the olive oil over medium heat. Add the onion, red peppers, tomatoes, ⅛ teaspoon (0.5 mL) of the salt, and a few cracks of pepper, and cook, stirring occasionally, for 5 minutes.

2. Add the cauliflower to the skillet with ¼ cup (60 mL) of the water. Increase the heat to medium-high and cover the skillet for 5 minutes to steam the vegetables.

3. Remove the lid from the skillet and reduce the heat to medium. Add the garlic, the remaining ⅛ teaspoon (0.5 mL) salt, tomato paste, the remaining 2 tablespoons (30 mL) water, and cannellini beans. Simmer until the liquid is fully absorbed, stirring occasionally, about 5 minutes. Remove from the heat.

4. Stir in the parsley, olives, lemon zest and juice, and bread crumbs. Taste and adjust seasoning with salt, pepper, and a bit more lemon juice, if needed.

5. Serve this hearty sauté on its own or with millet or brown rice (if using).

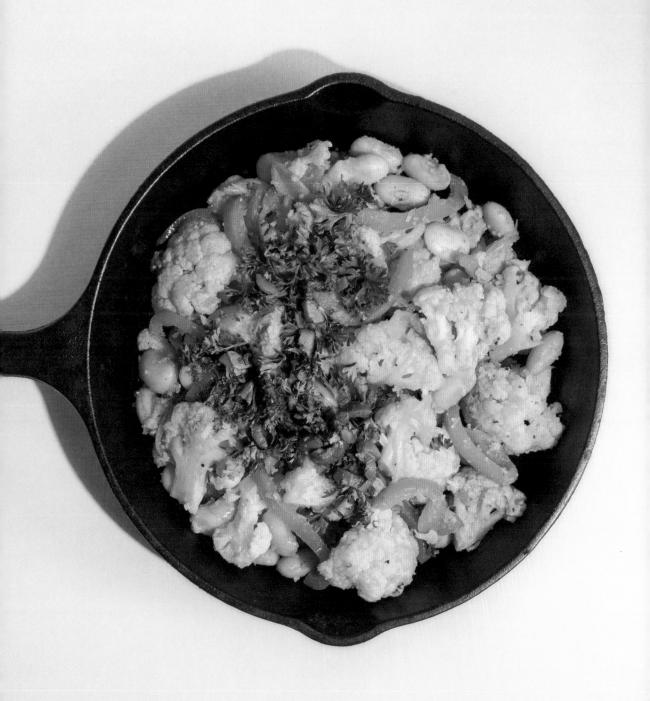

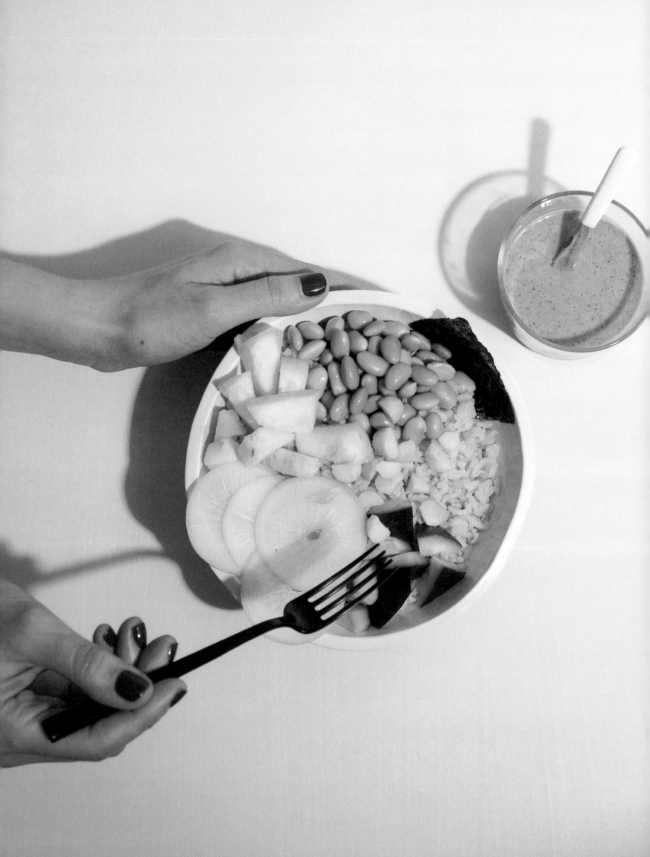

# Edamame Hula Bowl with Almond Miso Sauce

DAIRY-FREE | GLUTEN-FREE | NUT-FREE | VEGAN | VEGETARIAN

**SERVES 4**

I am always inspired by the sights and tastes of Kauai, Hawaii—one of my favourite places on earth. Sitting in the sunshine, relaxing, and eating healthy homegrown produce is my idea of a good time. Poke, a Hawaiian-Asian fusion of raw marinated fish, is everywhere on the island, as are the poke bowls they have inspired back at home. This is my take on building a hearty grain bowl, inspired by the Asian-Hawaiian vibes of poke. Edamame, immature green soybeans, are high in protein and isoflavones, anti-inflammatory flavonoid compounds that are also thought to be beneficial to gut health.

1. **Make the Almond Miso Sauce** In a wide-mouthed jar or medium bowl, whisk together the almond butter, water, miso, lime juice, ginger, tamari, and maple syrup until blended. Blend with a handheld immersion blender for a creamier, silkier texture.

2. **Assemble the Edamame Hula Bowl** Divide the edamame, cucumber, pineapple, brown rice, avocado, and radish evenly among 4 bowls. Drizzle with the Almond Miso Sauce and top with nori strips, sesame seeds, and macadamia nuts.

Tip  I am a big fan of including whole organic soy foods in the diet; if you are intolerant to soy, feel free to substitute green chickpeas.

## Almond Miso Sauce

¼ cup (60 mL) raw almond butter

½ cup (125 mL) water

3 tablespoons (45 mL) white miso

1 tablespoon (15 mL) freshly squeezed lime juice

1 teaspoon (5 mL) freshly grated peeled ginger

1 teaspoon (5 mL) gluten-free tamari

1 teaspoon (5 mL) pure maple syrup

## Edamame Hula Bowl

2 cups (500 mL) shelled frozen edamame, cooked according to package instructions

2 cups (500 mL) chopped cucumber

1½ cups (375 mL) chopped fresh pineapple

1 cup (250 mL) cooked brown rice

2 avocados, pitted, peeled, and sliced

½ cup (125 mL) thinly sliced lo bok or daikon radish

## Garnish

Nori strips or crushed seaweed snacks

Black sesame seeds

Chopped roasted macadamia nuts

# Mayo-Roasted Carrots with Curried Millet

DAIRY-FREE | GLUTEN-FREE | NUT-FREE | VEGAN | VEGETARIAN

SERVES 4

Most mayonnaise is made from seed oils high in omega-6 fats, so if you love it like I do, you will need a healthy alternative such as my Turmeric Mayonnaise (page 259). Roasting carrots with mayonnaise instead of oil results in a beautifully caramelized, blistered exterior that makes for a satisfying side dish on its own or becomes the star of the show on a bed of curried millet. Packed with energizing minerals like copper and manganese, millet is a nutrient-dense whole grain that is fluffy and flavourful with a little spice.

## Mayo-Roasted Carrots

3 tablespoons (45 mL) vegan mayonnaise

½ teaspoon (2 mL) ground sumac

¼ teaspoon (1 mL) salt

⅛ teaspoon (0.5 mL) ground cumin

1 pound (450 g) carrots, cut on the diagonal into ½-inch (1 cm) slices

## Curried Millet

¼ cup (60 mL) extra-virgin olive oil

½ cup (125 mL) diced shallots

1 teaspoon (5 mL) spicy curry powder or 2 teaspoons (10 mL) mild curry powder

1 cup (250 mL) uncooked millet

2½ cups (625 mL) water

1 can (14 ounces/398 mL) chickpeas, drained and rinsed

½ teaspoon (2 mL) salt

1. Preheat the oven to 425°F (220°C). Line a baking sheet with parchment paper.

2. **Make the Mayo-Roasted Carrots** In a large mixing bowl, combine the mayonnaise, sumac, salt, and cumin. Add the carrots, toss to coat, and spread evenly on the prepared baking sheet. Bake until golden brown and blistered, about 15 minutes for new carrots and 20 minutes for large, mature carrots.

3. **Make the Curried Millet** In a medium saucepan, heat the olive oil over medium heat. Add the shallots and curry powder and cook, stirring often, for 3 to 5 minutes until softened. Add the millet and stir for 1 minute to coat the millet with oil.

4. Add the water, chickpeas, and salt and bring to a boil over high heat. Reduce the heat to low and simmer, covered, for 15 to 20 minutes until all the water is absorbed and the millet is chewy and fluffy.

5. Divide among 4 plates, top with the Mayo-Roasted Carrots, and serve.

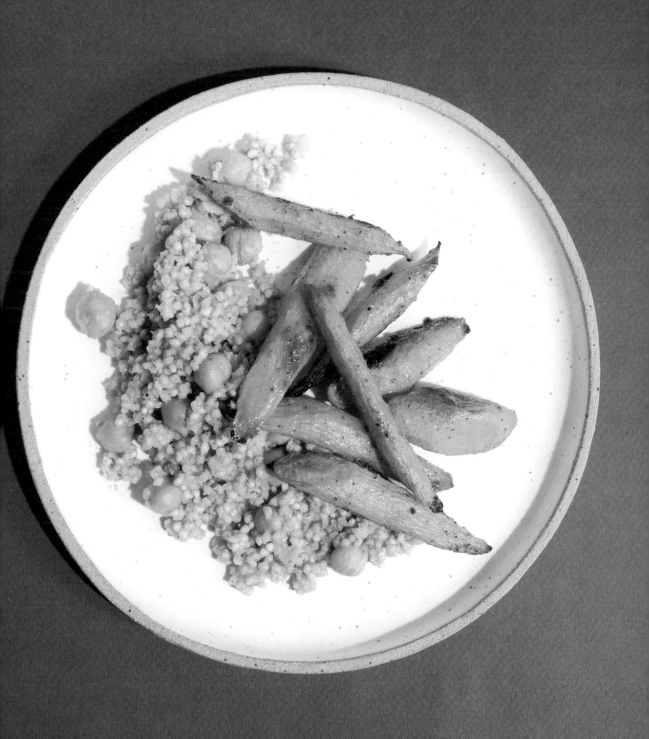

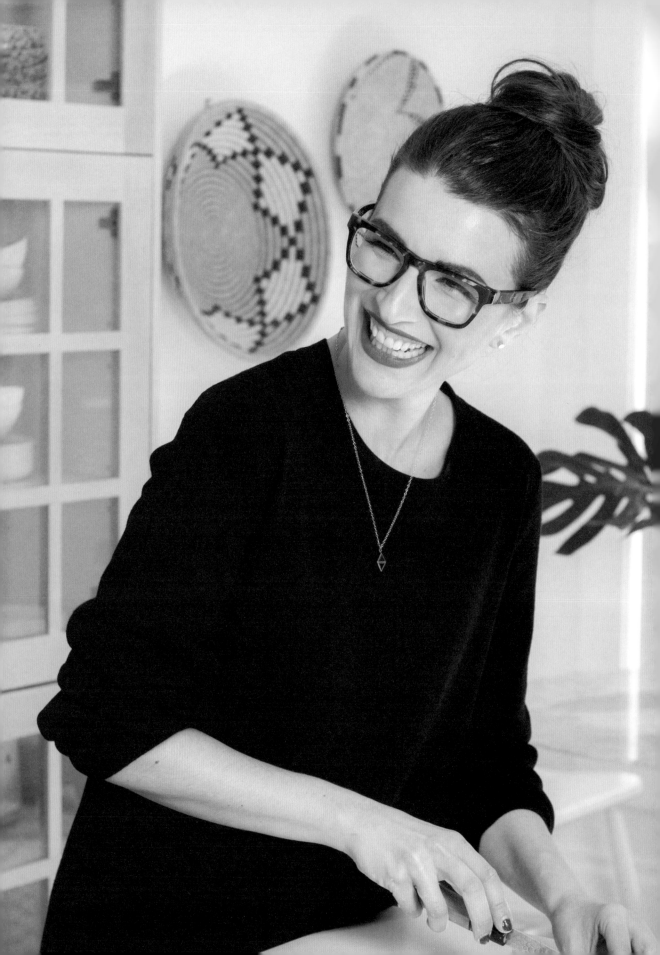

# Miso-Roasted Taro and Black Beans

DAIRY-FREE | GLUTEN-FREE | VEGAN | VEGETARIAN

**SERVES 4 TO 5**

Sheet pan dinners are weeknight perfection. Put all the good stuff on one pan and let it roast. To be honest, a bunch of roasted stuff is my go-to dinner when I do not know what to make, so I thought I would make a fancier version of my kitchen sink supper for you. This recipe uses a small, furry round taro known as eddoe, which has a clean, sweet taste kind of like potato. Eddoes have a lower glycemic index than potatoes and beneficial polysaccharides. The skin of eddoes has high levels of oxalate that can irritate your skin, so parboiling them makes them easy to peel and quicker to roast.

Paired with high-protein, high-fibre black beans—the black skin is your clue that these beans contain anti-inflammatory anthocyanins—and savoury red miso, this is a delicious meal that comes together in about 40 minutes, including cleanup!

1¼ pounds (565 g) eddoes (4 to 5 medium eddoes)

⅓ cup (75 mL) avocado oil

¼ cup (60 mL) red miso

2 tablespoons (30 mL) pure maple syrup

2 tablespoons (30 mL) water

3 cloves garlic, crushed or grated on a microplane

1 teaspoon (5 mL) unseasoned rice vinegar

2 cans (14 ounces/398 mL each) black beans, drained and rinsed

2 sweet red peppers, cut into 1-inch (2.5 cm) chunks

1 cup (250 mL) sugar snap peas, sliced ½ inch (1 cm) thick on the diagonal

⅓ cup (75 mL) unsalted redskin peanuts

**Tip** No eddoes at your local store? Use baby potatoes, cut in half. No parboiling necessary, but you might need to roast them for 10 minutes more.

1. Preheat the oven to 425°F (220°C). Line a baking sheet with parchment paper.

2. Bring a medium pot of water to a boil. Place the eddoes, skin on, into the boiling water and parboil for 10 minutes. Drain the hot water, pour cold water over the eddoes to cover, and add a tray of ice cubes so the eddoes can cool enough to handle quickly.

3. Meanwhile, in a small bowl, whisk together the avocado oil, miso, maple syrup, water, garlic, and rice vinegar.

4. Peel the cooled eddoes and rinse them under cold water to make them less slippery. Carefully slice into ½-inch (1 cm) slices and then cut into bite-sized chunks.

5. In a large bowl, toss the eddoe slices with the black beans, red peppers, and half of the miso dressing. Spread the mixture on the prepared baking sheet and roast until the eddoes are fork-tender but not mushy, 15 to 18 minutes.

6. Add the snap peas and peanuts to the baking sheet and drizzle with the remaining dressing. Divide among plates and serve.

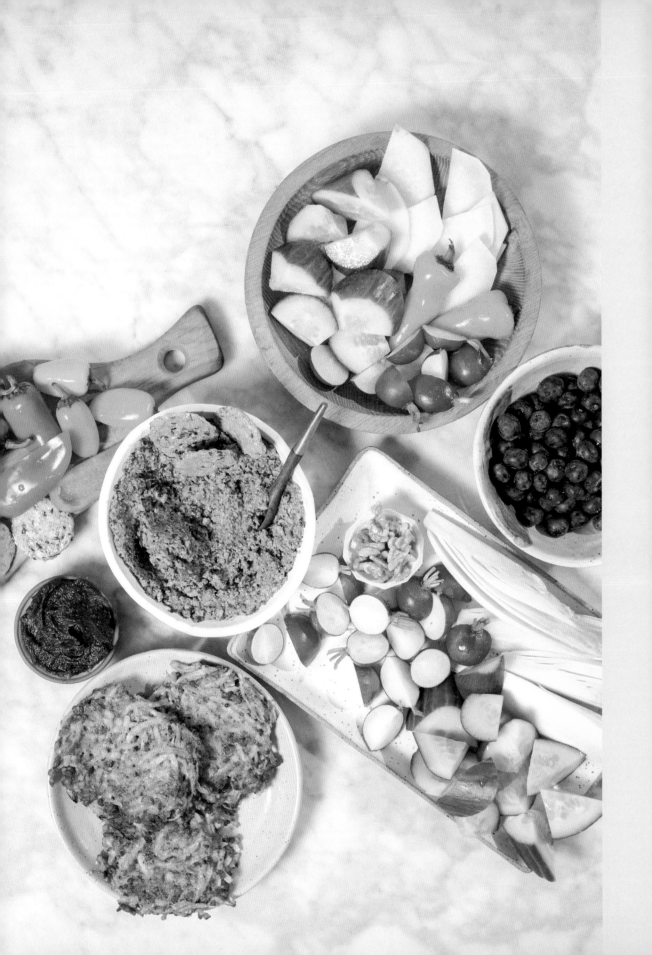

# 8

# Super-Powered Starters, Snacks, and Sides

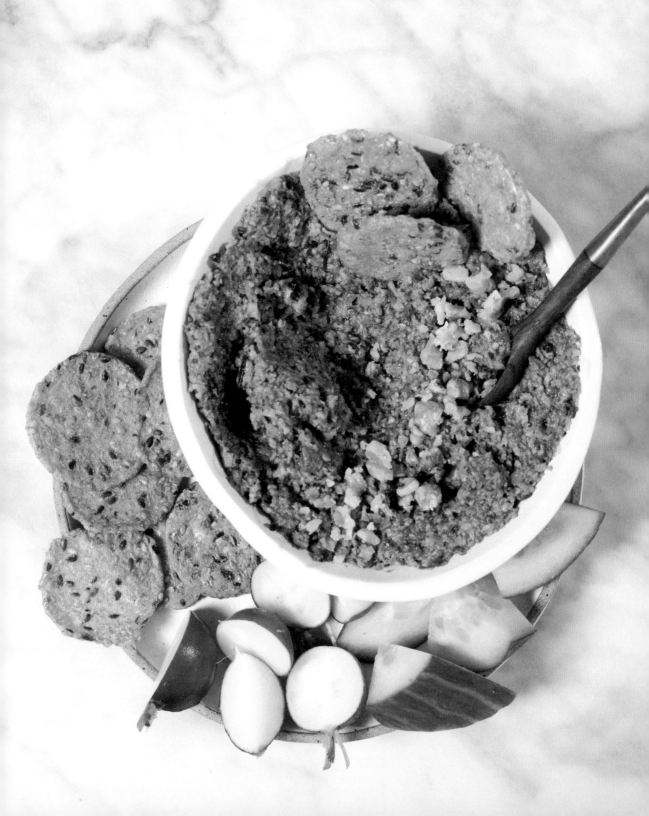

# Truffled Mushroom Pâté

DAIRY-FREE | GLUTEN-FREE | NUT-FREE | PALEO-FRIENDLY | VEGAN | VEGETARIAN

MAKES 1½ CUPS (375 ML)

I love a good dip. Sometimes, though, you want something a little fancier. This delicious spread will make people think twice about what plant-based food is.

It can be easy to forget how phenomenally healthy mushrooms are in our eat the rainbow world. They contain polysaccharides known as beta-glucans that are thought to have immune-modulating and perhaps even anti-cancer properties. Shiitake mushrooms have been the best researched in this regard, but do not discount the humble brown button and cremini—they boast impressive amounts of minerals like copper and antioxidant selenium, too.

---

1. Soak the dried mushrooms in ½ cup (125 mL) hot water for 5 minutes. Drain the mushrooms and reserve the liquid.

2. In a medium frying pan, heat 2 tablespoons (30 mL) of the olive oil over medium-high heat. Add the onion and sauté for 3 to 5 minutes until glossy. Add the fresh mushrooms and sauté until they begin to brown, 5 to 7 minutes. Try not to stir them too much so they can caramelize a bit.

3. Add the garlic and sauté, stirring constantly, for about 3 minutes. Then add the lentils and a bit of water to deglaze the pan. Season to taste with salt and pepper. Remove from the heat.

4. Place the vegetable mixture in a food processor and add the hydrated mushrooms, parsley, the remaining 2 tablespoons (30 mL) olive oil, lemon juice, thyme, rosemary, and truffle salt. Purée until well combined. Add the reserved mushroom soaking liquid to reach the desired consistency (I like my pâté well puréed but not paste-like). You should still see the ingredients. Taste and adjust seasoning, if necessary.

5. Serve with Seedy Crackers, Real Deal Gluten-Free Bread, and sliced vegetables. Store the pâté in a resealable container in the fridge for up to 3 days.

¾ ounce (20 g) dried mushrooms (porcini or a mixture)

4 tablespoons (60 mL) olive oil, divided

½ yellow onion, roughly chopped

½ pound (225 g) assorted fresh mushrooms, sliced (shiitake, cremini, chanterelle)

3 cloves garlic, roughly chopped

½ cup (125 mL) cooked or canned French lentils

Salt and freshly cracked pepper

¼ cup (60 mL) lightly packed chopped fresh flat-leaf parsley

2 teaspoons (10 mL) freshly squeezed lemon juice

2 teaspoons (10 mL) fresh thyme leaves

1 teaspoon (5 mL) chopped fresh rosemary

1 teaspoon (5 mL) truffle salt or salt

*For serving*

Seedy Crackers (page 265) or your favourite gluten-free crackers

Real Deal Gluten-Free Bread (page 267) or your favourite gluten-free bread

Sliced vegetables (kohlrabi, jicama, fennel, sweet red pepper)

# Grilled Avocado in Black Bean Broth

DAIRY-FREE | GLUTEN-FREE | NUT-FREE | VEGAN | VEGETARIAN

SERVES 4

1 can (14 ounces/398 mL) black beans

¼ cup (60 mL) extra-virgin olive oil, plus more for grilling

2 cloves garlic, grated on a microplane

1 teaspoon (5 mL) dried oregano

1 teaspoon (5 mL) ground cumin

⅛ teaspoon (0.5 mL) hot smoked paprika

½ jalapeño pepper, seeded and finely diced

½ teaspoon (2 mL) salt

1 teaspoon (5 mL) tomato paste

2 avocados, halved, pitted, and peeled

**For serving**

Handful of fresh cilantro

Fresh lime wedges

Tip  1. The heat level of jalapeño peppers varies considerably; before I add them to a recipe, I always try a little nibble. If the flesh is very mild, I will use more or add the seeds. If the flesh is spicy, I use less or omit the seeds. 2. Traditionalist? Purée the beans and liquid for a blended soup. Garnish with cilantro and sliced avocado.

This recipe was inspired by an epic meal I had in Mexico City. Amid the many courses, I was served this simple grilled avocado, floating in a black bean broth. Not a thick soup, but a broth. Obsessed is an understatement. This is such a lovely first course to serve your guests; the buttery richness of the avocado is so satisfying that no one will think about how healthy it is.

Avocado is primarily a monounsaturated fat, just like olive oil is, but we forget about all the tummy-taming soluble fibre it contains. In addition, avocado is rich in folate and anti-inflammatory vitamin K. Now, that is what I call the good kind of fat.

1. Prepare a grill for direct cooking over medium-high heat.

2. Drain the black beans in a strainer placed over a bowl to capture the soaking liquid. Rinse the beans over the bowl with 1 can of water. This liquid is your broth base. Set the beans aside.

3. To prepare the broth, in a small saucepan over medium heat, heat the olive oil with the garlic, oregano, cumin, paprika, and jalapeño and let it sizzle, stirring often, for 2 minutes.

4. Add the black bean liquid, salt, and tomato paste. Let it come to a boil, add the beans, and then reduce the heat to medium-low and simmer for 10 minutes while you grill the avocado.

5. Brush the cut sides of the avocado with olive oil and grill cut side down until grill marks appear, 3 to 4 minutes. (If not using a barbecue, you can grill the avocado on a stovetop grill pan or simply pan-fry over medium heat until they turn golden.) Carefully lift off the grill and slice.

6. To serve, arrange half an avocado in the base of 4 bowls. Ladle the broth and black beans around the avocado. Top with cilantro and a squeeze of fresh lime juice.

Make It Faster  You can make the broth ahead of time, storing it in the fridge for up to 1 day, and the flavours will deepen over time.

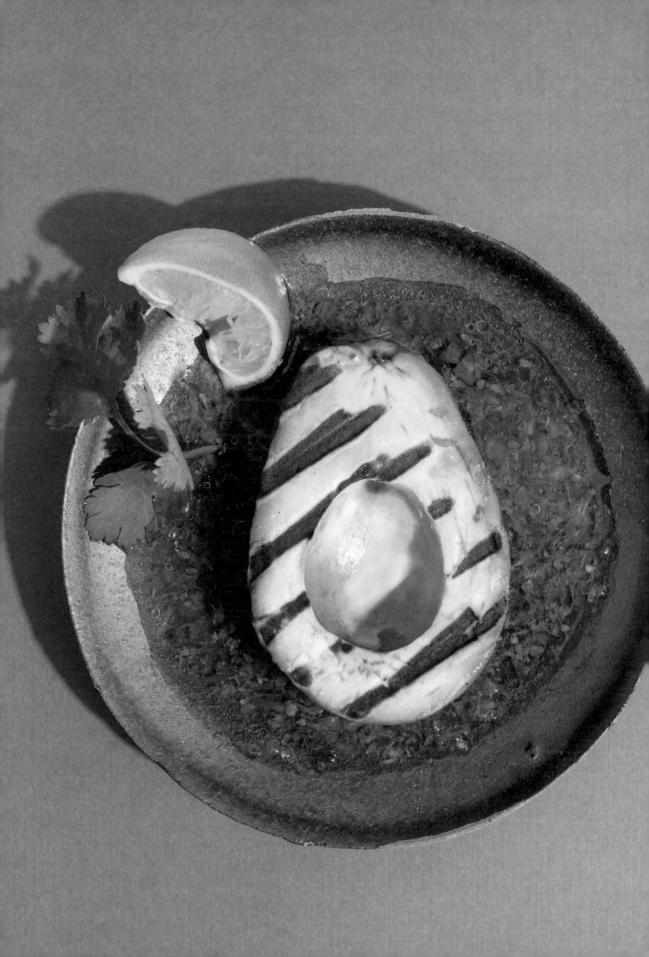

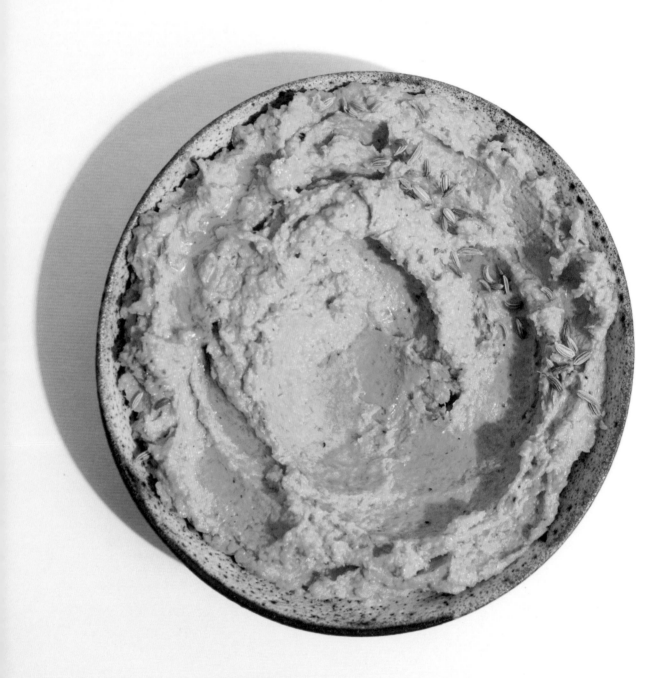

# Spiced Carrot Dip

DAIRY-FREE | GLUTEN-FREE | NUT-FREE | PALEO-FRIENDLY | VEGAN | VEGETARIAN

MAKES 2 CUPS (500 ML)

Carrots are affordable, available year-round, and packed with anti-oxidant beta-carotene, lutein, and zeaxanthin; they deserve a starring role in an anti-inflammatory kitchen. Carotenoids like beta-carotene are fat-soluble nutrients, so enjoying them with healthy fats from olive oil and tahini is key to improve their bioavailability.

I wanted to create a delicious dip that also counts as eating your veggies and, in the process, make carrots exciting again. Caramelizing the carrots in a skillet is much faster than roasting and when combined with tahini, the result is a luscious *I cannot believe this is healthy* dip inspired by the flavours of the Mediterranean. It also makes a delicious sandwich spread in place of hummus—try it with my Green Machine Burgers (page 140).

¼ cup (60 mL) extra-virgin olive oil

1 pound (450 g) carrots, scrubbed and sliced thinly

1 tablespoon (15 mL) grated peeled fresh ginger

½ teaspoon (2 mL) ground cumin

¼ teaspoon (1 mL) fennel seed

½ cup (125 mL) raw tahini

3 tablespoons (45 mL) freshly squeezed lemon juice

1 clove garlic, crushed or grated on a microplane

¾ teaspoon (4 mL) salt

½ teaspoon (2 mL) fresh thyme leaves

1 teaspoon (5 mL) pure maple syrup

*For serving*

Seedy Crackers (page 265) or your favourite gluten-free crackers

Real Deal Gluten-Free Bread (page 267) or your favourite gluten-free bread

Sliced vegetables (kohlrabi, radishes, celery, fennel, sweet red pepper)

1. In a large skillet, heat the olive oil over medium-high heat, then add the carrots. Let them sizzle for 5 minutes.

2. Add the ginger, cumin, and fennel seed to the skillet, reduce the heat to medium, and cook for 3 to 5 minutes until the spices are fragrant and the carrots starting to caramelize.

3. Add the carrot-spice mixture to a food processor with the tahini, lemon juice, garlic, salt, thyme, and maple syrup and process for 2 minutes until smooth. Scrape down the sides of the bowl halfway through processing.

4. Serve with Seedy Crackers, Real Deal Gluten-Free Bread, and sliced vegetables. Store in a resealable container in the fridge for up to 4 days.

# Beet Tartare

DAIRY-FREE | GLUTEN-FREE | NUT-FREE | PALEO-FRIENDLY | VEGAN | VEGETARIAN

SERVES 4

I love giving veggies the starring role in traditional, meat-centric dishes. This is a cheeky take on a dish I have not eaten in its original form, but it always represented old-school sophistication to me because I remember seeing it on the menus of fancy restaurants when I was younger. Packed with anti-inflammatory plant pigments like betalains and flavonoids, beets also contain the antioxidant minerals manganese and copper. This simple, flavourful appetizer proves that health food can be elegant, too.

2½ cups (625 mL) finely diced peeled cooked red beets

2 tablespoons (30 mL) finely diced shallot (about 1 small shallot)

1 tablespoon (15 mL) finely chopped fresh dill

2 teaspoons (10 mL) vegan prepared horseradish

1 teaspoon (5 mL) balsamic vinegar

½ teaspoon (2 mL) salt

For serving

Seedy Crackers (page 265) or your favourite gluten-free crackers

Real Deal Gluten-Free Bread (page 267) or your favourite gluten-free bread

Belgian endive

1. Combine the beet, shallot, dill, horseradish, balsamic vinegar, and salt in a large bowl and stir to distribute the ingredients.

2. Scoop the beet mixture into a serving dish or onto a plate using a ring mould for a more elegant look and serve with Seedy Crackers, Real Deal Gluten-Free Bread, and Belgian endive.

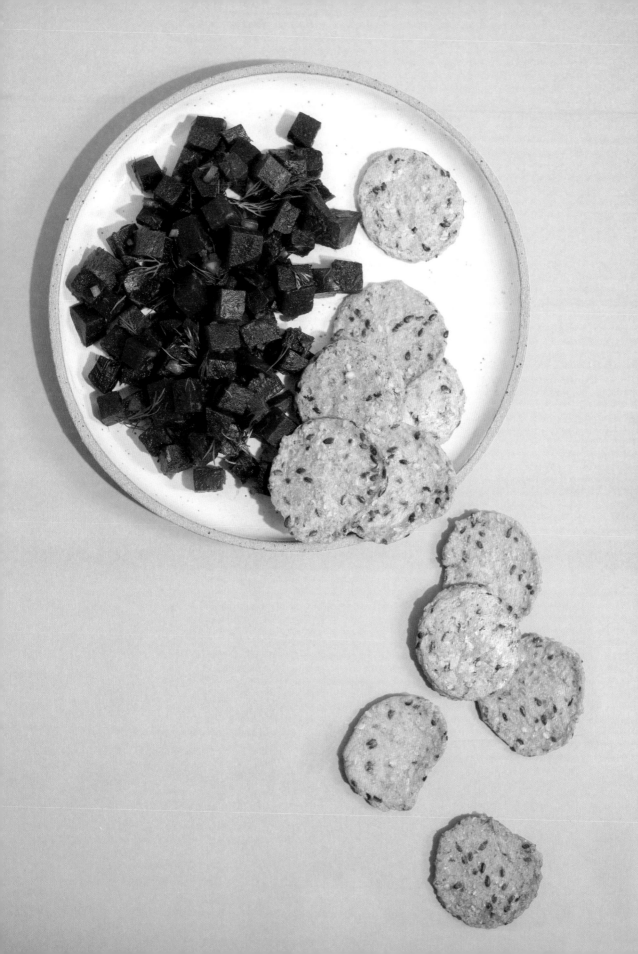

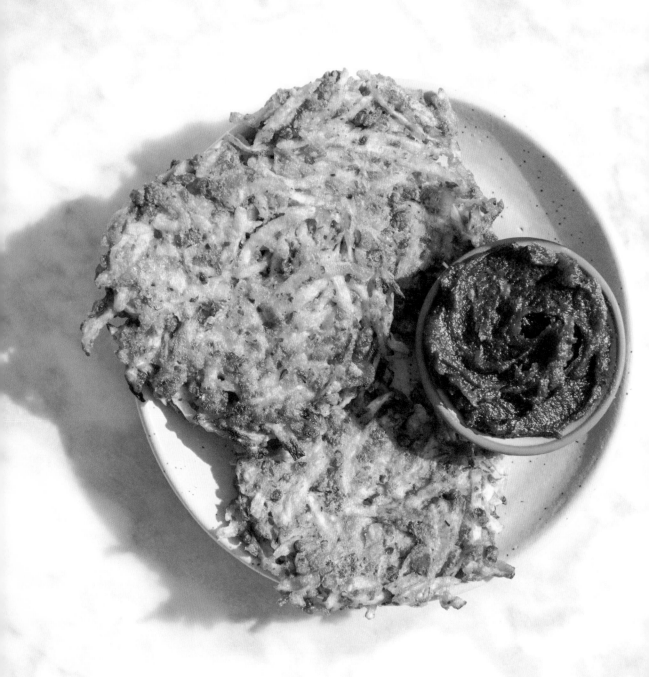

# Celeriac Lentil Fritters with Date Jam

DAIRY-FREE | GLUTEN-FREE | NUT-FREE | VEGAN | VEGETARIAN

**MAKES 8 FRITTERS**

Snack foods are typically just starch, sugar, and salt, but not these! These fritters are kind of like nutrient-dense latkes. Celeriac (celery root) has a wonderfully mellow flavour that pairs well with savoury spices and an addictive chili-spiked date jam. Think lower glycemic impact, higher protein, but still as satisfying as a fried pillow of potato. These are wonderful served as an appetizer or side dish, or try them as the base for vegan "eggs" Benedict, topped with a slice of smoked tofu and sautéed greens.

1. **Make the Celeriac Lentil Fritters** In a medium bowl, whisk together the flour, flaxseed, za'atar, salt, and cumin. Add the celeriac, lentils, onion, and water and mix.

2. In a large skillet, heat the coconut oil over medium heat. Drop ½ cup (125 mL) of the batter into the oil and use the back of the measuring cup to press it into a ½ inch (1 cm) thick fritter. Cook until a golden-brown crust forms, 2 to 3 minutes. Flip carefully and cook for 2 to 3 minutes until brown. Remove from the pan and place on a plate lined with paper towel. Add more coconut oil as needed to maintain a thin coating in the skillet. Repeat with the remaining batter.

3. **Make the Date Jam** In a small saucepan, combine the dates, water, balsamic vinegar, and chili flakes and bring to a boil over medium-high heat. Reduce the heat to medium-low and simmer, stirring occasionally, for 5 to 7 minutes or until the dates are very soft. Remove from the heat and, using a handheld immersion blender, purée into a smooth consistency. Season with a pinch of salt.

4. Serve the Celeriac Lentil Fritters with a generous smear of Date Jam. The Date Jam will keep in a resealable container in the fridge for up to 1 week.

**Tip** Za'atar is a Middle Eastern spice blend of thyme, oregano, and sesame seeds that you can find in the imported foods section of major supermarkets and gourmet stores.

## Celeriac Lentil Fritters

¾ cup (175 mL) gluten-free all-purpose flour

2 tablespoons (30 mL) ground flaxseed

1 teaspoon (5 mL) za'atar

¾ teaspoon (4 mL) salt

½ teaspoon (2 mL) ground cumin

4 cups (1 L) grated celeriac (about 1 large celeriac)

1 can (14 ounces/398 mL) green or brown lentils, drained and rinsed

½ cup (125 mL) grated yellow onion

½ cup (125 mL) water

Refined coconut oil, for frying

## Date Jam

1 cup (250 mL) Medjool dates, pitted

⅓ cup (75 mL) water

1 tablespoon (15 mL) balsamic vinegar

½ teaspoon (2 mL) red chili flakes

Salt

**Make It Faster** These fritters freeze well between sheets of parchment paper in a resealable plastic bag for up to 1 month. Reheat in a 375°F (190°C) oven for 15 to 20 minutes until warmed through.

# Sweet Potato Jackfruit Sliders

DAIRY-FREE | GLUTEN-FREE | NUT-FREE | PALEO-FRIENDLY | VEGAN | VEGETARIAN

MAKES 12 SLIDERS

2 large sweet potatoes

1 teaspoon (5 mL) +
   2 tablespoons (30 mL)
   extra-virgin olive oil, divided

Salt and freshly cracked
   pepper

2 cans (14 ounces/398 mL
   each) jackfruit in brine

½ cup (125 mL) tomato sauce

1 tablespoon (15 mL)
   blackstrap molasses

2 teaspoons (10 mL) vegan
   Worcestershire sauce

1 teaspoon (5 mL) chili powder

½ teaspoon (2 mL) ground
   cumin

½ teaspoon (2 mL) sweet
   paprika

1 teaspoon (5 mL) apple
   cider vinegar

1 teaspoon (5 mL) pure
   maple syrup

1 small yellow onion,
   finely diced

1 sweet red pepper,
   finely diced

4 cloves garlic, minced

1 cup (250 mL) water

Tip These sliders are
substantial; 12 will satisfy
6 people as a snack or starter.
If you are cooking for 2, this
recipe is easily halved, and
you will still have some left
over for tomorrow's lunch!

Jackfruit is perhaps the most enjoyable dish to serve to meat lovers because it looks and chews so much like meat. It is also simple to prepare. High in fibre and rich in antioxidant carotenoids, these sliders are a tangy, sweet, and savoury treat. I like to serve them bun style with two slices of sweet potato, but you can also serve them open-faced—and this recipe will serve a whole cocktail party. If you want to turn this into dinner, cube and roast the sweet potatoes and serve them as a base for the Sloppy Joe–style jackfruit or just pile the jackfruit onto gluten-free hamburger buns. If you opt for buns, my Celeriac Mash (page 215) is a delish and hearty side dish that boosts the protein of the meal.

1. Preheat the oven to 400°F (200°C). Line a baking sheet with parchment paper.

2. Slice the sweet potatoes into twenty-four ½-inch (1 cm) thick slices. Toss with 1 teaspoon (5 mL) of the olive oil, a generous pinch of salt, and a few cracks of pepper and arrange slices on the prepared baking sheet. Bake for 15 minutes, flip, then bake for 10 minutes more. Set aside.

3. Drain and rinse the jackfruit. Slice the chunks into bite-sized pieces.

4. In a small bowl, whisk together the tomato sauce, molasses, Worcestershire, chili powder, cumin, paprika, apple cider vinegar, and maple syrup.

5. In a medium skillet, heat the remaining 2 tablespoons (30 mL) olive oil over medium heat. Add the onion and red pepper, cook, stirring occasionally, until soft and glossy, 5 to 7 minutes. Add the garlic and stir for 30 seconds, then add the jackfruit, molasses mixture, and water. Cover with a lid and simmer for 15 minutes.

6. Remove the lid and mash the jackfruit with a potato masher or shred using 2 forks.

7. To serve, place a generous scoop of jackfruit on a slice of sweet potato. Top with another slice of sweet potato.

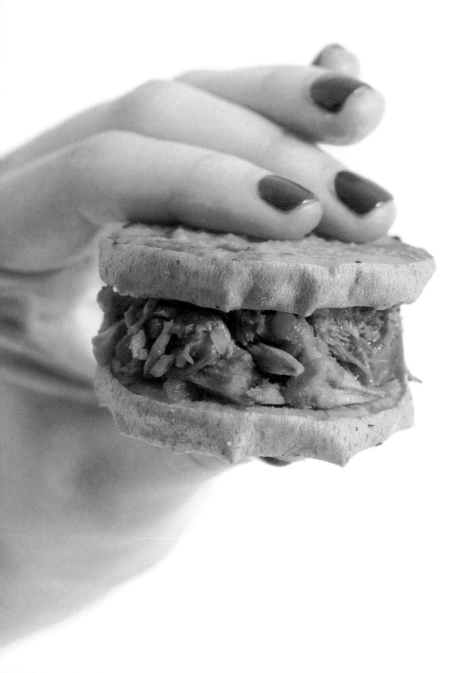

**Make It Faster**  You can make both the sweet potato buns and the jackfruit in advance. The jackfruit will hold its flavour well for 2 days in the fridge; for best texture, make the sweet potato buns up to 4 hours in advance. Just reheat and serve.

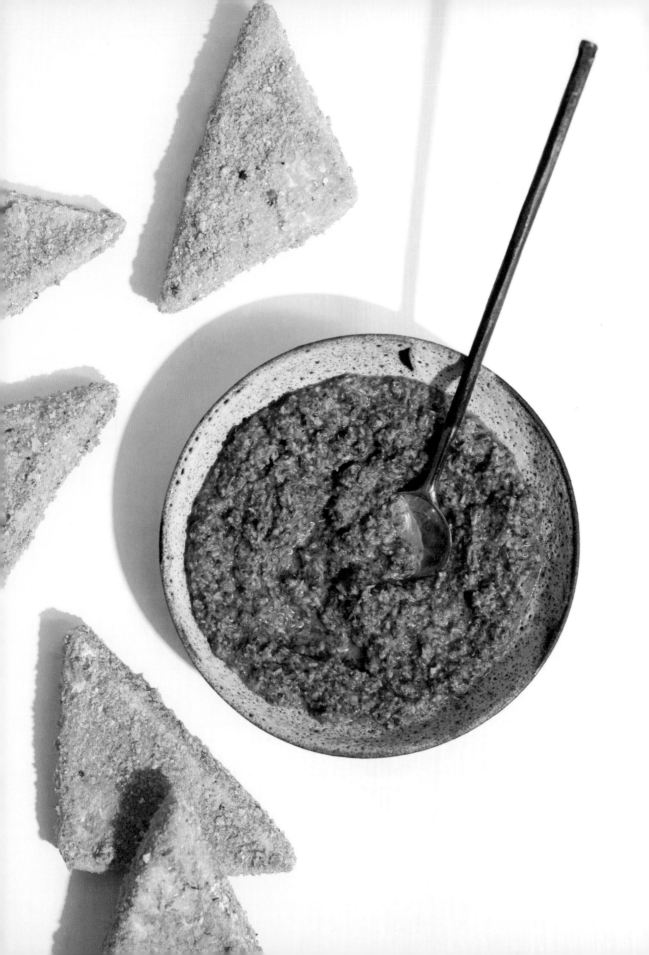

# Baked Tofu Paneer with Mint Chutney

DAIRY-FREE | GLUTEN-FREE | NUT-FREE | VEGAN | VEGETARIAN

SERVES 4

Full disclosure: tofu is not my family's favourite food! Therefore, every time I discover a method of cooking tofu that they wholeheartedly love, I am over the moon. This is one of them. Loosely inspired by one of my old faves, paneer pakoras, these baked tofu triangles are great as a protein-rich snack or a protein-rich sandwich filling. Protein is critical in a plant-based anti-inflammatory diet both to keep blood sugars balanced and to support immune system function. When you are new to plant-based eating, it can be so easy to default to starchy meals and snacks. These will help! Both the baked tofu and the chutney will come together in less than an hour. It is worth making a double batch of the tofu to snack on all week! Any leftover chutney is lovely on grain bowls or sandwiches. Try it on Real Deal Gluten-Free Bread (page 267) layered with Spiced Carrot Dip (Page 193).

1.  Preheat the oven to 425°F (220°C). Line a baking sheet with parchment paper.

2.  **Make the Baked Tofu Paneer** Set up 3 small bowls for breading the tofu on the counter. In the first bowl, combine the arrowroot starch, ¼ teaspoon (1 mL) of the salt, and pepper. In the second bowl, add the soy milk. In the third bowl, combine the bread crumbs, nutritional yeast, the remaining ¼ teaspoon (1 mL) salt, garlic powder, garam masala, and pepper.

3.  Cut the block of tofu in half to create 2 squares and slice those squares horizontally to create 2 thinner squares. Cut the squares in half crosswise so you have 8 triangles.

4.  Dredge the tofu triangles in the arrowroot mixture, dip them in the soy milk, and finally dredge them in the bread crumb mixture. Place them on the prepared baking sheet.

5.  Bake for 15 minutes, then carefully flip. Bake for 12 to 14 minutes more so that both sides have crisped and the tofu starts to look a bit puffed up.

## Baked Tofu Paneer

½ cup (125 mL) arrowroot starch

½ teaspoon (2 mL) salt, divided

Freshly cracked pepper

½ cup (125 mL) unsweetened soy milk

⅓ cup (75 mL) gluten-free bread crumbs

⅓ cup (75 mL) nutritional yeast

½ teaspoon (2 mL) garlic powder

¼ teaspoon (1 mL) garam masala

1 package (12 ounces/350 g) extra-firm tofu

## Mint Chutney

¾ cup (175 mL) packed fresh cilantro leaves

¾ cup (175 mL) packed fresh mint leaves

1 teaspoon (5 mL) grated peeled fresh ginger

½ jalapeño pepper, with or without seeds

2 tablespoons (30 mL) unsweetened flaked coconut

1 clove garlic, crushed or grated on a microplane

1 tablespoon (15 mL) freshly squeezed lime juice

1 teaspoon (5 mL) hemp oil

2 tablespoons (30 mL) water

⅛ teaspoon (0.5 mL) salt

*recipe continues*

6. **Make the Mint Chutney**  In a small food processor, add the cilantro, mint, ginger, jalapeño, coconut, garlic, lime juice, hemp oil, water, and salt. Blend to form a loose paste, drizzling in another 1 tablespoon (15 mL) of water as needed to reach the desired consistency.

7. Serve the Baked Tofu Paneer on a serving dish with the Mint Chutney drizzled on top.

Tip  Always taste your jalapeño pepper! Some are very hot, so ¼ jalapeño without seeds will add spice to the chutney. For others, ½ jalapeño with the seeds will not add much bite. So, slice a tiny piece off the end; if the flesh is mild, adjust the amount used accordingly. You want heat in the chutney without causing a four-alarm blaze.

# Fried Eggplant with Chili and Pomegranate Molasses

DAIRY-FREE | GLUTEN-FREE | NUT-FREE | PALEO-FRIENDLY | VEGAN | VEGETARIAN

SERVES 4

I spent a week in Spain eating variations of this dish almost every day. While it tasted a bit different everywhere I tried it, it was always delicious. Eggplant is something you have to get just right; it can get slimy or rubbery but when lightly pan-fried, it takes on the silkiest, most decadent texture. Rich in soothing soluble fibre, the dark purple skin is filled with anti-inflammatory anthocyanin pigments. Traditionally served with cane syrup or honey, I love the sweet-tart kick of pomegranate molasses. It is so yummy, I could easily eat a whole eggplant by myself! This would make a delicious part of a tapas spread, alongside my Spiced Carrot Dip (page 193) and Celeriac Lentil Fritters with Date Jam (page 197).

1. Trim the ends off the eggplant and cut into ½-inch (1 cm) thick slices. Place on a baking sheet lined with parchment paper and season with salt. Let rest for 30 minutes, then rinse the eggplant slices and pat dry with paper towel.

2. In a small bowl, mix the brown rice flour with a pinch of salt and freshly cracked pepper. Dredge each slice of eggplant in the flour mixture, tapping off excess.

3. In a large skillet, heat 2 tablespoons (30 mL) coconut oil over medium-high heat. Test the temperature with the edge of an eggplant slice; it should sizzle immediately. Place the eggplant in a single layer in the pan. Do not crowd.

4. Fry until the eggplant turns light golden, about 1 to 2 minutes. Flip and fry for 1 to 2 minutes more. Keep adding coconut oil by the spoonful as it gets absorbed or you won't get a nice colour on the eggplant.

1 large eggplant (8 to 10 inches/20 to 25 cm long)

1 teaspoon (5 mL) salt, plus more for seasoning

⅓ cup (75 mL) brown rice flour

Freshly cracked pepper

Refined coconut oil or avocado oil, for frying

Red chili flakes

¼ cup (60 mL) pomegranate molasses

*recipe continues*

5.  Transfer the cooked eggplant to a plate lined with paper towel and sprinkle with the salt and a generous pinch of chili flakes. When the last batch is done, place all the eggplant on a serving platter, drizzle with the pomegranate molasses, and serve immediately.

Tip 1. Virgin coconut oil, like extra-virgin olive oil, may smoke when frying. Look for coconut oil that has been naturally refined, making it better for high heat. If sediment gathers on the frying pan in between batches, it might burn and smoke. Carefully wipe it out with a damp cloth, then return the pan to the heat, add more coconut oil, and fry the next batch. 2. There is a debate about whether you need to salt eggplant. When frying like this, I definitely recommend salting the eggplant, as the texture will be better— silky and light.

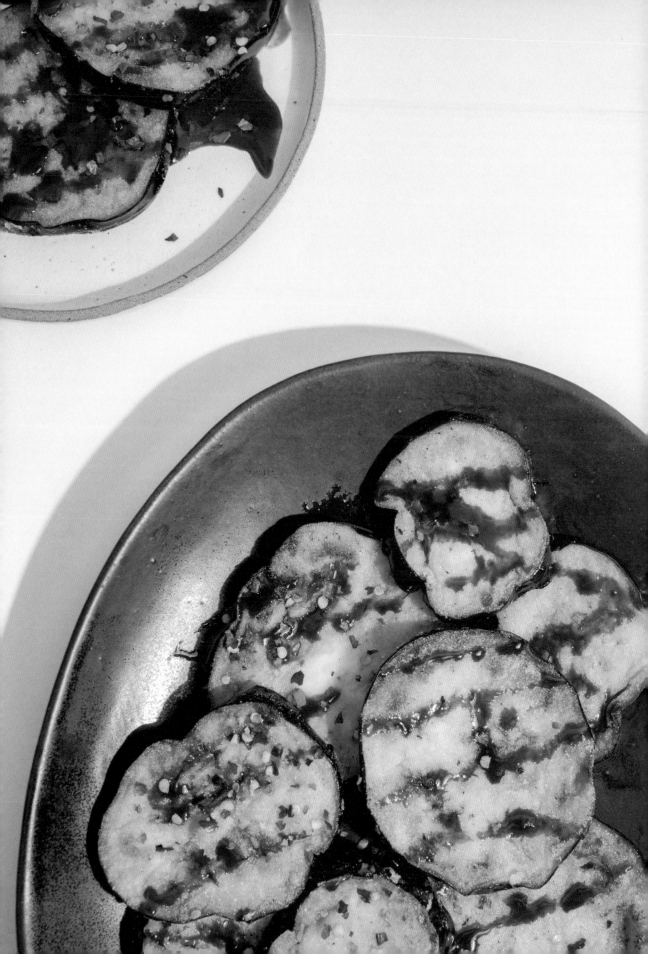

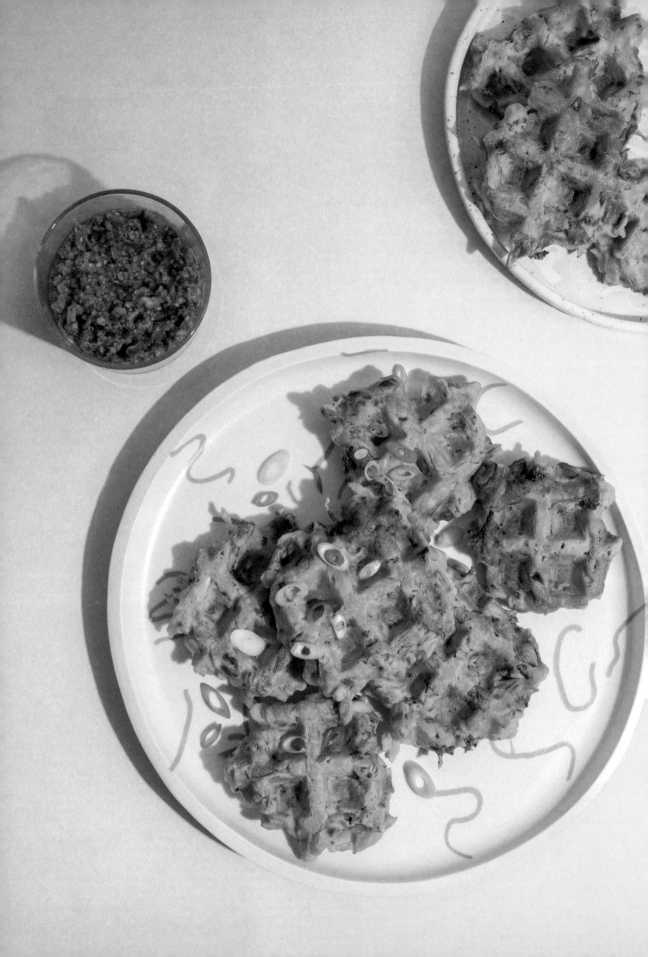

# Green Onion Pancakes with XOXO Sauce

DAIRY-FREE | GLUTEN-FREE | NUT-FREE | VEGAN | VEGETARIAN

**MAKES 7 TO 8 PANCAKES**

I am happy when I can get more vegetables into snacks. Pancakes are a treat, so I wanted to create a truly healthy version with extra veggies and a kick of high-protein flour. Parsley is one of my secret weapons. High in anti-inflammatory pigments like chlorophyll, parsley is a budget-friendly herb that we should treat like a vegetable more often. The sauce is a version of the famous XO sauce, an umami-bomb typically made with dried seafood. Dried mushrooms stand in quite nicely. These pancakes are great all on their own: salty, oniony, and satisfying. With a dab of sauce, they are unforgettable.

1. In a large bowl, whisk together the brown rice flour, chickpea flour, and salt. Add the green onion, parsley, coleslaw, tamari, Sriracha, lemon juice, sesame oil, and water and stir until mixed. Let sit for 10 minutes for the chickpea flour to hydrate.

2. In a large skillet, heat a heaping tablespoon (18 mL) of coconut oil over medium heat. Be patient; if the oil is not hot enough, the pancakes will be greasy and not brown. Make 2 pancakes at a time, dropping a scant ⅓ cup (75 mL) of batter in the skillet for each. Use the back of the cup to pat down the batter into 3- or 4-inch (8 to 10 cm) pancakes.

3. Cook the pancakes for 2 minutes, watching for the edges to turn golden brown and bubbles to form. Gently lift; if a crust has formed, carefully flip and cook for 2 minutes more. Add 1 tablespoon (15 mL) coconut oil so the pancakes are always sizzling.

4. Transfer the cooked pancakes to a plate lined with paper towel. Repeat with the remaining batter.

5. Slice the pancakes in half and serve with XOXO Sauce.

Tip You can also enjoy these as waffles; I recommend adding 2 tablespoons (30 mL) of coconut oil to the batter. The batter produces a wonderful, crisp texture when waffled.

¾ cup (175 mL) brown rice flour

¾ cup (175 mL) chickpea flour

1 teaspoon (5 mL) salt

4 green onions (white and light green parts only), thinly sliced

1 cup (250 mL) lightly packed chopped fresh curly parsley

1 cup (250 mL) lightly packed coleslaw mix

1 tablespoon (15 mL) gluten-free tamari

1 teaspoon (5 mL) Sriracha

1 tablespoon (15 mL) freshly squeezed lemon juice

1 tablespoon (15 mL) toasted sesame oil

1 cup (250 mL) water

Refined coconut oil or avocado oil, for frying

1 batch XOXO Sauce (page 208)

# XOXO Sauce

DAIRY-FREE | GLUTEN-FREE | NUT-FREE | VEGAN | VEGETARIAN

MAKES ABOUT 1½ CUPS (375 ML)

This sauce is essentially a quartet of anti-inflammatory superfoods: shiitake mushrooms, shallot, garlic, and ginger. It is the extra touch that takes my Green Onion Pancakes (page 207) to another level! The recipe makes a big batch, but you can (and should) use any leftovers as a sauce for ramen or soba noodles, to top grilled tofu and burgers, or to add to grain bowls and wraps. Try it as a condiment for the Spicy Miso Soba Bowl (page 155), Edamame Hula Bowl (page 181), or Green Machine Burgers (page 140). It keeps well in the refrigerator for a couple of weeks but because it is made with coconut oil, it solidifies when cold and needs to be warmed to at least room temperature for the best texture and taste.

1 package (¾ ounce/20 g) dried shiitake mushrooms

1 large shallot, quartered

3 cloves garlic, peeled

1-inch (2.5 cm) piece fresh ginger, peeled and halved

¼ cup (60 mL) virgin coconut oil

¼ cup (60 mL) gluten-free tamari

3 tablespoons (45 mL) unseasoned rice vinegar

1 tablespoon (15 mL) toasted sesame oil

1 teaspoon (5 mL) cane sugar

¾ teaspoon (4 mL) five-spice powder

⅛ teaspoon (0.5 mL) red chili flakes

1. In a small bowl, soak the shiitake mushrooms in ½ cup (125 mL) boiling water for 10 minutes. Squeeze the water out of the mushrooms and reserve the soaking liquid.

2. In a small food processor, add the mushrooms, shallot, garlic, and ginger. Pulse until uniform and finely chopped but not a paste.

3. In a small saucepan, melt the coconut oil over medium-low heat. Add the pulsed vegetables and tamari and simmer for 5 to 7 minutes to soften the vegetables.

4. Stir in the rice vinegar, sesame oil, sugar, five spice, chili flakes, and 2 tablespoons (30 mL) of the reserved mushroom liquid. Reduce the heat to low as soon as the mixture comes to a boil and let simmer for 10 minutes.

Tip You can make this sauce before you start making the Green Onion Pancakes (page 207) and keep it warm on the stove until ready to use.

# Mexican Street Corn

DAIRY-FREE | GLUTEN-FREE | NUT-FREE | VEGAN | VEGETARIAN

SERVES 4

This is perhaps my favourite way to serve fresh corn. The chili lime sauce adds a bit of sass to a barbecue staple that is positively addictive. This is so good you will want to eat all four cobs. Forget sharing!

And if you're wondering what sweet corn is doing in an anti-inflammatory cookbook, you might be surprised to learn that corn contains small amounts of important phytochemicals like lutein and zeaxanthin, along with manganese. Manganese is a mineral that fuels the activity of a form of superoxide dismutase, a master antioxidant enzyme in the body. A plant-based diet does not have to be all kale—all plants deserve a place at the table.

1. Prepare a grill for direct cooking over high heat.

2. Put the corn on the grill, close the lid, and grill until lightly charred on all sides, 6 to 8 minutes, turning often.

3. To make the sauce, in a small bowl combine the mayonnaise, chili powder, garlic, cumin, cayenne, and salt to taste. Add the lime juice, 1 teaspoon (5 mL) at a time, to reach the desired consistency. You want the sauce thick enough that it sticks to the corn.

4. Serve the grilled corn immediately, slathered with sauce and sprinkled with Almond Ricotta Cheese (if using). Serve each cob with a lime wedge, if desired.

Tip No barbecue? Just boil the corn as usual. It will not be quite the same, but it will do!

4 cobs fresh sweet corn, husks removed

3 tablespoons (45 mL) vegan mayonnaise

½ teaspoon (2 mL) Mexican chili powder

½ clove garlic, crushed or grated on a microplane

⅛ teaspoon (0.5 mL) ground cumin

⅛ teaspoon (0.5 mL) cayenne pepper

Salt

2 teaspoons (10 mL) freshly squeezed lime juice

For serving (optional)

Almond Ricotta Cheese (page 260)

4 lime wedges

# Tomato Jam Tartines

DAIRY-FREE | GLUTEN-FREE | NUT-FREE | VEGAN | VEGETARIAN

SERVES 8

4 cups (1 L) cherry tomatoes or chopped Roma tomatoes

1 clove garlic, minced

2 tablespoons (30 mL) cane sugar

1 teaspoon (5 mL) curry powder

½ teaspoon (2 mL) salt

⅛ teaspoon (0.5 mL) ground turmeric

⅛ teaspoon (0.5 mL) red chili flakes

⅛ teaspoon (0.5 mL) ground cumin

⅛ teaspoon (0.5 mL) garam masala

1 tablespoon (15 mL) freshly squeezed lemon juice

Freshly cracked pepper

For serving

Real Deal Gluten-Free Bread (page 267) or your favourite gluten-free bread

Pea shoots

Sunflower sprouts

Chopped fresh flat-leaf parsley

When having guests over and you want a little something to serve, this is it. You place all the ingredients in a pot and 30 minutes later have the most incredible sweet, tart, savoury, and spicy jam. Lycopene-rich tomatoes accented by anti-inflammatory spices in a spread too delicious to be healthy! Dollop it on thin slices of toast or crackers with a bit of greenery, and you are done. It is a great way to use an abundance of tomatoes that are nearing the end of their freshness. This is a large batch, but you will want to use it on everything: grain bowls, sandwiches, pasta, and salads.

1. In a medium pot, stir together the tomatoes, garlic, sugar, curry powder, salt, turmeric, chili flakes, cumin, and garam masala over medium heat. Bring to a boil.

2. Once boiling, reduce the heat to low and simmer for 30 minutes until the tomatoes burst and the liquid reduces to produce a loose jam-like texture. Adjust the heat as necessary to keep the mixture simmering but not boiling as it reduces.

3. Remove from the heat, taste, and add the lemon juice. Depending on the acidity of the tomatoes, you may want to add up to 1 tablespoon (15 mL) more. Season to taste with salt and pepper. Store in a resealable container in the fridge for up to 2 weeks.

4. To assemble the toasts, thinly slice the bread and toast until crisp. Cut any large slices into smaller 3- to 4-inch (8 to 10 cm) pieces. Place a generous dollop of tomato jam on the toasts and sprinkle with the greens of your choice.

Tip If your tomatoes are super sweet, start with 1 tablespoon (15 mL) cane sugar and adjust sweetness at the end if necessary. You may need a little more sugar when using imported tomatoes in the middle of winter.

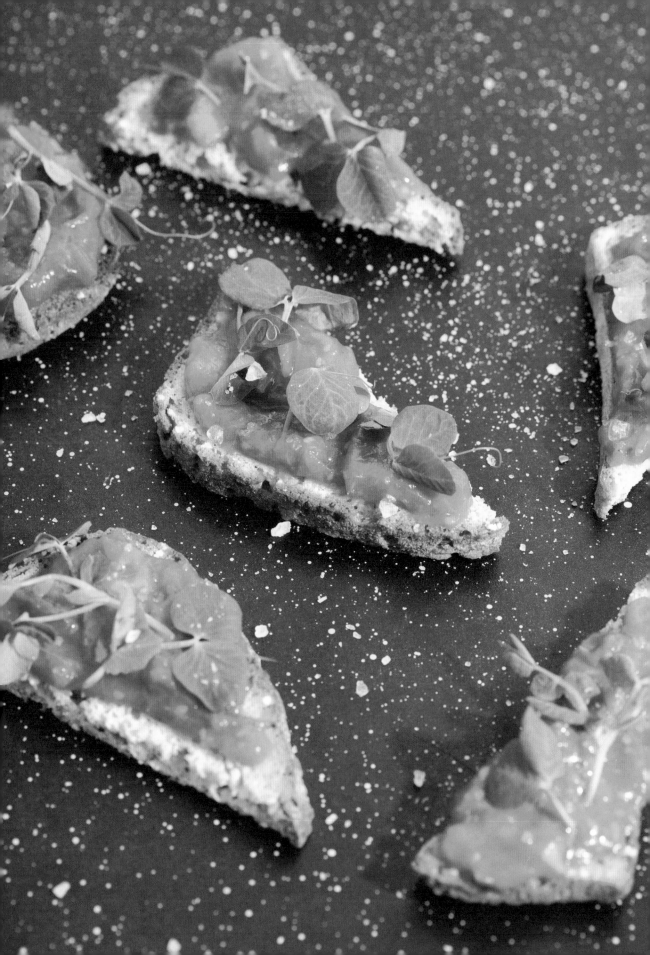

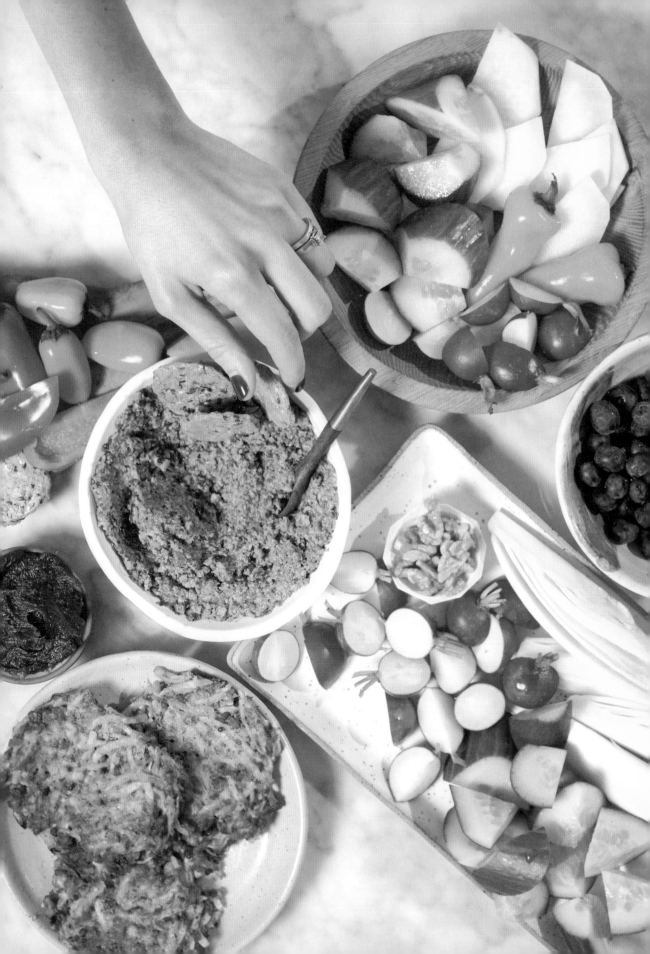

# Plant-Powered Charcuterie Board

FOR 6 PEOPLE, SERVE 1 TO 2 VARIETIES OF EACH FOOD; FOR 12 PEOPLE,
SERVE 2 TO 3 VARIETIES OF EACH FOOD

When I struck out on my own, I could always be counted on for a stacked charcuterie board. It was an easy way to entertain because I picked up everything at the Italian shop. Going plant-based means you need to branch out a little! I have put some of my favourite recommendations for plant-based meat and dairy alternatives in the Favourite Suppliers section (page 279).

Of course, if you are feeling ambitious, you can make it all yourself! It is easier than you think, since almost everything can be made well in advance of party time. For an epic platter, I like to serve a mix of the following foods.

---

## Grains and Starches

Real Deal Gluten-Free Bread (page 267)
Seedy Crackers (page 265)
Celeriac Lentil Fritters (see page 197)

## Spreads and Dips

Date Jam (see page 197)
Truffled Mushroom Pâté (page 189)
Spiced Carrot Dip (page 193)
Beet Pesto (page 262)
Tomato Jam (see page 210)

## Fruit

Grapes
Sliced pear or apple
Persimmon
Fresh figs
Seasonal berries (strawberries,
blackberries, blueberries)
Sliced plum
Kumquats
Sliced kiwi

## Vegetables

Raw jicama straws
Sliced kohlrabi
Sliced fennel
French breakfast radishes, served with sea salt
Chili Garlic Brussels Sprouts (page 214)
Fried Eggplant with Chili and Pomegranate
    Molasses (page 203)
Beet Tartare (page 194)

## Raw Nuts and Dried Fruit

Almonds
Macadamia nuts
Walnuts
Apricots
Figs
Tart cherries

## Cheeses

Almond Ricotta Cheese (page 260), drizzled
    with chili oil
Fermented Cashew Cream Cheese (page 271)

# Chili Garlic Brussels Sprouts

DAIRY-FREE | GLUTEN-FREE | NUT-FREE | PALEO-FRIENDLY | VEGAN | VEGETARIAN

SERVES 4

Brussels sprouts are easily one of my top five favourite vegetables of all time. As a member of the cruciferous family, they contain all of the sulphur-based phytochemicals that are foundational to an anti-inflammatory diet. Extremely high in vitamins K and C, Brussels sprouts even boast small amounts of omega-3 fats. They are also delicious, when you do not boil them into oblivion. Salty, spicy, and sweet, these sprouts are great as a side or a snack. I have been known to eat a pound all by myself. These are wonderful served with my Green Onion Pancakes with XOXO Sauce (page 207) or as side with Green Machine Burgers (page 140).

---

2 tablespoons (30 mL) gluten-free tamari

2 teaspoons (10 mL) unseasoned rice vinegar

1 teaspoon (5 mL) pure maple syrup

2 cloves garlic, crushed or grated on a microplane

1 teaspoon (5 mL) Sriracha

1 tablespoon (15 mL) refined coconut oil, for cooking

1 pound (450 g) Brussels sprouts, trimmed and halved

1. In a small bowl, whisk together the tamari, rice vinegar, maple syrup, garlic, and Sriracha.

2. In a large skillet, melt the coconut oil over high heat. Place the Brussels sprouts cut side down in a single layer and fry until crisp, about 2 minutes. Pour the sauce over the Brussels sprouts and cook for 2 minutes, so the sauce reduces and coats the Brussels sprouts.

3. Place the Brussels sprouts in a medium serving dish and serve immediately.

# Celeriac Mash

DAIRY-FREE | GLUTEN-FREE | NUT-FREE | VEGAN | VEGETARIAN

SERVES 4

Creamy and comforting, what is not to like about a mash? Here, celeriac and buttery white beans create a dreamy high-fibre, high-protein mash that will not require a post-meal nap. Prebiotic oligosaccharides in beans help feed beneficial bacteria in the gut, helping to keep inflammation at bay. White beans are my go-to when I want a creamy texture, and this garlic-infused mash will not disappoint. If cooking for one or two people, this recipe halves easily.

---

1. Preheat the oven to 450°F (230°C). Line a baking sheet with parchment paper.

2. In a large bowl, toss the celeriac with 2 tablespoons (30 mL) of the olive oil, thyme, salt, and pepper to taste and spread evenly on the baking sheet. Tuck the garlic in the centre of the vegetables to avoid burning.

3. Roast for 15 minutes, then sprinkle the white beans on the baking sheet and roast for 5 minutes more.

4. Carefully remove the garlic from the vegetables and let cool. Add the vegetables and beans to a food processor with the remaining 2 tablespoons (30 mL) olive oil, ¼ cup (60 mL) reserved bean liquid, nutritional yeast, and roasted garlic, squeezed out of the skin, and process until smooth.

5. Taste and adjust seasoning with salt and freshly cracked pepper, as desired.

Tip You can also mash the celeriac by hand with a potato ricer for a more rustic mash.

4 cups (1 L) diced celeriac (about 1 large celeriac)

¼ cup (60 mL) extra-virgin olive oil, divided

½ teaspoon (2 mL) fresh thyme leaves

¼ teaspoon (1 mL) salt

Freshly cracked pepper

5 cloves garlic, skin on

2 cans (14 ounces/398 mL each) butter beans, cannellini, or other white bean (reserve ¼ cup/60 mL liquid)

1 tablespoon + 1 teaspoon (20 mL) nutritional yeast

# Cheesy Lentil Grits

DAIRY-FREE | GLUTEN-FREE | NUT-FREE | VEGAN | VEGETARIAN

**SERVES 4 TO 6**

Creamy and starchy, grits are comfort food par excellence. I have added savoury, satisfying lentils to boost protein, fibre, and minerals and add an anti-inflammatory slant to this classic side dish.

Distinct from polenta, grits are made from ground white corn rather than the standard yellow corn used to make polenta. If you cannot find traditional white grits, polenta or coarse cornmeal will work in this recipe, too! These grits are so creamy and comforting, I will often eat a big helping of this topped with sautéed kale or my Chili Garlic Brussels Sprouts (page 214) for a quick and delicious dinner.

---

¼ cup (60 mL) extra-virgin olive oil

3 cloves garlic, minced

2 cans (14 ounces/398 mL each) green or brown lentils

2 teaspoons (10 mL) gluten-free tamari

2 cups (500 mL) unsweetened soy milk

2 cups (500 mL) water

1 cup (250 mL) gluten-free white corn grits (I use Bob's Red Mill)

½ teaspoon (2 mL) salt

2 tablespoons (30 mL) nutritional yeast

1. In a large pasta pot, heat the olive oil over medium heat. Using a large pot will help protect you from splatters because grits spit as they cook.

2. Add the garlic and cook until soft, about 2 minutes, stirring often so the garlic does not burn. Stir in the lentils and tamari, then add the soy milk and water. Increase the heat to high and bring to a boil.

3. Once boiling, reduce the heat to medium-high and add the grits and salt. Stir constantly to minimize spitting as the grits cook, 10 to 15 minutes. If spitting is an issue, turn down the heat slightly.

4. Remove from the heat, stir in the nutritional yeast, taste, and adjust seasoning if necessary. Transfer to a medium serving bowl and serve immediately.

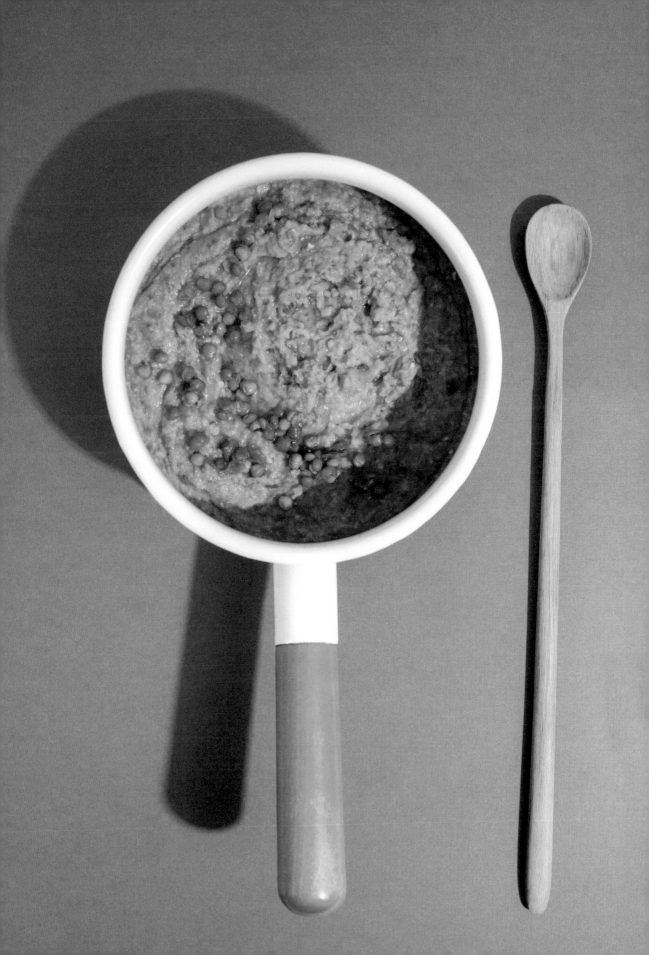

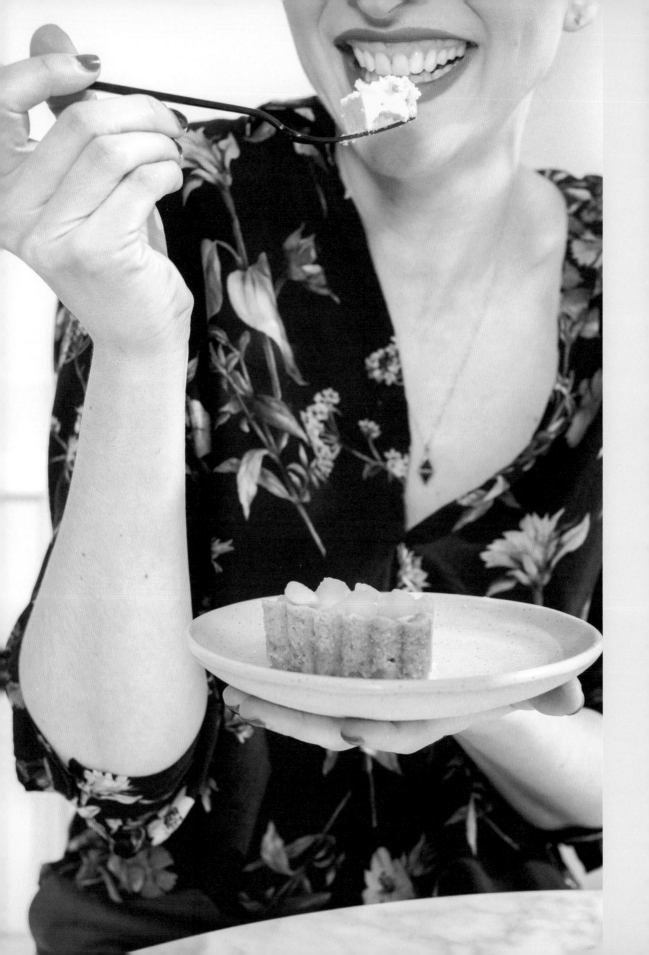

# 9

# Sweets with Benefits

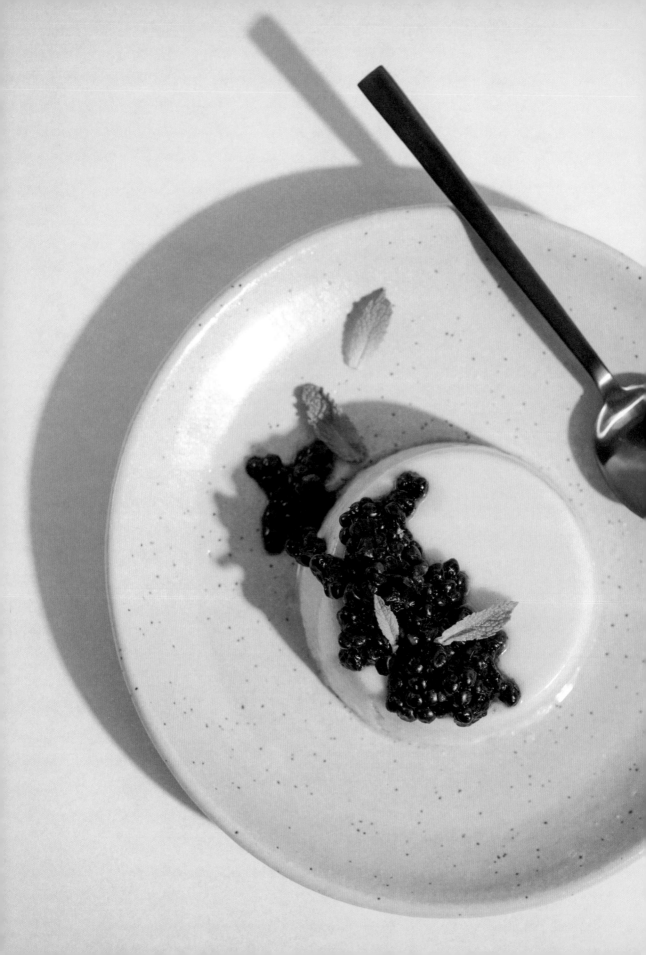

# Avocado Panna Cotta with Tequila Smashed Blackberries

DAIRY-FREE | GLUTEN-FREE | NUT-FREE | PALEO-FRIENDLY | VEGAN | VEGETARIAN

SERVES 4

I ate a transcendent sorrel panna cotta at a magical restaurant called Pilgrimme on Galiano Island, British Columbia, and when I got home, all I could think about was how to replicate it so I could eat it all the time. Sorrel is essentially a forest weed, with a light green, citrusy taste. But it can be hard to find. My mom suggested using avocado instead, which was genius!

Inspired by avocado margaritas, these are so good they make me giddy. I literally jumped up and down when I nailed this recipe.

---

1. In a small saucepan, whisk together the agar, orange juice, and lime juice until combined. Bring the mixture to a boil over medium-high heat. Reduce the heat to low, simmer for 1 minute, stirring often, and ensure that the agar does not settle in the bottom of the pan or your dessert will not gel. Remove from the heat and let cool for 3 to 5 minutes, whisking occasionally so the mixture does not set.

2. In a small blender, add the soy milk, avocado, maple syrup, cardamom, and a pinch of salt and blend until smooth. Add to the agar mixture and give it a quick mix.

3. Divide the mixture into 4 ramekins or decorative glasses. Let cool for 10 minutes, then refrigerate for at least 2 hours to set. Serve in the ramekins or carefully loosen the panna cotta from the ramekins, top with a plate, and gently turn over onto the plate for the classic presentation.

4. For serving, smash the blackberries and taste for sweetness. If they are juicy sweet, you don't need to do anything more. If they're a bit tart, add maple syrup ½ teaspoon (2 mL) at a time, to your taste. Sprinkle with a dash of tequila (if using) and serve overtop the panna cotta.

**Tip** Agar powder is a plant-based gelatin. It can be hard to find, but it is available in gourmet stores, health food stores, and online.

½ teaspoon (2 mL) agar powder

½ cup (125 mL) freshly squeezed orange juice

⅓ cup (75 mL) freshly squeezed lime juice

½ cup (125 mL) sweetened soy milk

⅓ cup (75 mL) ripe avocado (about ½ large avocado)

¼ cup (60 mL) pure maple syrup

⅛ teaspoon (0.5 mL) cardamom

Sea salt

### For serving

1 cup (250 mL) fresh or thawed frozen blackberries

Pure maple syrup, to taste

Pure agave tequila (optional)

# Almond Snickerdoodle Cookies

DAIRY-FREE | GLUTEN-FREE | PALEO-FRIENDLY | VEGAN | VEGETARIAN

MAKES 24 COOKIES

These cookies are magic and so easy to make. Everyone in my family gobbles these up, with the exception of my almond-intolerant husband! Almond flour is such an incredible ingredient because it is high in fibre and protein, helping you keep your blood sugars in check even while enjoying a treat. Pillowy soft, with just the right hint of sweetness and somehow tasting as if they are made with dairy butter, these cookies are living proof that plant foods like to party.

½ cup (125 mL) raw almond butter

⅓ cup (75 mL) pure maple syrup

1½ teaspoons (7 mL) pure vanilla extract

2 cups (500 mL) almond flour

¼ cup (60 mL) arrowroot powder

1 teaspoon (5 mL) cinnamon

½ teaspoon (2 mL) baking powder

½ teaspoon (2 mL) salt

1. Preheat the oven to 350°F (180°C). Line a baking sheet with parchment paper.

2. In a medium mixing bowl, combine the almond butter, maple syrup, and vanilla using an electric mixer.

3. Add the almond flour, arrowroot powder, cinnamon, baking powder, and salt and blend until well combined.

4. Using about 1 tablespoon (30 mL) of the mixture at a time, roll between your hands into balls. Gently press the balls to ¼-inch (5 mm) thickness.

5. Bake for 8 to 9 minutes. The tops should be soft but not feel raw. Place the baking sheet on a cooling rack; leave the cookies on the baking sheet to cool completely, as they will firm once cool.

6. Store in an airtight container on the counter for up to 3 days or in the freezer for up to 1 month.

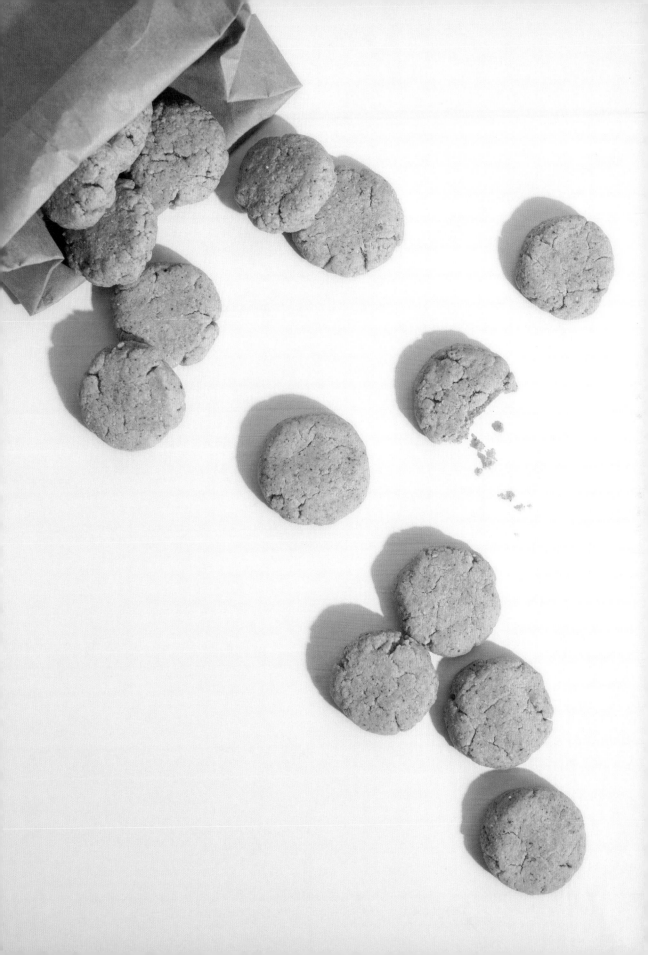

# Chocolate Hummus

DAIRY-FREE | GLUTEN-FREE | NUT-FREE | VEGAN | VEGETARIAN

**MAKES 1¾ CUPS (425 ML)**

I was skeptical about chocolate hummus, until I tried it! You may not think that chocolate and hummus are a natural combination, but trust me, if you like hummus, you will love this dip! This is a sweet, but not too sweet, take on my all-time favourite dip. It is high in fibre, a plant-based protein, and contains anti-inflammatory minerals, so you can enjoy a dollop on muffins or eat it as a dip with crackers or fruit. It is a good excuse to eat chocolate every day.

---

2 cups (500 mL) chickpeas, rinsed and drained

½ cup (125 mL) unsweetened vanilla almond milk or cashew milk

¼ cup (60 mL) raw tahini

¼ cup (60 mL) cocoa powder

¼ cup (60 mL) pure maple syrup

1 teaspoon (5 mL) pure vanilla extract

½ teaspoon (2 mL) cinnamon

⅛ teaspoon (0.5 mL) salt

1. In a in a food processor or high-speed blender, combine the chickpeas, almond milk, tahini, cocoa, maple syrup, vanilla, cinnamon, and salt and purée. Store in a resealable container in the fridge for up to 5 days.

Tip The better quality your ingredients, the more transcendent this dip will taste. If you have the time, cook your own chickpeas and then try this genius hack. Add 1 teaspoon (5 mL) baking soda to the cooking water. This is what we are taught not to do because it mushes up the chickpeas. However, if you are making hummus, this is exactly what you want for a crazy-smooth hummus.

# Salted Caramel Almond Blondies

DAIRY-FREE | GLUTEN-FREE | VEGAN | VEGETARIAN

MAKES 16 BLONDIES

I love a chickpea brownie. The boost of fibre and protein you get from chickpeas means a sweet treat that actually feels filling and satisfying, without the blood sugar crash. Of course, a little date caramel never hurt anyone either. Dates are rich in natural sugars, but they also come packed with potassium and trace amounts of minerals like calcium and magnesium.

These blondies are a very grown-up, richly flavoured treat and perhaps the closest I have come to re-creating the texture of a traditional blondie. My Masala Chai Almond Butter (page 261) is a delicious alternative to raw almond butter.

---

1. Preheat the oven to 350°F (180°C). Lightly grease an 8-inch (2 L) square baking dish with coconut oil.

2. **Make the Almond Blondies Batter** In a food processor, combine the chickpeas, reserved chickpea liquid, almond butter, maple syrup, vanilla, cinnamon, and salt. Blend until smooth.

3. Add the flour and baking powder and process until just blended.

4. Spread the batter evenly in the baking dish using a spatula.

5. **Make the Date Caramel** Drain the softened dates and add to a small bowl with the milk, vanilla, and salt. Using a handheld immersion blender or in a small food processor, purée until a smooth paste forms.

6. Spread the Date Caramel on top of the almond blondies batter and, using a spatula or knife, gently swirl the caramel through the top of the batter.

7. Bake for 18 to 20 minutes or until a toothpick inserted into the centre comes out clean. The Date Caramel does not fully set, so the toothpick may have a bit of date residue. Let cool completely before removing from the baking dish.

8. The blondies will keep, loosely covered, on the counter for up to 2 days.

## Almond Blondies

Coconut oil, for greasing the baking dish

1 can (14 ounces/398 mL) chickpeas (reserve 2 tablespoons/30 mL chickpea liquid)

½ cup (125 mL) raw almond butter

⅓ cup (75 mL) pure maple syrup

2 teaspoons (10 mL) pure vanilla extract

¾ teaspoon (4 mL) cinnamon

½ teaspoon (2 mL) salt

1 cup (250 mL) gluten-free all-purpose flour

½ teaspoon (2 mL) baking powder

## Date Caramel

½ cup (125 mL) Medjool dates, pitted and soaked in hot water to soften

¼ cup (60 mL) unsweetened oat milk or cashew milk

¼ teaspoon (1 mL) pure vanilla extract

⅛ rounded teaspoon (0.5 mL) salt

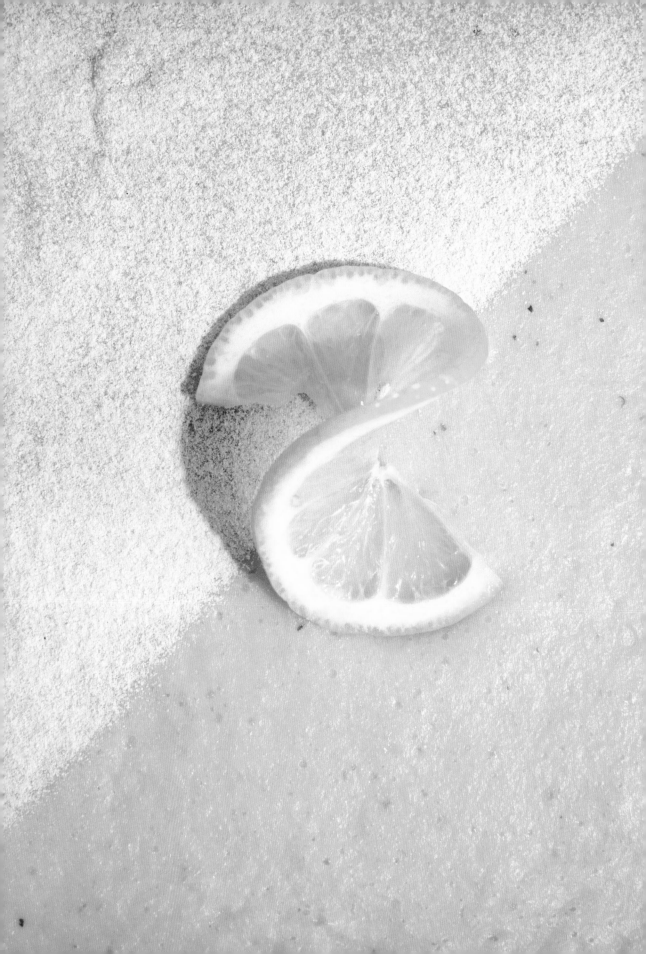

# Lemon Coconut Zinger Squares

DAIRY-FREE | GLUTEN-FREE | NUT-FREE | VEGAN | VEGETARIAN

**MAKES 16 SQUARES**

A few foods really give you a zing when eaten. Curly parsley is one of them and so is lemon peel. If you really want to embrace the health benefits of lemon, like vitamin C and bioflavonoids, you cannot just squeeze a bit into water. You have to eat the whole fruit, so these tart bars are made with puréed whole lemon. Yes, the whole thing. These bars have a coconut shortbread layer topped by silky soft (yet spiky!) lemon cream.

---

1.  Preheat the oven to 350°F (180°C). Grease an 8-inch (2 L) square baking dish with coconut oil and line the bottom with a piece of parchment paper.

2.  **Make the Coconut Shortbread Crust** In a medium bowl, whisk together the flour, coconut, lemon zest, and salt. Using your fingers, mix the coconut oil into the flour mixture until well distributed and it looks like tiny pebbles.

3.  Mix in the maple syrup and soy milk to form a dough. Press the dough into the baking dish and bake for 15 to 16 minutes or until the edges just start to turn golden.

4.  **Make the Lemon Coconut Filling** Meanwhile, remove the peel and white pith from the reserved lemon you partially zested for the crust. Cut into 3 slices and toss into a blender. Cut the second lemon with the skin on into quarters, toss into the blender, and process until puréed.

5.  Add the maple syrup and water to the blender and purée until smooth.

6.  Pour the lemon mixture into a small saucepan with the coconut milk, arrowroot starch, agar, and salt and whisk thoroughly. Heat the mixture over medium heat, whisking constantly once it comes to a boil until thickened, about 1 minute. Pour the lemon mixture over the baked crust and smooth the top.

7.  Bake for 12 to 15 minutes. The filling should look gently set and large bubbles should be forming at the edges. Remove and let cool completely on a rack before cutting into squares.

8.  Store in a resealable container in the fridge for up to 3 days.

## Coconut Shortbread Crust

1 cup (250 mL) gluten-free all-purpose flour

1 cup (250 mL) unsweetened shredded coconut

Zest of ½ lemon (reserve the lemon for the filling)

⅛ teaspoon (0.5 mL) salt

⅓ cup (75 mL) virgin coconut oil, plus more for greasing the baking dish

¼ cup (60 mL) pure maple syrup

¼ cup (60 mL) unsweetened soy milk or almond milk

## Lemon Coconut Filling

1 lemon, scrubbed and ends trimmed

6 tablespoons (90 mL) pure maple syrup

¼ cup (60 mL) water

⅔ cup (150 mL) full-fat coconut milk

¼ cup (60 mL) arrowroot starch

½ teaspoon (2 mL) agar powder

⅛ teaspoon (0.5 mL) salt

# Pineapple Ginger Cream Tart

DAIRY-FREE | GLUTEN-FREE | VEGAN | VEGETARIAN

MAKES ONE 9-INCH (23 CM) ROUND TART; SERVES 8 TO 10

I feel like eating pineapple is a mini holiday for your soul. It is also enormously soothing for your digestion, particularly when paired with plenty of fresh ginger. This creamy, dreamy tart is nestled on a macadamia cookie base that is rich in healthy fats and soluble fibre from the oat flour.

## Macadamia Cookie Crust

1 cup (250 mL) raw macadamia nuts

½ cup (125 mL) gluten-free oat flour

½ cup (125 mL) brown rice flour

¼ cup (60 mL) coconut oil, plus more for greasing the pan

3 tablespoons (45 mL) pure maple syrup

½ teaspoon (2 mL) baking powder

¼ teaspoon (1 mL) ground ginger

⅛ teaspoon (0.5 mL) salt

## Pineapple Ginger Cream

2 cups (500 mL) roughly chopped fresh pineapple

1 cup (250 mL) raw cashews, soaked for at least 2 hours, drained, and rinsed

¼ cup (60 mL) pure maple syrup

2 tablespoons (30 mL) freshly squeezed lemon juice

2 tablespoons (30 mL) water

1 tablespoon (15 mL) minced fresh ginger

¼ teaspoon (1 mL) ground turmeric

2 cups (500 mL) finely diced pineapple

1. Preheat the oven to 350°F (180°C). Grease a 9-inch (23 cm) round pie plate or tart pan with a bit of coconut oil.

2. **Make the Macadamia Cookie Crust** In a food processor, combine the macadamia nuts, oat flour, brown rice flour, coconut oil, maple syrup, baking powder, ginger, and salt and pulse until a thick paste forms. Pat into the pie plate, including up the sides, and chill the dough in the freezer for 15 minutes.

3. Prick the crust with a fork and bake until golden, 12 to 14 minutes. Let cool completely before topping with the Pineapple Ginger Cream.

4. **Make the Pineapple Ginger Cream** Meanwhile, combine the chopped pineapple, cashews, maple syrup, lemon juice, water, ginger, and turmeric in a high-speed blender and blend until smooth.

5. Sprinkle the diced pineapple over the Macadamia Cookie Crust and pour the Pineapple Ginger Cream overtop. Freeze for at least 30 minutes to set.

Make It Faster You can make this tart up to 3 days in advance and store it in the freezer, tightly wrapped with foil.

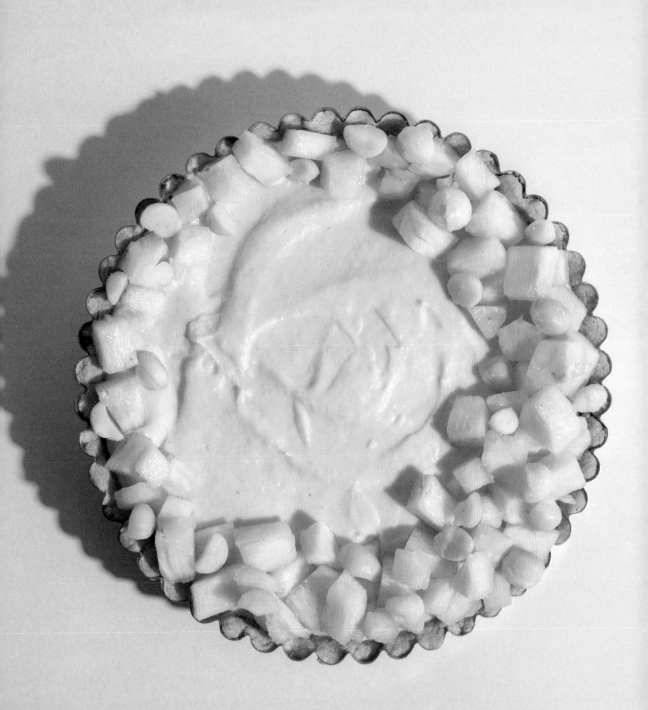

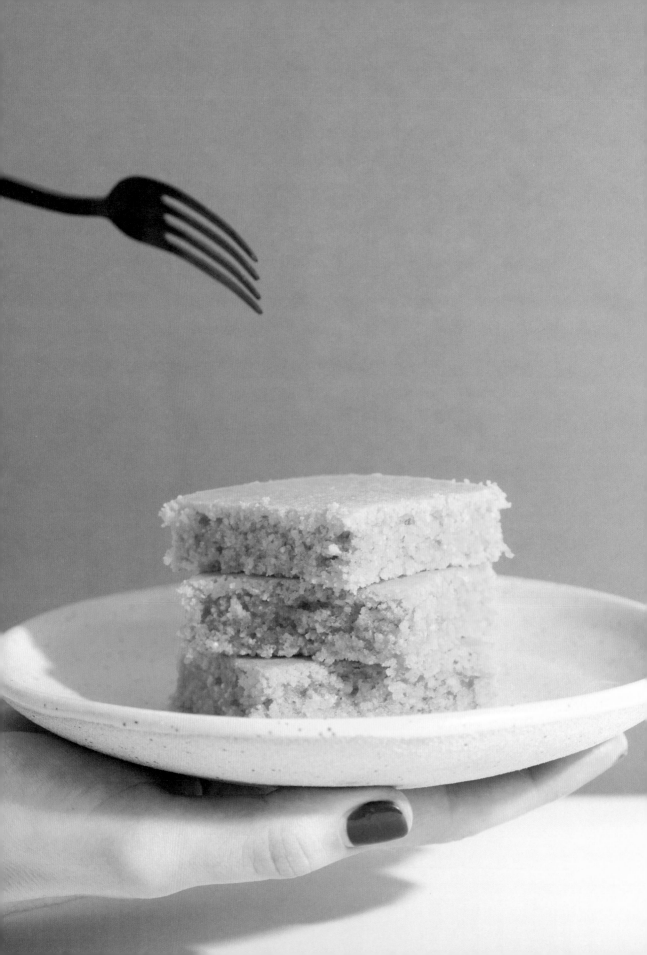

# Lebanese Turmeric Cake

DAIRY-FREE | GLUTEN-FREE | NUT-FREE | VEGAN | VEGETARIAN

MAKES ONE 9- × 13-INCH (23 × 33 CM) CAKE; SERVES 16

I love this cake made with turmeric—my favourite anti-inflammatory ingredient! This is my version of a traditional Lebanese snack cake, typically made with semolina. I have replaced that delicate crunch with cornmeal and drastically lowered the sugar content so that the turmeric is not drowned by a massive spike in blood sugar.

The rosewater and ground aniseed create a distinct and exotic perfume that makes you feel happy as soon as you open the oven door. As a fan of not-too-sweet sweets, I find this cake is perfect to enjoy with an afternoon cup of tea.

---

1. Preheat the oven to 350°F (180°C). Grease a 9- × 13-inch (23 × 33 cm) baking dish with the tahini and set aside.

2. In a large bowl, whisk together the cornmeal, flour, sugar, turmeric, baking powder, aniseed, and ginger.

3. In a medium bowl, mix the olive oil, soy milk, and rosewater. Add to the cornmeal mixture and mix to combine.

4. Pour the batter into the baking dish and bake until the edges just start to pull away from the dish and the top is firm, 33 to 35 minutes. Remove the dish to a rack and let cool at least 15 minutes before slicing. The cake is delicious served warm or at room temperature.

5. The cake will keep on the counter, loosely covered, for up to 3 days. It also freezes well, tightly wrapped in a double layer of plastic wrap, for up to 1 month.

Tip Rosewater comes in varying strengths; I prefer a strongly flavoured variety. Some supermarkets carry rosewater; however, it's more reliably found at gourmet stores, Mediterranean and Middle Eastern markets, and online.

3 tablespoons (45 mL) raw tahini, for greasing the dish

1½ cups (375 mL) medium grind cornmeal

1½ cups (375 mL) gluten-free all-purpose flour

½ cup (125 mL) cane sugar

1 tablespoon (15 mL) ground turmeric

2 teaspoons (10 mL) baking powder

1 teaspoon (5 mL) ground aniseed

½ teaspoon (2 mL) ground ginger

1 cup (250 mL) extra-virgin olive oil

1 cup (250 mL) unsweetened soy milk or almond milk

2 tablespoons (30 mL) rosewater

# Cocoa Cherry Brownies

**MAKES 12 BROWNIES**

Olive oil or coconut oil,
for greasing the pan

2½ cups (625 mL) cauliflower
florets

1 can (14 ounces/398 mL)
chickpeas, drained
and rinsed (reserve
2 tablespoons/30 mL
chickpea liquid)

5 chopped Medjool dates,
pitted

⅓ cup (75 mL) pure maple
syrup

¼ cup (60 mL) extra-virgin
olive oil

2 teaspoons (10 mL)
pure vanilla extract

½ cup (125 mL) gluten-free
all-purpose flour

½ cup (125 mL) cocoa powder

½ cup (125 mL) almond meal

2 teaspoons (10 mL) cinnamon

1 teaspoon (5 mL) baking
powder

½ teaspoon (2 mL) salt

¼ teaspoon (1 mL) allspice

¼ cup (60 mL) dairy-free mini
bittersweet chocolate chips
or cacao nibs

½ cup (125 mL) unsweetened
dried cherries

Yes, I put vegetables in these brownies. I promise, though, that they do not taste like salad. In fact, they are fudgy, chocolatey pillows of goodness. High in fibre and protein and rich in minerals, these brownies include a trio of anti-inflammatory power players: cauliflower, cocoa, and cherries. If you can find dried tart cherries, even better. Tart cherries have high levels of anthocyanins, a known anti-inflammatory phytochemical. You will not want to skip the chocolate chips; they give you a tiny burst of straight-up chocolatey goodness that really makes these brownies a treat.

1.  Preheat the oven to 350°F (180°C). Grease an 8-inch (2 L) square cake pan with a bit of olive oil or coconut oil.

2.  In a food processor, process the cauliflower until it resembles rice, then add the chickpeas, reserved chickpea liquid, dates, maple syrup, olive oil, and vanilla and purée.

3.  Add the flour, cocoa, almond meal, cinnamon, baking powder, salt, and allspice and pulse until just combined.

4.  Remove the blade from the food processor and stir in the chocolate chips and dried cherries.

5.  Spread the batter into the cake pan, tapping a bit to even it out. Bake until fully set, 30 to 32 minutes. The brownies will have a soft, fudgy texture that will set further as they cool. A toothpick will not come out clean, but the batter should not be goopy.

6.  Let the brownies cool completely, as they are very soft when warm and will firm up when cool. Brownies will keep, loosely covered, on the counter for up to 2 days or in the freezer, tightly wrapped in a double layer of plastic wrap, for up to 1 month.

# Peanut Butter Energy Fudge

DAIRY-FREE | GLUTEN-FREE | VEGAN | VEGETARIAN

MAKES 16 SQUARES OR 24 BALLS

I have been known to eat peanut butter right off a spoon. This no-bake energy fudge is a single step up on the effort scale and worth it. Many energy balls are high in natural sugars, and sometimes I want something that will not just be a sugar rush. Natural peanut butter offers healthy fats and protein, in addition to anti-inflammatory and immune-supportive minerals like magnesium and zinc. Chickpeas add gut-friendly fibre and help keep your energy stable longer. Keep these on hand whenever you need a little something.

---

1. In a food processor, process the chickpeas into a rice-like consistency. Add the peanut butter, maple syrup, coconut oil, vanilla, and a pinch of salt and process until a smooth dough forms.

2. Spread into an 8-inch (2 L) square baking dish or roll between your hands into 1-inch (2.5 cm) diameter balls. Freeze for 2 hours to set.

3. Cut the fudge into 16 squares and store in an airtight container in the freezer for up to 1 month. Flavour is best when you let the fudge stand at room temperature for 5 minutes before eating.

1 cup (250 mL) cooked chickpeas

1½ cups (375 mL) natural peanut butter

⅓ cup (75 mL) pure maple syrup

⅓ cup (75 mL) virgin coconut oil, melted

1 teaspoon (5 mL) pure vanilla extract

Salt

# Carrot Tahini Granola Bars

DAIRY-FREE | GLUTEN-FREE | NUT-FREE | VEGAN | VEGETARIAN

MAKES 12 LARGE BARS OR 24 SMALL SQUARES

I seem almost compulsively drawn to putting some sort of nut, nut butter, or nut flour in my recipes. However, once you have a kid at a nut-free school, it is like bashing your head against the fridge because, once again, you made something they cannot bring to school.

I created these nut-free granola bars with creamy tahini instead of nut butter. I opted for crunchy, zinc-rich pumpkin seeds to support gut health and immunity. These are granola bars you can feel good about because they are packed with nutrition along with a bit of chocolate, for the kids (okay, for me!).

---

2 cups (500 mL) grated carrot (about 4 small carrots)

1½ cups (375 mL) gluten-free rolled oats

1 cup (250 mL) hemp seeds

½ cup (125 mL) raw pumpkin seeds

⅓ cup (75 mL) dairy-free bittersweet mini chocolate chips

1½ teaspoons (7 mL) cinnamon

¼ teaspoon (1 mL) salt

⅓ cup (75 mL) mashed ripe banana (1 small banana)

½ cup (125 mL) raw tahini

3 tablespoons (45 mL) pure maple syrup

2 teaspoons (10 mL) orange zest (from 1 large orange)

2 tablespoons (30 mL) freshly squeezed orange juice

1. Preheat the oven to 350°F (180°C). Line a baking sheet with parchment paper.

2. In a medium bowl, combine the carrot, rolled oats, hemp seeds, pumpkin seeds, chocolate chips, cinnamon, and salt.

3. In a small bowl, mix together the banana, tahini, maple syrup, orange zest and juice until well combined.

4. Add the banana mixture to the carrot mixture and then mix them together with your hands. It is a bit messy (and fun!), but it is the best method for this type of dough.

5. Press the dough onto the prepared baking sheet and spread evenly until about 1 inch (2.5 cm) thick; do not worry about pressing the dough to the edges of the pan.

6. Bake for 25 minutes, until the edges are firm and golden brown. The bars will still be soft in the middle. Place the baking sheet on a rack and let cool for 10 minutes. Then carefully transfer to a cutting board and cut into 12 bars or a size of your choice.

7. Let cool fully to firm up, then store loosely covered with plastic wrap on the counter for up to 5 days. These bars also freeze well, tightly covered with plastic wrap, for up to 1 month.

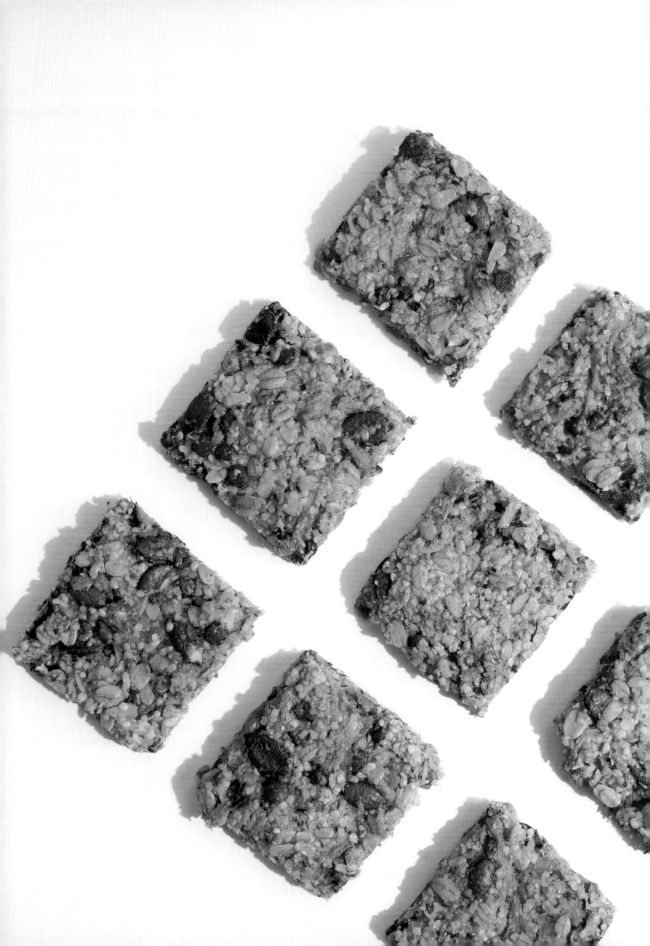

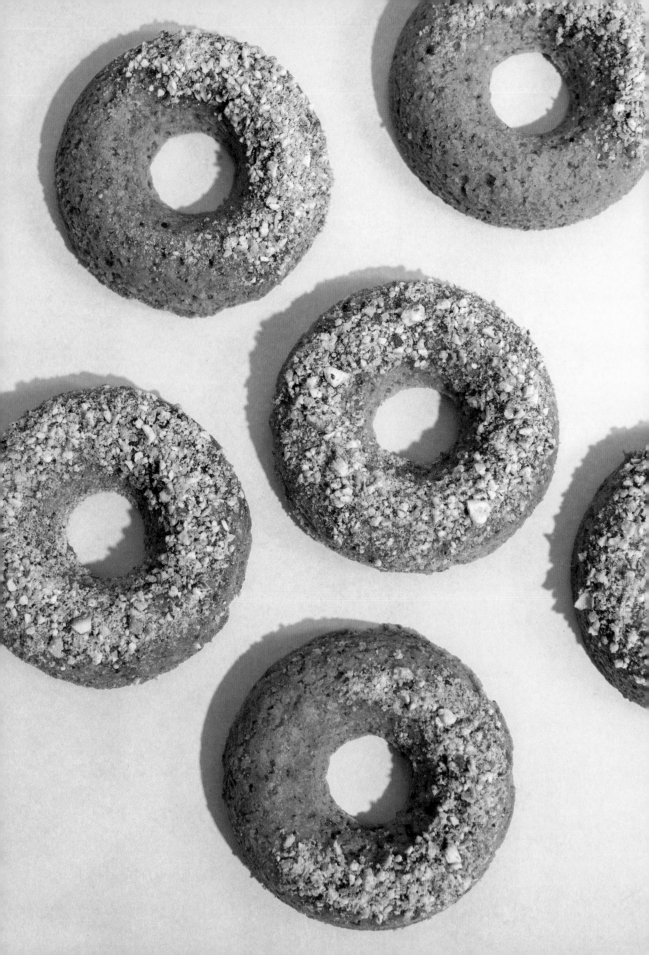

# Pistachio and Cardamom Doughnuts with Rosewater Glaze

DAIRY-FREE | GLUTEN-FREE | VEGAN | VEGETARIAN

MAKES 6 DOUGHNUTS

I never really understood the appeal of doughnuts. I even tried those gourmet ones, but they left me cold because they were all so sweet. Then I tried making my own doughnuts, and I fell in love with them.

Infused with the flavours of the Eastern Mediterranean, these are a delightful departure from the everyday jelly doughnut. Cardamom is, by far, my favourite sweet spice; traditionally used to ease digestion, it is also emerging as a potential anti-inflammatory. Like I needed an excuse! Instead of a traditional glaze, I created a rosewater syrup that acts as delicious glue for a sprinkling of crushed pistachio.

1. Preheat the oven to 350°F (180°C). Grease a 6-pocket doughnut pan with a bit of coconut oil.

2. **Make the Pistachio and Cardamom Doughnuts** In a medium bowl, whisk together ½ cup (125 mL) of the pistachios, almond flour, arrowroot, all-purpose flour, baking powder, and cardamom.

3. In a small bowl, whisk together the maple syrup, olive oil, chickpea liquid, and rosewater until frothy.

4. Tip the maple syrup mixture into the flour mixture and mix until combined.

5. Spoon the batter into the doughnut pan, spreading evenly among the 6 pockets. Bake for 20 to 22 minutes until a toothpick inserted into the centre comes out clean.

6. **Make the Rosewater Glaze** Meanwhile, in a small saucepan, mix together the maple syrup, rosewater, and coconut oil and heat over the lowest possible setting. Remove from the heat and cover the pot to keep it warm.

7. Remove the doughnuts from the oven and cool for 15 minutes in the pan set on a rack. Gently loosen the edges and flip out the doughnuts onto the rack. Once cooled, brush the doughnuts with the glaze and sprinkle with the remaining ¼ cup (60 mL) pistachios.

8. The doughnuts will keep on the counter, in a loosely covered resealable container, for up to 3 days.

### Pistachio and Cardamom Doughnuts

Coconut oil, for greasing the pan

¾ cup (175 mL) ground unsalted natural pistachios, divided

½ cup (125 mL) almond flour

3 tablespoons (45 mL) arrowroot

2 tablespoons (30 mL) gluten-free all-purpose flour

1 teaspoon (5 mL) baking powder

1 teaspoon (5 mL) ground cardamom

¼ cup (60 mL) pure maple syrup

¼ cup (60 mL) extra-virgin olive oil

2 tablespoons (30 mL) canned chickpea liquid

1 tablespoon (15 mL) rosewater

### Rosewater Glaze

3 tablespoons (45 mL) pure maple syrup

1 tablespoon (15 mL) rosewater

1 tablespoon (15 mL) coconut oil

# Raspberry Cacao Slice

DAIRY-FREE | GLUTEN-FREE | PALEO-FRIENDLY | VEGAN | VEGETARIAN

**MAKES 1 LOAF CAKE; SERVES 8**

### Cocoa Coconut Crust

¾ cup (175 mL) unsweetened shredded coconut

½ cup (125 mL) Medjool dates, pitted

¼ cup (60 mL) almond meal

2 tablespoons (30 mL) cocoa powder

⅛ teaspoon (0.5 mL) salt

1 to 2 tablespoons (15 to 30 mL) water, as needed

### Raspberry Cashew Cream Filling

1½ cups (375 mL) raw cashews, soaked in water for at least 4 hours, drained, and rinsed

2½ cups (625 mL) frozen raspberries, divided

¼ cup (60 mL) coconut oil, melted

3 tablespoons (45 mL) pure maple syrup

2 tablespoons (30 mL) freshly squeezed lemon juice

1 teaspoon (5 mL) pure vanilla extract

⅛ teaspoon (0.5 mL) salt

¼ cup (60 mL) water, as needed for blending

¼ cup (60 mL) cacao nibs

Raspberry and chocolate are a match made in anti-inflammatory heaven. Raspberries are one of the highest fibre fruits, keeping your tummy happy and your blood sugars balanced. Flavonoid-rich cocoa is at its most nutrient dense when you are eating the whole cocoa bean, also known as cacao nibs—nature's chocolate chip. Bursting with tart raspberry flavour and low in added sugar, this is a nearly perfect healthy indulgence.

1. Line an 8- × 4-inch (20 × 10 cm) loaf pan with a sheet of parchment paper. Cut it long enough so that extra hangs over the sides for easy removal of the frozen treats.

2. **Make the Cocoa Coconut Crust** In a food processor, combine the coconut, dates, almond meal, cocoa, and salt and blend until the dates are finely chopped and the mixture is well incorporated. Drizzle in water as needed to moisten the mixture so it starts to look like a uniform dough. The dough should stick together when pressed with your fingers but should not be wet.

3. Evenly press the dough into the loaf pan and set aside.

4. **Make the Raspberry Cashew Cream Filling** In a high-speed blender, combine the cashews, 1½ cups (375 mL) of the raspberries, coconut oil, maple syrup, lemon juice, vanilla, and salt and blend until smooth. Add the water, 1 tablespoon (15 mL) at a time, as needed to get the blender moving if the mixture becomes too thick to blend.

5. With the blender turned off, use a spatula to stir in the cacao nibs.

6. Pour the Raspberry Cashew Cream Filling overtop the Cocoa Coconut Crust. Sprinkle the remaining 1 cup (250 mL) raspberries on top. Cover the pan with foil and freeze until firm, at least 2 hours. For easy serving, I like to slice the cake before it is too frozen. Store the slices in an airtight container in the freezer for up to 1 month.

7. When ready to serve, remove from the freezer. The flavour will be best if you allow the slices to thaw slightly for 10 minutes before eating.

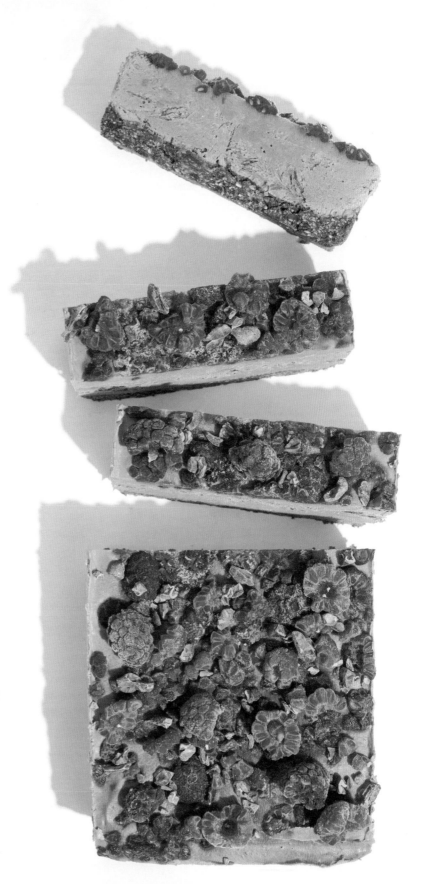

Tip  1. I like making this treat in a loaf pan so that you get a nice slice of thick raspberry cream accented by a smaller ridge of cocoa crust. You can also make it in an 8-inch (2 L) square baking dish and it is equally delicious. 2. Using a high-speed blender is important to get a light, smooth, and silky consistency for the Raspberry Cashew Cream Filling. In a pinch, you can use a food processor; it will still be delicious, but it will have a very heavy, dense texture.

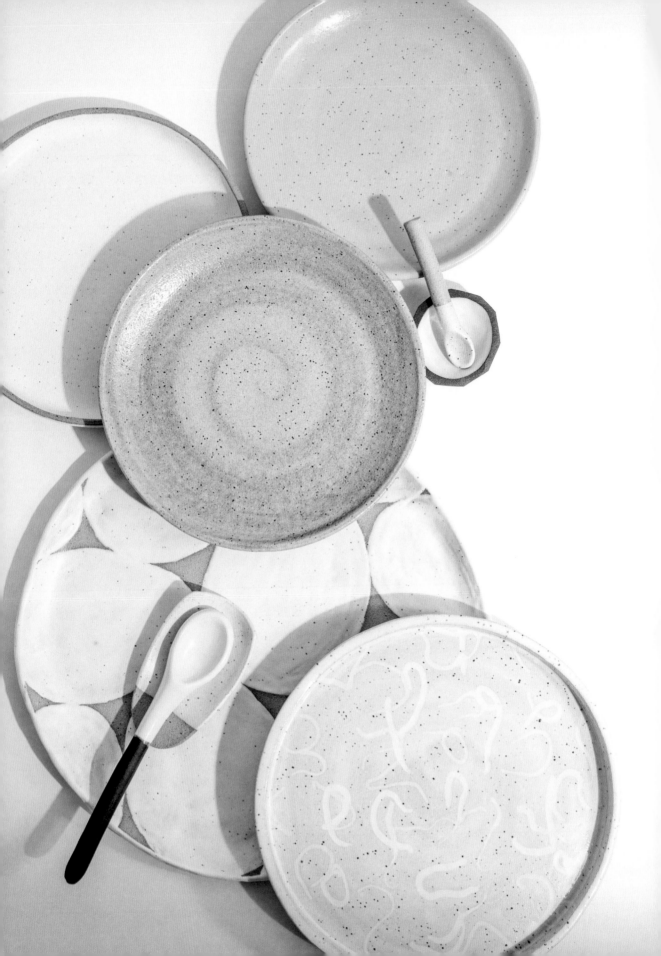

# Pumpkin Pie Energy Balls

DAIRY-FREE | GLUTEN-FREE | PALEO-FRIENDLY | VEGAN | VEGETARIAN

MAKES 12 ENERGY BALLS

My friend Melissa, who is a talented cook and has shot much of the food photography on my website, will go down in friendship history for famously saying, "The world really doesn't need another bliss ball." I totally get that, but these energy balls are delicious and definitely worth sharing. They are like little pumpkin pie truffles, packed with carotenoids, healthy fats, and anti-inflammatory spice. They are a great way to healthfully indulge a sweet tooth. And, Melissa likes them!

1. In a food processor, combine the dates and almonds and pulse into small pieces. Add the pumpkin purée, coconut butter, chia seeds, cinnamon, nutmeg, a pinch of allspice, and a pinch of cardamom. Pulse until well blended but with some ingredients still visible; you do not want a purée.

2. Using your hands, roll the mixture into twelve 1-inch (2.5 cm) diameter balls. In a small bowl, add the shredded coconut or cinnamon (if using) and roll the balls to coat. Store in a resealable container in the fridge for up to 1 week or in the freezer for up to 1 month.

Tip 1. Coconut butter, or coconut manna, is made from the flesh of the coconut, just like other nut butters. 2. You can also roll the energy balls in a mixture of equal amounts of cinnamon and almond meal so that they look like powdered doughnut holes.

10 Medjool dates, pitted

½ cup (125 mL) raw almonds

⅓ cup (75 mL) pure pumpkin purée

¼ cup (60 mL) coconut butter

1 tablespoon (15 mL) chia seeds

¼ teaspoon (1 mL) cinnamon

⅛ teaspoon (0.5 mL) ground nutmeg

Allspice

Ground cardamom

Finely shredded unsweetened coconut or cinnamon for rolling (optional)

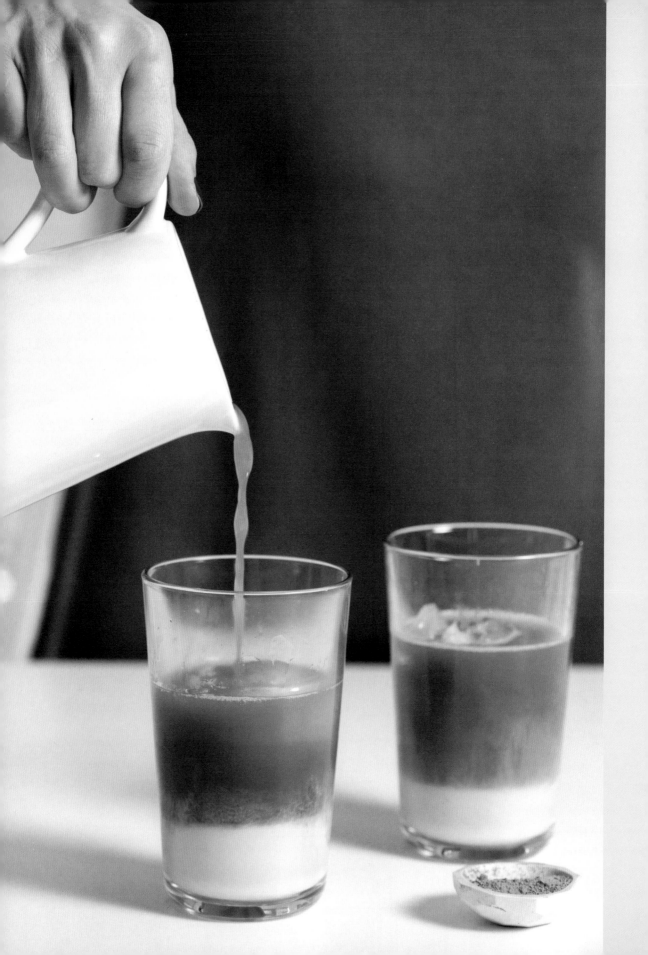

# 10
# Energizing Drinks

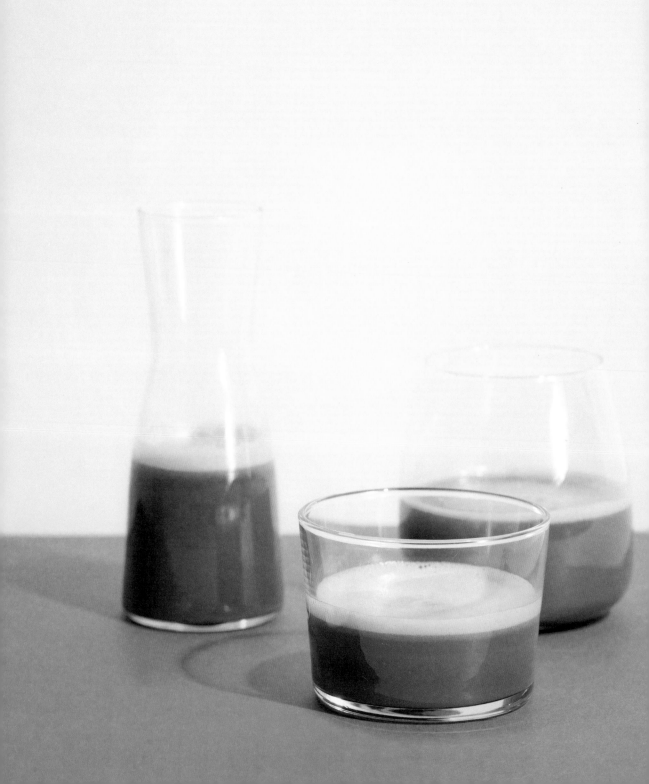

# Verdita

DAIRY-FREE | GLUTEN-FREE | NUT-FREE | PALEO-FRIENDLY | VEGAN | VEGETARIAN

MAKES 1 CUP (250 ML)

I am over the moon for all the flavours of Mexico, tequila included, which is where the inspiration for this drink came to me. Verdita means little green and is traditionally served as a chaser alongside tequila. It has savoury ingredients, but it is pleasantly sweet, with a side of sass. It is also extremely healthy. Cilantro and mint are packed with anti-inflammatory phytochemicals, yet we rarely eat them in meaningful amounts. You can take this as a wellness shot or add ¼ cup (60 mL) Verdita to 1 cup (250 mL) soda water. Friday fun times? Enjoy a shot alongside a shot of good tequila or shake up ¼ cup (60 mL) with 1 ounce (30 mL) of tequila or mezcal.

1. In a high-speed blender, add the cilantro, mint, jalapeño, pineapple chunks, lime juice, and cold water. Blend until smooth. If you want it really smooth, strain through a nut milk bag or a fine mesh sieve.

2. Serve cold. Store in the fridge for up to 3 days.

Tip Although most of the heat in a jalapeño is found in the seeds, the flesh varies in heat level, too. I like this juice with a bit of heat. So, cut off a tiny piece of the flesh and taste it. If it has some heat, go ahead and seed the pepper. If it is super mild, leave at least half the seeds on. The juice will not be too spicy, as the cilantro and mint cool it off nicely.

½ cup (125 mL) fresh cilantro leaves

⅓ cup (75 mL) fresh mint leaves

½ jalapeño pepper, seeded (see Tip)

1 cup (250 mL) fresh pineapple chunks

Juice of 2 limes (about ¼ cup/60 mL)

¼ cup (60 mL) cold water

# Iced Ginger Vanilla Matcha Latte

DAIRY-FREE | GLUTEN-FREE | NUT-FREE | PALEO-FRIENDLY | VEGAN | VEGETARIAN

SERVES 2

Green tea is one of the most researched anti-inflammatory and anti-cancer foods; epigallocatechin gallate is a green tea flavonoid that is super effective at squelching free radical damage. Matcha is specially grown green tea, ground into powder form, so you consume the whole leaf instead of throwing it away once you are done steeping. This means more anti-inflammatory power.

If you get caffeine jitters, matcha may be a better choice than coffee, as it contains L-theanine, an amino acid that helps to balance the effects of caffeine on the body. This is a lightly sweet drink perfect for beating the afternoon slump.

---

1 teaspoon (5 mL) matcha powder

½ cup (125 mL) near-boiling water

½ teaspoon (2 mL) ginger juice or ¼ teaspoon (1 mL) ground ginger

2 teaspoons (10 mL) pure maple syrup

1 teaspoon (5 mL) pure vanilla extract

1½ cups (375 mL) unsweetened vanilla almond milk or cashew milk

Ice

1. In a small bowl, whisk together the matcha and hot water until frothy.

2. Add the ginger, maple syrup, and vanilla and whisk again.

3. In a tall glass, pour the almond milk over ice and top with the matcha mixture.

Tip  As matcha becomes more popular, some manufacturers are offering regular green tea (Sencha) ground into powder, which has a more olive green colour than true matcha (Tencha), which should be very bright green. I recommend buying Japanese matcha, as there are concerns about lead contamination in matcha grown elsewhere.

Make It Faster  Ginger juice is super easy to make. Simply grate peeled fresh ginger on a microplane, then squeeze it between your fingers to release the juice. In a rush? Use ground ginger instead. It tastes great, too.

Make It Healthier  If you already love matcha, double the amount in the recipe for even more antioxidant power, but I recommend not drinking strong matcha after 3 p.m. or it might interfere with your sleep.

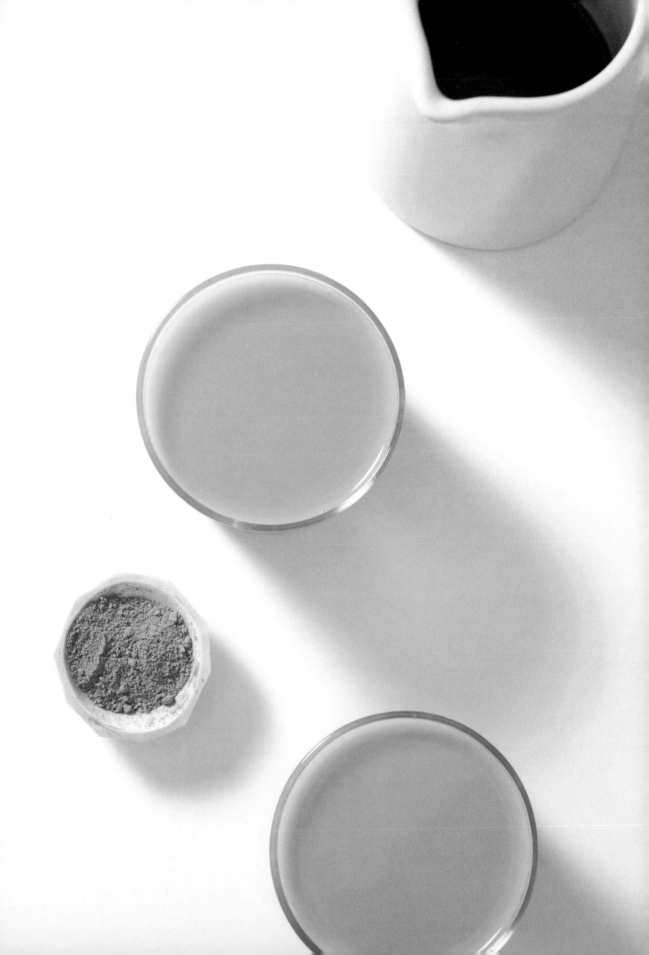

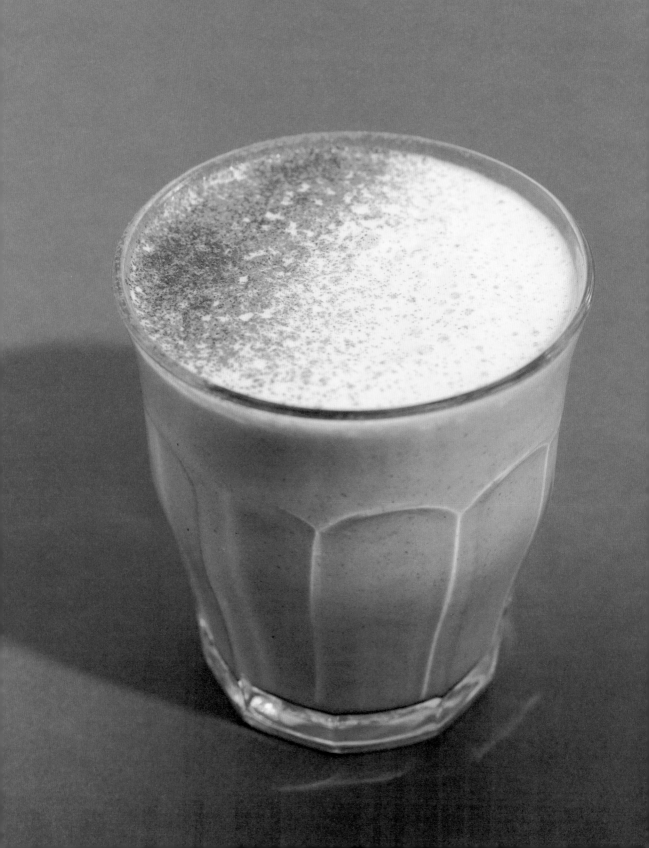

# Tahini Date Shake

DAIRY-FREE | GLUTEN-FREE | NUT-FREE | PALEO-FRIENDLY | VEGAN | VEGETARIAN

SERVES 2

A milkshake is a thing of beauty, especially when you still feel energized and vibrant after drinking it. Date shakes, the Palm Springs
staple, get a grown-up plant-based makeover with creamy, savoury,
mineral-rich tahini and soy milk instead of ice cream. Thick and rich,
using frozen banana makes this date shake even frostier. In a pinch,
just add a few ice cubes.

1.  In a high-speed blender, combine the dates, banana, soy milk, tahini,
    vanilla, nutmeg, cinnamon, and a pinch of salt. Blend until smooth.

2.  Add the ice cubes and blend again. The double blend really does
    make the milkshake extra smooth and frothy.

    Tip  Medjool dates are large fresh dates grown in the United
    States. Deglet Noor are smaller and typically imported but much
    softer and fruitier than the dried dates you might find on store
    shelves. Either one is delicious in this recipe.

4 large Medjool dates, soaked
in hot water for 5 minutes to
soften, drained, pitted, and
chopped

1 medium frozen peeled ripe
banana

1 cup (250 mL) unsweetened
soy milk

2 tablespoons (30 mL) raw
tahini

1 teaspoon (5 mL) pure vanilla
extract

⅛ teaspoon (0.5 mL) ground
nutmeg

⅛ teaspoon (0.5 mL) cinnamon

Salt

4 ice cubes

# Turmeric Chai

DAIRY-FREE | GLUTEN-FREE | PALEO-FRIENDLY | VEGAN | VEGETARIAN

**SERVES 1 (MAKES ENOUGH TURMERIC CHAI MIX FOR 12 SERVINGS)**

A warm, spicy cup of tea is heavenly. Inspired by both golden milk lattes and masala chai, I wanted a mix that I could keep in the pantry to make a soothing drink anytime I had a craving. Packed with anti-inflammatory turmeric and digestion-soothing spices, this is a wonderful lightly caffeinated drink, so you can enjoy a couple of cups in the afternoon without worrying you will be up all night. Sweetened with blackstrap molasses and boosted with my Masala Chai Almond Butter (page 261), this is a truly nourishing drink. The molasses adds a boost of minerals and the almond butter makes it creamier and improves the absorption of the turmeric.

---

**Turmeric Chai Mix**
**(enough for 12 cups of chai)**

4 teaspoons (20 mL) cinnamon

2 teaspoons (10 mL) ground turmeric

2 teaspoons (10 mL) ground cardamom

1 teaspoon (5 mL) ground fennel seeds

1 teaspoon (5 mL) ground ginger

⅛ teaspoon (0.5 mL) ground cloves

⅛ teaspoon (0.5 mL) freshly cracked pepper

Tea leaves from 2 Darjeeling black tea bags (about 3 teaspoons/15 mL loose tea leaves)

**For Each Cup of Turmeric Chai**

¾ cup (175 mL) unsweetened almond milk or cashew milk

1 teaspoon (5 mL) Turmeric Chai Mix (recipe above)

1 teaspoon (5 mL) blackstrap molasses

1 teaspoon (5 mL) Masala Chai Almond Butter (page 261) or raw almond butter

1. **Make the Turmeric Chai Mix** Combine the cinnamon, turmeric, cardamom, fennel seeds, ginger, cloves, pepper, and tea leaves in a 1-cup (250 mL) mason jar.

2. For each cup of Turmeric Chai, in a small saucepan simmer the almond milk and Turmeric Chai Mix over medium-low heat for 10 minutes, watching that it does not scorch.

3. Add the molasses and almond butter. Whisk vigorously, pour into your favourite mug, and serve.

4. The mixture settles over time, so stir occasionally as you sip. You can strain the tea prior to drinking, but I like to get all that spicy goodness into my belly!

Tip Love pumpkin? Try simmering the chai with 2 tablespoons (30 mL) pure pumpkin purée per serving and replace the blackstrap molasses with 1 teaspoon (5 mL) pure maple syrup.

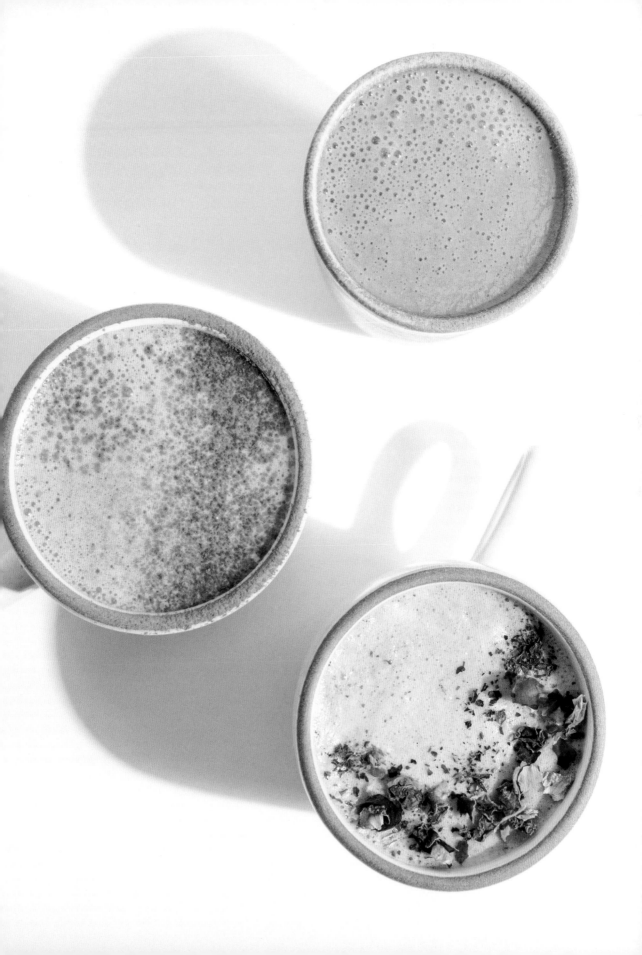

# Cardamom Rose Beet Latte

DAIRY-FREE | GLUTEN-FREE | NUT-FREE | PALEO-FRIENDLY | VEGAN | VEGETARIAN

SERVES 2

My spice drawer is total chaos. I am always buying stuff that I rarely use because some recipe calls for it. However, I use few spices as much as cardamom. It is sweet and peppery, and I cannot get enough of it. It is thought to be excellent for digestion. Cardamom pods, lightly crushed, make for a better pot of tea or coffee. Ground cardamom is my go-to for most sweets.

This latte is inspired by the flavours of the eastern Mediterranean. Rosewater and cardamom give it a unique perfume that is super soothing to the mind. When you want a warm, comforting beverage that is not coffee, curl up with one of these. Yes, there is an anti-inflammatory beet in there for good measure. It will make your drink look like a pink cloud.

---

2 cups (500 mL) unsweetened cashew milk or oat milk

⅔ cup (150 mL) peeled and chopped cooked red beet or ¼ cup (60 mL) beet juice

3 to 4 teaspoons (15 to 20 mL) pure maple syrup

2 teaspoons (10 mL) rosewater

½ teaspoon (2 mL) pure vanilla extract

¼ teaspoon (1 mL) ground cardamom

1. In a small saucepan, heat the cashew milk over medium heat until just steaming. Remove from the heat.

2. In a blender or using a handheld immersion blender in the saucepan, blend the cashew milk, beet, maple syrup, rosewater, vanilla, and cardamom until frothy and well combined.

Tip 1. You may be surprised to learn that most grocery stores sell beet juice. You usually can find it on the top shelf in the juice aisle in a little glass bottle, from a European company called Biotta.
2. Rosewater can pose its own challenges; it can vary greatly in aroma, with some being much more potent. Taste yours; if it is very mild, you may want to adjust the amount you use.

# Cinnamon Walnut Horchata

DAIRY-FREE | GLUTEN-FREE | VEGAN | VEGETARIAN

MAKES 4 CUPS (1 L)

I typically observe four major groups of drinkables: water, matcha, coffee, and wine. However, I occasionally make an exception for Horchata. Horchata is a cinnamon-infused plant-based milk that comes in many variations; typically, the base is nuts, seeds, and rice. I have chosen walnuts here for a more complex flavour and added omega-3 fats. Try using this Horchata to take your lattes to the next level.

1.  In a high-speed blender, combine the brown rice, white rice, walnuts, and cinnamon with 2 cups (500 mL) of the water. Pulse until a uniform slurry forms.

2.  Add the remaining 2 cups (500 mL) water, maple syrup, coconut butter, vanilla, and a pinch of salt. Blend to combine.

3.  Place the blender jar in the fridge for 24 hours to infuse, then reblend and strain through a nut milk bag over a bowl to remove solids. Pour into glass bottles with lids and store in the fridge for 3 to 4 days

    Tip  A bit of separation is normal because no stabilizers are used, so give the bottles a little shake before pouring.

½ cup (125 mL) brown basmati rice

½ cup (125 mL) white basmati rice

½ cup (125 mL) raw walnuts

3-inch (8 cm) cinnamon stick

4 cups (1 L) water, divided

¼ cup (60 mL) pure maple syrup

1 tablespoon (15 mL) coconut butter

1 tablespoon (15 mL) pure vanilla extract

Salt

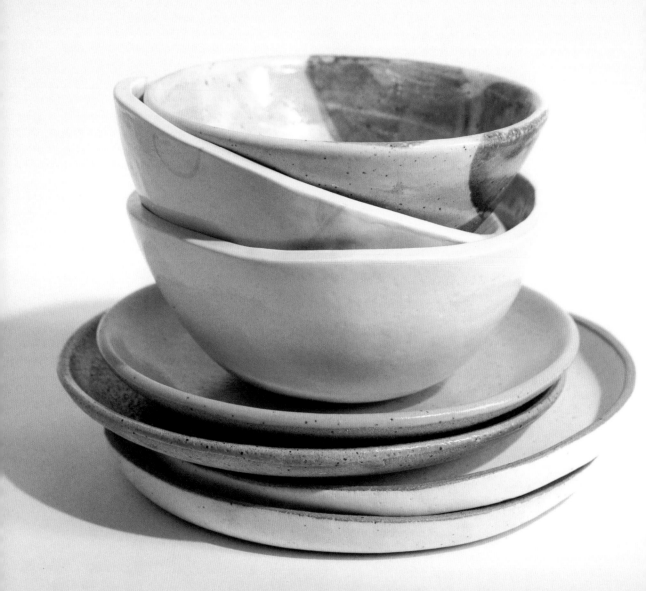

# Superfood Hot Chocolate

DAIRY-FREE | GLUTEN-FREE | PALEO-FRIENDLY | VEGAN | VEGETARIAN

SERVES 1

I grew up on packaged hot chocolate mix. When I discovered how easy it is to make from scratch and how much healthier that makes it, I never bought the packaged stuff again! Raw cacao or natural, non-Dutched cocoa powder are very high in flavonoids that help give your skin that glow and fight inflammation. This simple sipper was designed as a foil for my favourite adaptogen, ashwagandha, but it is delicious and good for you all on its own!

1. In a small saucepan, warm the cashew milk over medium heat. Remove from the heat; add the cacao, almond butter, cinnamon, maple syrup, vanilla and ashwagandha (if using) and blend with a handheld immersion blender.

2. Pour into a mug and enjoy.

Tip Making this a special treat? Top with coconut whip. Keep a can of full-fat coconut milk chilled in the fridge. Scoop out just the thick cream from the can and beat it like whipping cream.

Make It Faster If your blender has a heat setting, simply blend the cashew milk, cacao, almond butter, cinnamon, maple syrup, and vanilla until frothy and warm.

1 cup (250 mL) unsweetened cashew milk or almond milk

1 tablespoon (15 mL) raw cacao or pure baking cocoa

1 tablespoon (15 mL) raw almond butter

½ teaspoon (2 mL) cinnamon

1 to 2 teaspoons (5 to 10 mL) pure maple syrup

¼ teaspoon (1 mL) pure vanilla extract or powder

½ teaspoon (2 mL) ashwagandha or your favourite adaptogen powder (optional)

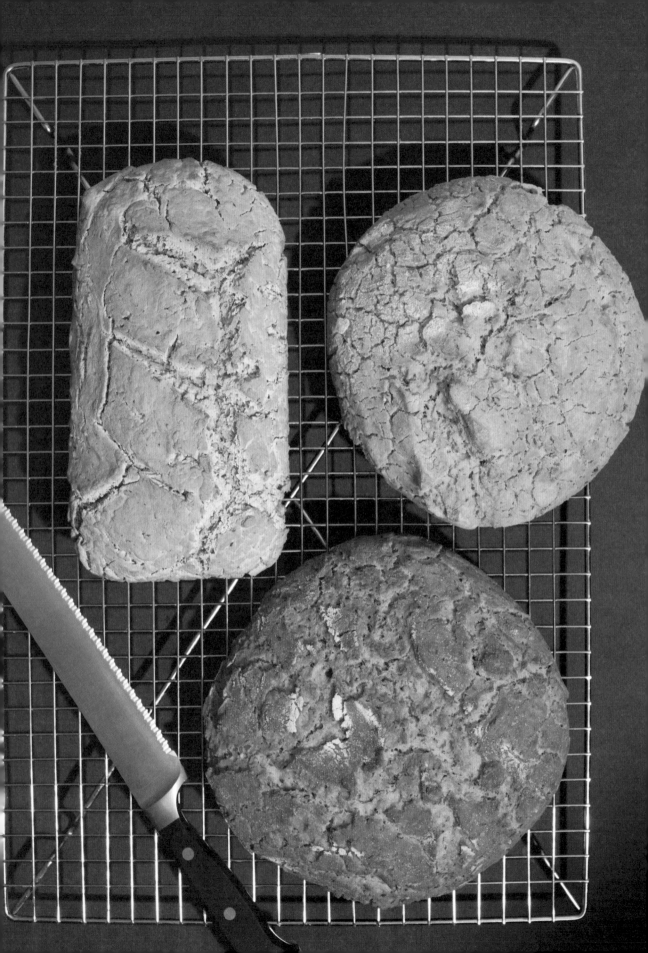

# 11

# Plant-Based Staples

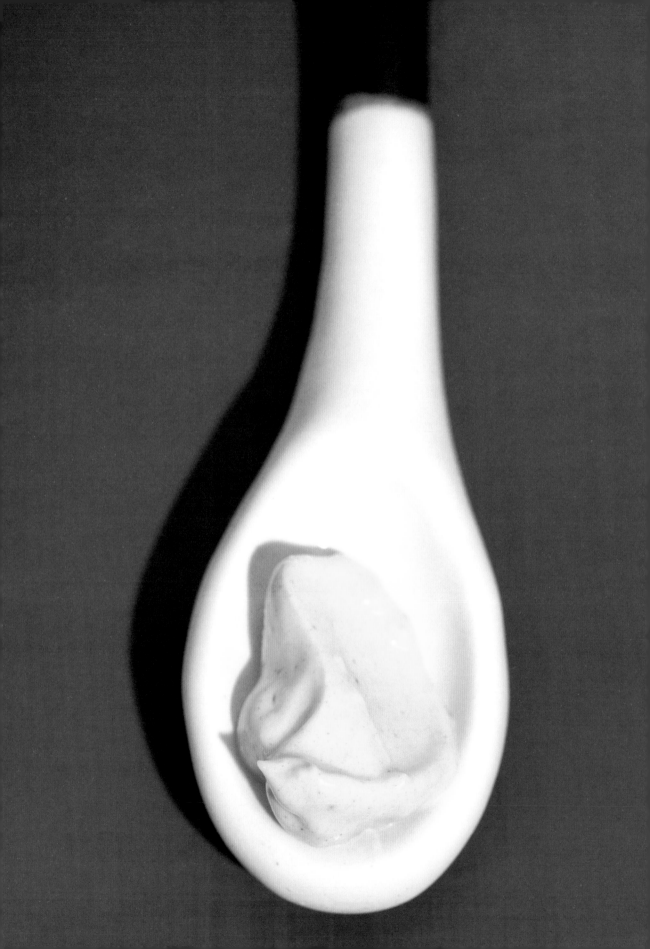

# Turmeric Mayonnaise

DAIRY-FREE | GLUTEN-FREE | NUT-FREE | VEGAN | VEGETARIAN

**MAKES ABOUT ½ CUP (125 ML)**

Mayonnaise is one of my favourite spreads, but I never understood why people think of it as unhealthy. Of course, its healthfulness hinges on the quality of oil you use. Filtered avocado oil contains the same primary fat as olive oil, monounsaturated oleic acid, and has a light taste that does not compete with the flavour of classic mayonnaise. Liquid from canned chickpeas (aquafaba) holds the key to making homemade mayonnaise a snap; unlike with traditional recipes, you do not have to worry about the emulsion breaking. This recipe is so simple that you may never need to buy mayonnaise again, and so delicious that you may not want to.

---

1. In a wide-mouthed jar, combine the avocado oil, chickpea liquid, lemon juice, mustard, garlic, salt, turmeric, sugar, and pepper. Using a handheld immersion blender, mix until a thick mayonnaise texture forms, about 30 seconds.

2. Store in the jar, covered with a lid, in the fridge for up to 5 days.

Tip  1. Filtered avocado oil is a better choice for this mayonnaise than unfiltered because it has a milder taste, and it is also wonderful for high-heat cooking. This is one recipe where I urge you not to use extra-virgin olive oil; it will taste funny, as the polyphenols in cold-pressed oil turn bitter at high friction. 2. If you want a milder flavoured white mayonnaise for everyday use, omit the turmeric and use just ½ a garlic clove.

½ cup (125 mL) filtered avocado oil

2 tablespoons (30 mL) liquid from canned chickpeas

1 tablespoon (15 mL) freshly squeezed lemon juice

1 teaspoon (5 mL) Dijon mustard

1 clove garlic, crushed or grated on a microplane

½ teaspoon (2 mL) salt

¼ teaspoon (1 mL) ground turmeric

¼ teaspoon (1 mL) cane sugar

Freshly cracked pepper

# Almond Ricotta Cheese

DAIRY-FREE | GLUTEN-FREE | PALEO-FRIENDLY | VEGAN | VEGETARIAN

MAKES 1½ CUPS (375 ML)

For many years, I thought I could not give up my love affair with cheese. Part of the reason was that what counted as vegan cheese had more in common with edible putty than actual food. Then some magical human figured out how beautifully nuts step in for cheese.

Almond Ricotta Cheese is high in gut-friendly fibre, protein, and two nutrients—calcium and magnesium—that are key when you are swapping out dairy. This is delish smothered over toast, as a creamy layer for a vegetable lasagna, or on salads.

1½ cups (375 mL) raw almonds, soaked in water for at least 4 hours or overnight, drained, and rinsed

¼ cup (60 mL) water

2 tablespoons (30 mL) freshly squeezed lemon juice

½ clove garlic

½ teaspoon (2 mL) salt

1. Rub the skin off the almonds. Soaking should help to remove the skin.

2. In a food processor, combine the almonds, water, lemon juice, garlic, and salt. Process for 2 to 3 minutes until the ingredients resemble ricotta cheese, loosely puréed with a bit of texture. The ricotta should form a soft ball when pressed in your hand.

3. Taste and adjust the salt and add a dash more lemon juice, if needed. Store in a resealable container in the fridge for up to 1 week.

**Make It Faster**  You can substitute soaked blanched natural almonds to eliminate the peeling step. Make this cheese ahead of time and refresh with a squeeze of lemon juice before serving, as it tends to dry out a bit.

# Masala Chai Almond Butter

DAIRY-FREE | GLUTEN-FREE | PALEO-FRIENDLY | VEGAN | VEGETARIAN

MAKES 1 CUP (250 ML)

Turmeric aside, spices are probably the most underrated anti-inflammatory food. In larger amounts, cinnamon supports blood sugar balance. Ginger can ease an unsettled stomach and fight inflammation. Clove is antibacterial. While many of us in North America are light handed with spices, many food cultures around the world lavish their meals with spice. In that spicy spirit, I have infused homemade almond butter so it is reminiscent of a cup of chai tea. It is so easy to make almond butter, but it does take a bit of patience. A hint of maple syrup helps bring out the flavours of the spices without adding too much actual sugar.

---

1.  In a food processor, combine the almonds, almond oil, cinnamon, cardamom, allspice, cloves, ginger, fennel seeds, salt, and pepper and process until a rich, thick, creamy-looking butter forms and no visible nut texture remains. Scrape the sides of the bowl if the blending stalls or builds up, which will be more frequent in the first 10 minutes of processing. It takes time for the oils to start releasing, and both the food processor and the almond butter will warm up. A silky almond butter should form in 15 to 20 minutes.

2.  Stir in the maple syrup (if using), 1 teaspoon (5 mL) at a time, once the almond butter is smooth. If you add the maple syrup too soon, the butter will seize up and take extra time to process. Store in a resealable container in the fridge for up to 2 weeks.

2 cups (500 mL) raw almonds

2 tablespoons (30 mL) almond oil or avocado oil

1 teaspoon (5 mL) cinnamon

½ teaspoon (2 mL) ground cardamom

½ teaspoon (2 mL) allspice

¼ teaspoon (1 mL) ground cloves

¼ teaspoon (1 mL) ground ginger

⅛ teaspoon (0.5 mL) ground or crushed fennel seeds

¼ teaspoon (1 mL) salt

Freshly cracked pepper

1 to 3 teaspoons (5 to 15 mL) pure maple syrup (optional)

# Beet Pesto

DAIRY-FREE | GLUTEN-FREE | PALEO-FRIENDLY | VEGAN | VEGETARIAN

MAKE 1¼ CUPS (300 ML)

You love beets, but you do not eat a lot of them. I get it. They take time to prepare, and they are not easy to snack on or the kind of vegetable you put in a stir-fry. This sweet and earthy pesto will remove all excuses for not getting more beets in your diet. I like to spread this beet pesto on crackers or toast, dollop it on a salad or grain bowl, or toss it with pasta. Using cooked beets, it takes 30 seconds to make! Filled with powerful plant pigments and omega-3 fats, it has never been this easy to eat your veggies.

---

1 cup (250 mL) chopped peeled cooked red beet

½ cup (125 mL) raw walnuts

1 clove garlic, crushed or grated on a microplane

2 tablespoons (30 mL) freshly squeezed lemon juice

½ teaspoon (2 mL) salt

Ground fennel seed

Ground thyme

⅓ cup (75 mL) olive oil

1. In a small food processor, purée the beet, walnuts, garlic, lemon juice, salt, and a pinch each of fennel seed and thyme. With the processor running, drizzle in the olive oil until just combined.

2. Store in a resealable container in the fridge for up to 1 week.


Tip  Buying pre-cooked beets at the grocery store is a godsend. No prep, no waste. Of course, if you have beets kicking around, you can always roast them yourself. Peel and quarter a large red beet, drizzle with olive oil and salt, and roast tightly wrapped in foil for 35 to 45 minutes or until fork-tender.

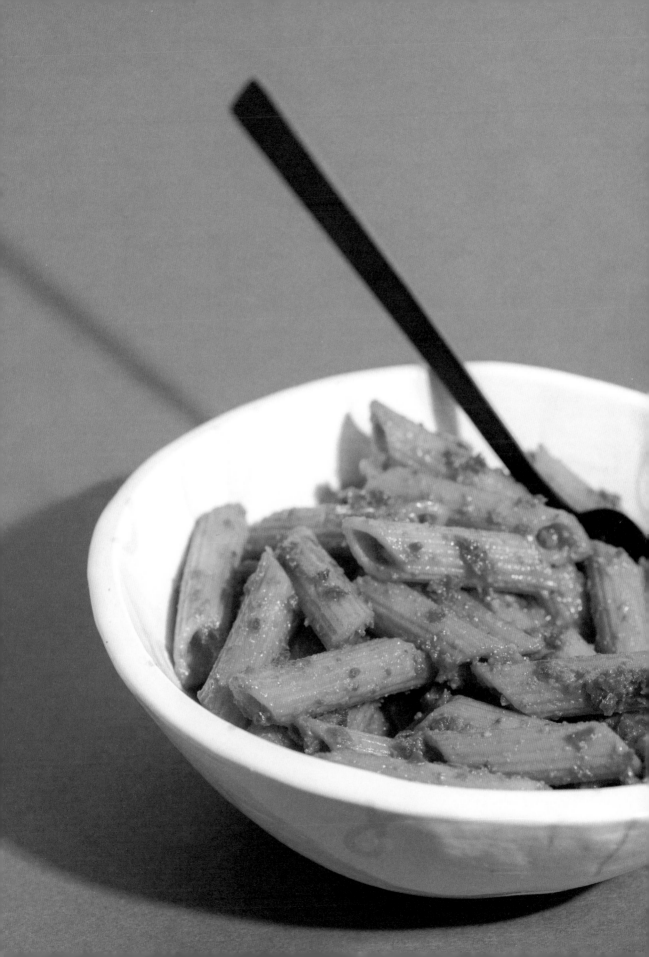

# Queso Dip

DAIRY-FREE | GLUTEN-FREE | NUT-FREE | VEGAN | VEGETARIAN

SERVES 4 TO 6

## Basic Queso

3 tablespoons (45 mL) extra-virgin olive oil

1 medium sweet onion, chopped

2 medium carrots, scrubbed and diced

2 cloves garlic, sliced

1 cup (250 mL) plain unsweetened soy milk

½ cup (125 mL) nutritional yeast

¼ cup (60 mL) chopped pickled jalepeño peppers

2 tablespoons (30 mL) freshly squeezed lemon juice

1 tablespoon (15 mL) tomato paste

1 tablespoon (15 mL) Dijon mustard

1 teaspoon (5 mL) jalapeño pepper pickling liquid

½ teaspoon (2 mL) chili powder

½ teaspoon (2 mL) ground cumin

½ teaspoon (2 mL) salt

Queso is life. Poured over chips, it is nachos. Served with veggies, a cheesy dip can make anyone excited to eat more plants. You can even toss it with pasta for a spunky mac and cheese. Queso is often made with butternut squash, which I find too sweet, but I have kept the veggies in with plenty of phytochemical-rich onion, carrot, garlic, and tomato paste. I like to pour this sauce over a plate of tortilla chips loaded with chopped tomato, green pepper, sliced olives, and black beans for a healthier nacho night.

The heart of any queso is nutritional yeast, which is protein-rich, high in B vitamins for energy metabolism, and packed with umami. B vitamins are a great support in times of stress, so eating this queso is practically therapeutic.

1. In a medium skillet, heat the olive oil over medium-high heat. Add the onion and sauté for 3 minutes, stirring occasionally. Add the carrot and cook until fork-tender and the onion is golden, about 7 minutes. Add the garlic and cook for 1 minute more.

2. Add the onion mixture, soy milk, nutritional yeast, jalapeño, lemon juice, tomato paste, mustard, jalapeño liquid, chili powder, cumin, and salt to a high-speed blender and blend on high until smooth.

3. Pour the blended queso into the skillet and gently heat to the desired temperature (or keep warm in a fondue pot).

## Variations

**Roasted Tomato and Black Bean** Omit the tomato paste and jalapeño pepper and juice. Once blended, stir ½ cup (125 mL) canned fire-roasted tomatoes and ¾ cup (175 mL) cooked black beans into the queso. Taste and adjust seasoning with salt and lemon juice.

**Chipotle** Swap ¼ cup (60 mL) chipotle peppers packed in adobo sauce for the pickled jalapeño. Taste and adjust seasoning with salt and lemon juice.

# Seedy Crackers

DAIRY-FREE | GLUTEN-FREE | NUT-FREE | VEGAN | VEGETARIAN

MAKES TWENTY-FOUR 2-INCH (5 CM) CRACKERS

I have eaten so many little dehydrated seed crackers that I should probably buy stock in the company, or make my own. How easy is it to make your own crackers? It takes just 10 minutes!

Instead of being nutrient-poor and blood sugar–spiking, these seed crackers are packed with fibre, protein, and omega-3 fatty acids—tasty, crispy, feel-good food. They are delicious with any topping you can imagine; I recommend trying them with my Truffled Mushroom Pâté (page 189), Spiced Carrot Dip (page 193), or a thick spread of Almond Ricotta Cheese (page 260) and a drizzle of balsamic glaze.

---

1. Preheat the oven to 350°F (180°C). Line a baking sheet with parchment paper and set aside an additional piece of parchment paper.

2. In a medium bowl, whisk together the chickpea flour, water, chia seeds, salt, garlic, lemon juice, and a pinch of chili flakes and soak for 5 minutes. Mix in the sunflower seeds, hemp seeds, and pumpkin seeds to form a moist, thick dough.

3. Spread the cracker dough onto the prepared baking sheet. Lay the second piece of parchment paper on top. With a rolling pin, evenly roll out the cracker dough to ¼-inch (5 mm) thickness. Remove the top layer of parchment paper and discard. Smooth the top of the cracker dough with wet hands, if necessary.

4. Bake for 20 minutes or until golden brown. Lift the parchment paper onto a cutting board and, using a pizza cutter, score the crackers, forming 2-inch (5 cm) square crackers. Let cool completely and store in an airtight container for up to 1 week.

Tip  If the crackers lose their crispness, simply reheat in a 350°F (180°F) oven for 10 minutes.

½ cup (125 mL) chickpea flour

½ cup + 1 tablespoon (140 mL) water

¼ cup (60 mL) chia seeds

2 teaspoons (10 mL) salt

½ clove garlic, crushed or grated on a microplane

1 teaspoon (5 mL) freshly squeezed lemon juice

Red chili flakes

1 cup (250 mL) raw sunflower seeds

½ cup (125 mL) hemp seeds

½ cup (125 mL) raw pumpkin seeds

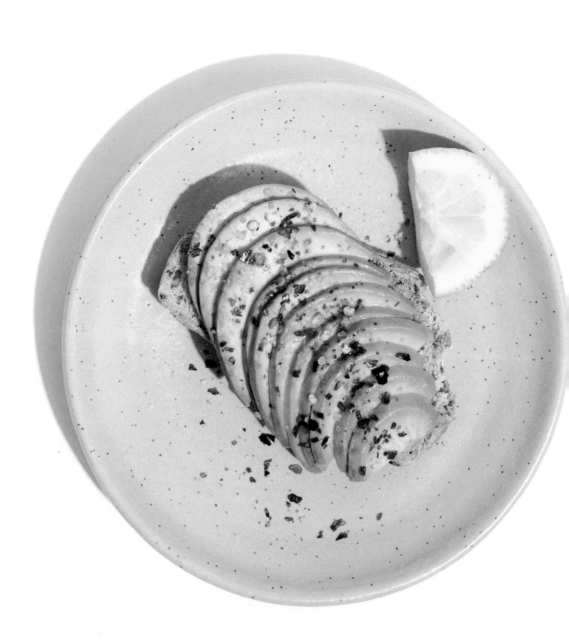

# Real Deal Gluten-Free Bread

DAIRY-FREE | GLUTEN-FREE | NUT-FREE | VEGAN | VEGETARIAN

MAKES 1 LOAF

When I was about halfway through recipe development, I asked my community what recipes they would like to see in the book. Overwhelmingly, the answer was "good bread!" I am a novice baker, so I was a bit worried, but I had one ace up my sleeve. I knew how to make Jim Lahey's No-Knead Bread. However, could I take inspiration from Lahey and create a gluten-free version?

I did my research on flours and found that Bob's Red Mill All Purpose Flour (not the 1-to-1 blend) seemed to have the best protein content. I adapted the method slightly to acknowledge that gluten-free bread is not going to rise like the regular stuff. Then I gave it a go and it worked. I actually teared up when I ate this bread. It looks like a real deal bakery loaf. The chickpea-based flour gives it a very savoury and rich flavour. It is great for making sandwiches like the Shiitake BLT Sandwich (page 139) or serving alongside soups and stews like the Red Grape, Chickpea, and Pine Nut Stew (page 149). It is so much better than store-bought! Not quick, but it is easy to make and worth every minute.

1. In a large bowl, whisk together the flour, yeast, flaxseed, and salt. Add the water and stir until blended. It will look more like a thick cake batter and not like bread dough at this point, but do not worry. Cover the bowl with plastic wrap and wrap a clean kitchen towel around the bowl to keep it cozy and warm.

2. Let the dough rest for 12 hours. If your kitchen is not warm, I highly recommend storing it in your oven with the light turned on.

3. Lightly flour a large cutting board and place the dough on it, using just enough flour to make it possible to knead gently until the dough feels slightly drier and more dough-like. Work into a round dough ball, with the seam side down. Sprinkle a bit more flour on the ball and place a clean kitchen towel over it, letting it rest for 2 hours.

4. Place a 7¼-quart (6.9 L) cast iron or enamel pot in the oven and preheat to 450°F (230°C).

3 cups (750 mL) gluten-free all-purpose flour, plus more for preparation

1 teaspoon (5 mL) traditional yeast (not instant)

¼ cup (60 mL) ground flaxseed

1½ teaspoons (7 mL) salt

1⅔ cup (400 mL) water

*recipe continues*

5.  When the dough is ready, if it has flattened and spread out, give the dough a couple more kneads and re-form it into a ball with the seam side down. Carefully remove the pot from the oven and place the dough ball into the pot, giving it as much height as possible, since it will not rise much in cooking. Place the lid on the pot and bake for 30 minutes until the loaf is golden brown.

6.  Remove the lid and bake for 5 to 10 minutes more until the loaf is a deep golden brown. Remove the bread from the pot and cool on a rack. Slice when completely cooled. Bread will keep in a paper bag on the counter for up to 2 days. You can also slice and freeze whatever you will not use immediately, tightly wrapped in plastic wrap, for up to 1 month.

# DIY Alternative Flour

DAIRY-FREE | VEGAN | VEGETARIAN

MAKES 2 CUPS (500 ML)

There is nothing worse than running out of flour when you are making something. Just ask a gal who tests recipes for a living. I feel like I wore out the sidewalk between my house and the grocery store while writing this book.

If you do run out, or if you find yourself with limited supplies at your local store, it is super easy to make your own alternative flours. Simply grind nuts such as blanched almonds or walnuts, dried chickpeas, lentils, millet, or rolled oats in a food processor or high-speed blender until it turns into flour. Yes, it is that easy, and it takes about 60 seconds.

---

1. In a food processor or high-speed blender, add the nuts, chickpeas, lentils, or whole grains and process to a flour-like consistency.

2. Sift the flour into a bowl to capture any large unprocessed pieces. Return these pieces to the food processor or high-speed blender and process until fine. Use immediately or store in a resealable container in the fridge for up to 2 weeks or in the freezer for up to 1 month.

2 cups (500 mL) nuts, dried chickpeas, lentils, or whole grains

# DIY Nut Milk

DAIRY-FREE | GLUTEN-FREE | VEGAN | VEGETARIAN

MAKES ABOUT 4 CUPS (1 L)

If you have never made your own nut milk, you may be surprised at how easy and how delicious it is. Not as easy as buying a 2-quart (2 L) carton at the store, but still quite easy!

You can make your own nut milk from almost any nut, including macadamia nuts, cashews, almonds, hazelnuts, walnuts, or a combination of these.

---

**Basic Recipe**

1 cup (250 mL) raw nuts

4 cups (1 L) water

Salt

**Sweetener Options**
(choose one)

2 to 3 Medjool dates, pitted

1 tablespoon (15 mL) pure maple syrup

**Flavour Options**
(choose one or all)

½ teaspoon (5 mL) pure vanilla extract

¼ teaspoon (1 mL) cinnamon

¼ teaspoon (1 mL) cardamom

1 cup (250 mL) fresh berries (strawberries, blueberries, or blackberries)

1. Soak the nuts in the water for 8 to 12 hours or overnight. Rinse, drain, and place them in a high-speed blender with a pinch of salt and any desired sweeteners or flavours. Blend on high for 1 to 2 minutes until smooth.

2. You can drink the nut milk as is, especially if you are going to use it in a smoothie, but for a less gritty and more milk-like experience, you will want to strain it using a nut milk bag.

3. To strain, place a nut milk bag over a large bowl and pour the milk, in batches, into the bag. Wring out the bag until all that is left is the dry nut pulp. Pour the nut milk into a resealable bottle or mason jar and store in the fridge for up to 2 to 3 days for best flavour and texture.

Tip Save the nut pulp and dry it out in a 200°F (100°C) oven for 1 to 2 hours, checking every 15 minutes after the first hour, until completely dry. You can process it in a food processor to make it extra fine if you wish. Store in a reusable container in the freezer for up to 3 months and use it like flour in recipes for crackers, muffins, or pancakes.

# Fermented Cashew Cream Cheese

DAIRY-FREE | GLUTEN-FREE | PALEO-FRIENDLY | VEGAN | VEGETARIAN

MAKES 2 CUPS (500 ML)

Cashews are a clever stand-in for dairy for a couple of reasons: high in protein, magnesium, iron, and zinc, cashews help replace nutrients commonly found in animal products. They also have a sprinkling of the anti-inflammatory minerals copper and selenium. Cashew cheese is lovely, but when fermented it takes on that fresh, tangy flavour that makes cream cheese so dreamy. Because it takes time to ferment, this recipe makes a big batch, but it will keep in the fridge for a couple of weeks. Try slathering this creamy spread on Seedy Crackers (page 265) or Green Machine Burgers (page 140) or use it as a second layer for the Tomato Jam Tartines (page 210).

---

**2 cups (500 mL) raw cashews**

**¼ cup (60 mL) water**

**½ teaspoon (2 mL) salt, divided**

**1 fifty billion–CFU probiotic capsule (I use Bio-K+)**

**1 teaspoon (5 mL) freshly squeezed lemon juice**

1. In a medium bowl, soak the cashews in water for 4 to 12 hours. Drain and rinse well.

2. In a high-speed blender, combine the soaked cashews, water, and ¼ teaspoon (1 mL) of the salt and blend until very smooth but not liquid, 2 to 3 minutes. If the mixture is too thick, add more water, 1 tablespoon (15 mL) at a time, to assist with the blending.

3. Place the cashew cream in a medium glass bowl or large jar and stir in the contents of the probiotic capsule. Cut a round piece of parchment paper to fit over the cashew cream to help prevent it from drying out, then cover the bowl with plastic wrap and let it sit for 24 to 28 hours on the counter.

4. Stir in the remaining ¼ teaspoon (1 mL) salt and lemon juice. Store in a resealable container in the fridge for up to 2 weeks.

Tip  You can easily make a half-portion of this recipe, using the same strength of probiotic.

## Variation

Try flavouring the cream cheese with different flavours, depending on your taste: cinnamon and maple syrup make a lovely sweet version, or try savoury fresh dill with a bit of grated garlic or hot sauce and roasted garlic.

# Fermented Ketchup

DAIRY-FREE | GLUTEN-FREE | PALEO-FRIENDLY | VEGAN | VEGETARIAN

MAKES 1¼ CUPS (300 ML)

I may be the only person on the planet who did not like ketchup as a kid. I was staunchly in the mayonnaise camp. I am always on the lookout for savoury over sweet, so I wanted to try my hand at making my own ketchup.

Tomato paste is the most concentrated source of anti-inflammatory lycopene. With a bit of garlic and spice, you can legitimately think of this condiment as a health food. This still has that sweet acidity you associate with store-bought varieties, but it is not as sweet. A light fermentation gives it that tang that makes it extra special.

1 cup (250 mL) tomato paste

¼ cup (60 mL) raw apple cider vinegar

3 tablespoons (45 mL) pure maple syrup

2 tablespoons (30 mL) fermented vegetable brine (such as from sauerkraut)

1 clove garlic, crushed or grated on a microplane

1 teaspoon (5 mL) salt

⅛ teaspoon (0.5 mL) ground cardamom

Ground cloves

Allspice

1.  In a medium bowl, whisk together the tomato paste, apple cider vinegar, maple syrup, vegetable brine, garlic, salt, cardamom, and a pinch each of cloves and allspice. Let sit on the counter, covered with cheesecloth or paper towel secured by a rubber band, for 8 hours.

2.  Transfer the fermented ketchup to a resealable container and store in the fridge for up to 3 weeks.

Tip This ketchup has a tendency to thicken after 3 or 4 days without any loss of quality. If it thickens, remove a portion and reblend with 1 to 2 tablespoons (15 to 30 mL) of water to loosen it up.

# Lacto-Fermented Beet Noodles

DAIRY-FREE | GLUTEN-FREE | NUT-FREE | PALEO-FRIENDLY | VEGAN | VEGETARIAN

MAKES 1¼ CUP (300 ML)

Pickled beets go well with everything, so you will want to keep a jar of these on hand in the fridge for an instant veggie boost. Unlike onions, beets create their own brine, which is cool to watch. If you do not have a spiralizer, you can use a veggie peeler to make long, thin ribbons.

1. Wash a 2-cup (500 mL) mason jar with a lot of hot, soapy water and dry with a clean kitchen towel to avoid contamination.

2. Spiralize the beets and place them in a medium bowl. Sprinkle with the salt and massage the beets with your hands for 2 to 3 minutes, until they visibly wilt and start to release at least 2 to 3 tablespoons (30 to 45 mL) of juice.

3. Pack the spiralized beets into the clean mason jar and pour the beet brine on top, pressing the beets down to submerge them in their brine. Use a fermentation weight or a small resealable plastic bag filled with water to keep the beets under the brine. Loosely seal the lid on the jar. You want to protect the beets from dirt, while allowing some oxygen to reach the mixture to avoid promoting the growth of dangerous microbes.

4. Let sit in a warm area, away from direct sunlight, to ferment for 3 to 4 days. To test, give the beets a taste; if they have a nice pickled tang, they are ready! If not, make sure they are in a warm spot, wrap the jar with a clean kitchen towel to insulate, and let them ferment for up to 7 days to achieve the right flavour.

5. Once fermented, remove the weight, tightly seal the lid on the mason jar, and store in the fridge for up to 2 weeks.

2 large red beets, trimmed and peeled

1 teaspoon (5 mL) salt

# Lacto-Fermented Turmeric Onions

DAIRY-FREE | GLUTEN-FREE | NUT-FREE | PALEO-FRIENDLY | VEGAN | VEGETARIAN

MAKES 2 CUPS (500 ML)

When you multiply the gut and immune benefits of raw onion with turmeric and fermentation, they become a very worthy addition to any meal. Their sulphur-based compounds have anti-cancer and anti-microbial effects and also support the growth of beneficial bacteria in the gut with their prebiotic fructans. Enjoy these pickled onions as a condiment on grain bowls, sandwiches, wraps, and salads. The fermenting liquid gives a nice little kick to salad dressings and sauces. You can also swap in these onions for the quick pickle version in my Lentil and Walnut Tacos (page 143).

Fermentation is super simple, but there are a few tricks to master. The first is temperature. In the winter, your kitchen may not be warm enough to allow fermentation to happen. If so, place the jar on top of the refrigerator or in the oven with the light turned on, wrapped in a kitchen towel. Be sure to keep the onions submerged in brine with fermentation weights or a resealable plastic bag filled with water.

---

1 medium sweet yellow onion

1 teaspoon (5 mL) salt

½ teaspoon (2 mL) ground turmeric

¾ cup (175 mL) water

1. Wash a 2-cup (500 mL) mason jar with a lot of hot, soapy water and dry with a clean kitchen towel to avoid contamination.

2. Using a mandolin, thinly slice the onion. Pack the onions into the clean mason jar and add the salt, turmeric, and water.

3. Cover and tighten the lid, then shake well to mix the brine. Remove the lid and press the onions under the brine. Use a fermentation weight or a small resealable plastic bag filled with water to keep the onions under the brine. Loosely seal the lid on the jar. You want to protect the onions from dirt, while allowing some oxygen to reach the mixture to avoid promoting the growth of dangerous microbes.

4. Let sit in a warm area, away from direct sunlight, to ferment for 3 to 4 days. To test, give the onions a taste; if they have a nice pickled tang, they are ready! If not, make sure they are in a warm spot, wrap the jar with a clean kitchen towel to insulate, and let them ferment for up to 7 days to achieve the right flavour.

5. Once fermented, remove the weight, tightly seal the lid on the mason jar, and store in the fridge for up to 2 weeks.

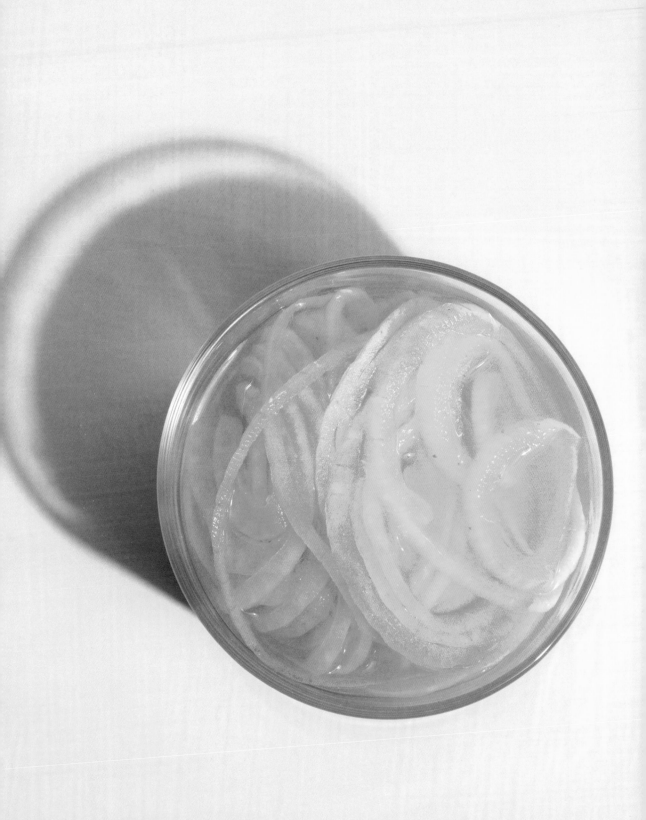

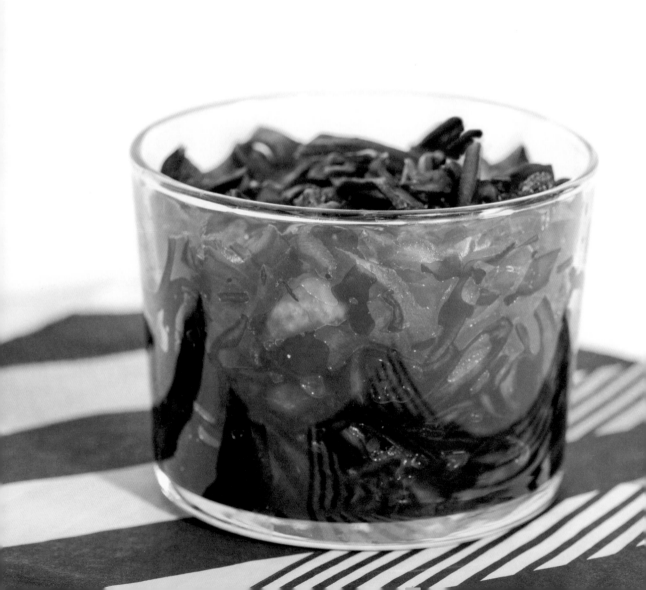

# Red Cabbage Sauerkraut

DAIRY-FREE | GLUTEN-FREE | PALEO-FRIENDLY | VEGAN | VEGETARIAN

MAKES 5 CUPS (1.25 L)

This jewel-toned sauerkraut is delicious and a wonderful way to get started with fermenting vegetables. All you need is cabbage, salt, and a jar. Fermentation harnesses the natural lactobacillus bacteria all around us; as it ferments the cabbage, it releases lactic acid and a host of other beneficial compounds. Cabbage is a particularly gut-friendly ferment because of its natural L-glutamine content. L-glutamine is an amino acid that helps feed gut cells and supports the integrity of your digestive tract. I use sauerkraut as a condiment on grain bowls, sandwiches, wraps, and salads. Try it on the Jicama Avocado Tacos (page 144) or on the Spicy Miso Soba Bowl (page 155).

---

1. Wash a 2-quart (2 L) flip-top mason jar with a lot of hot, soapy water and dry with a clean kitchen towel to avoid contamination.

2. Shred the cabbage using a mandolin or food processor so that it is very fine and place in a large bowl.

3. Sprinkle the salt on the cabbage, add your variation ingredients (Variation 1 or 2 at right), and massage the mixture until it releases enough brine that you can submerge the sauerkraut. It is a good workout that will take at least 5 minutes.

4. Pack the sauerkraut, with its brine, into the mason jar. Use a fermentation weight or a resealable plastic bag filled with water to keep the cabbage under the brine. Loosely top the jar with the lid to protect it from dirt, while allowing some oxygen to reach the mixture to avoid promoting the growth of dangerous microbes. Place the jar in a warm spot in your kitchen, away from direct sunlight and wrapped in a kitchen towel for temperature control, and let the sauerkraut ferment.

5. Check your ferment daily. Remove the lid and the weight, taste with a clean utensil, then replace and press down on the weight to release carbon dioxide bubbles. When it tastes tart to your liking, remove the weight, tightly seal the lid, and place it in the fridge. This can take 3 to 10 days, depending on the temperature. The sauerkraut will keep in the fridge for up to 1 month.

2 pounds (900 g) red cabbage

1 tablespoon (15 mL) salt

### Variation 1

½ Granny Smith apple, peeled and thinly sliced

1 teaspoon (5 mL) caraway seeds

### Variation 2

1 clove garlic, minced

1 teaspoon (5 mL) whole black peppercorns

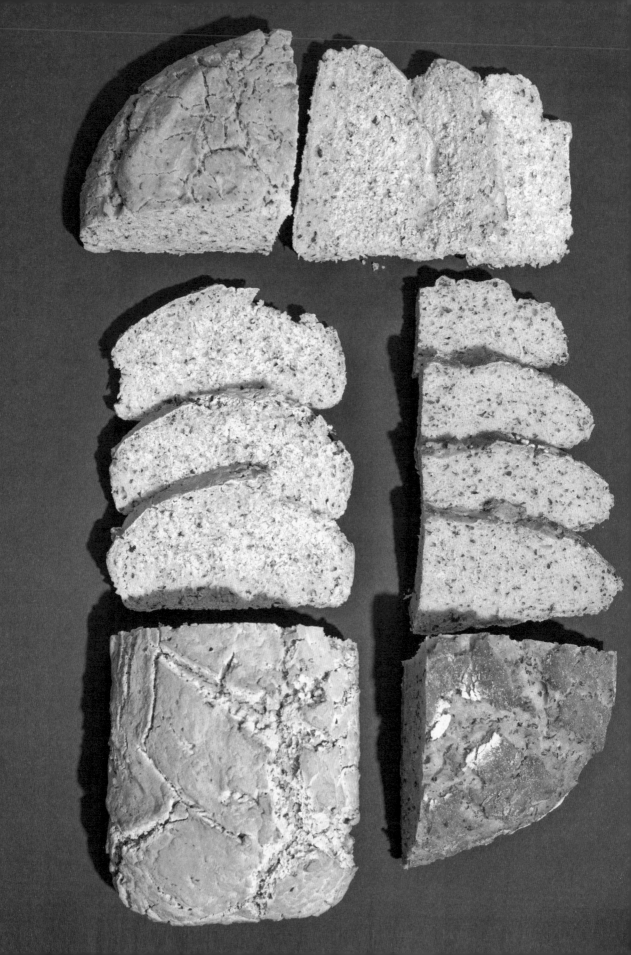

# Favourite Suppliers

## Adaptogens

The quality of herbal products varies widely and affects their effectiveness. I like the powder formulations from Sun Potion and use them regularly. They are available online and in specialty stores in the United States and Canada. I also love the fermented herbal tinctures from Botanica, a Canadian company; they are widely available in health food stores across Canada and online.

**WWW.SUNPOTION.COM**
**WWW.BOTANICAHEALTH.COM**

## Dairy Alternatives

I use primarily Earth's Own plant-based milk alternatives; this company offers almost every variety you can imagine, including oat milk. Earth's Own is a Canadian company and its products are widely available across Canada in health food stores, supermarkets, and warehouse clubs.

**WWW.EARTHSOWN.COM**

For those looking for an allergen-friendly alternative, I like Veggemo. It is made from a pea protein base, making it nut- and soy-free. Available at health food stores and supermarkets in Canada and health food stores in the United States.

**WWW.VEGGEMO.COM**

I tend not to use many butter alternatives, as the flavour of national brands isn't quite the same and they are often made from more inflammatory oils. However, I find Melt Organic products to be one of the best for flavour and nutrition.

**WWW.MELTORGANIC.COM**

My absolute favourite plant-based yogurt is Forager Cashewgurt because it contains simple ingredients, is delicious unsweetened, and contains a bit of protein. It is widely available at health food stores in the United States. In Canada, I find that the plain coconut yogurt from Silk is the best tasting and most widely available plant-based yogurt at both health food stores and supermarkets.

**WWW.FORAGERPROJECT.COM**
**WWW.DRINKSILK.CA**

## Fermented Foods

My favourite large-scale suppliers of sauerkraut and kimchi are Farmhouse Culture and Firefly Kitchens. Their products taste fresh and flavourful and are widely available at health food stores across Canada and the United States.
WWW.FARMHOUSECULTURE.COM
WWW.FIREFLYKITCHENS.COM

I also encourage you to search out locally produced fermented foods from small-scale producers at the farmers' market or health food store. In Vancouver, we have Pure Earth Superfoods, which is a woman-owned company.
WWW.PUREEARTHSUPERFOODS.CA

For clinical probiotics, I recommend Bio-K+, which comes in a fresh fermented liquid and capsules. It is a Canadian, family-owned company whose products are of the highest quality and potency. Available at pharmacies, supermarkets, and health food stores across Canada and the United States.
WWW.BIOKPLUS.COM

## Flours and Baking Supplies

Whenever I call for gluten-free all-purpose flour, I have used Bob's Red Mill gluten-free all-purpose—not its 1-to-1 blend. I have chosen this product because it is chickpea-based and therefore more nutritious than primarily starch blends and it is widely available across Canada and the United States at supermarkets, health food stores, and online. Bob's Red Mill has a dedicated gluten-free facility, so it is a good resource.
WWW.BOBSREDMILL.COM

I also use many Cuisine Soleil products. It is a Canadian company with a 100 percent gluten-free production facility that is also certified organic. Its all-purpose blend is also chickpea-based and available at health food stores across Canada.
WWW.CUISINESOLEIL.COM

Everland is a Canadian company that offers certified organic baking supplies, such as nutritional yeast and baking powder. It also has my favourite refined organic coconut oil, which has zero coconut scent and performs beautifully. Available at supermarkets and health food stores in Canada.
WWW.EVERLAND.CA

Camino is a Canadian, cooperatively owned company that sells fair trade cocoa and sugar. It offers a natural, non-Dutched cocoa. Available in health food stores in Canada.
WWW.CAMINO.CA

Wholesome Sweeteners offers organic sweeteners and is widely available at health food stores in Canada and the United States.
**WWW.WHOLESOMESWEET.COM**

Nutiva makes my favourite coconut butter and excellent-quality hemp and coconut oil products. Available at supermarkets and health food stores across Canada and the United States and online.
**WWW.NUTIVA.COM**

NOW Foods is a reliable source for agar powder. You can find it at health food stores in Canada and the United States and online.
**WWW.NOWFOODS.COM**

## Grains and Beans

Nature's Path is a Canadian, family-owned company that produces certified organic and gluten-free foods in a dedicated facility. Its gluten-free oats and ground flaxseed are my go-to products. Available at supermarkets, health food stores, and wholesale clubs across Canada and the United States.
**WWW.NATURESPATH.COM**

If you are not celiac or diagnosed gluten intolerant, my favourite grain and dried bean supplier is GRAIN. A woman-owned company, it sources traceable, Canadian-grown products that are incredibly fresh and taste better than just about anything you have ever tried. It ships direct from its website to both the United States and Canada.
**WWW.EATGRAIN.CA**

All my recipes have been developed using no-salt-added beans. I typically use either San Remo Organic or Eden Organic, which is more widely available in supermarkets and health food stores across the United States and Canada.
**WWW.SANREMOFOODS.COM**
**WWW.EDENFOODS.COM**

## Oils and Condiments

Chosen Foods makes an excellent naturally refined, high-heat avocado oil that I like to use for frying and in the occasional recipe where the flavour of olive oil will not work. Available at supermarkets, health food stores, and warehouse clubs across Canada and the United States.
**WWW.CHOSENFOODS.COM**

Maison Orphée is my favourite national brand for high-quality extra-virgin olive oil, including one that is properly refined for cooking (it is actually labelled "for everyday cooking"). It makes great Dijon, too. Available at health food stores across Canada.
**WWW.MAISONORPHEE.COM**

Spectrum Organics is another reliable brand for high-quality cooking oils that is more widely available at health food stores and supermarkets across the United States and Canada.
**WWW.SPECTRUMORGANICS.COM**

Amano Foods makes my favourite gluten-free tamari and miso. Kikkoman is widely available in Canada and the United States and offers a gluten-free soy sauce and gluten-free panko crumbs.
**WWW.AMANOFOODS.CA**
**WWW.KIKKOMANUSA.COM**

## Nuts and Seeds

Prana is a Canadian company whose products are all organic, vegan, and gluten-free, which is a huge bonus because it can be difficult to source gluten-free bulk nuts. Its products are widely available at supermarkets across Canada and via its website, where it ships to the United States. It also sells large-format packages on its website.
**WWW.PRANA.BIO**

If you use nuts in large quantities like I do, Costco offers large-format shipments of gluten-free nuts from Yupik on its website. You will save a lot of money as long as you have room to store the bags!
**WWW.COSTCO.CA or WWW.COSTCO.COM**

I use Nuts To You raw nut butters and tahini, which are widely available in health food stores and supermarkets in Canada and online. In the United States, Justin's makes excellent-quality nut butters. I love its portable squeeze packets you can take for travel!
**WWW.NUTS-TO-YOU.COM**
**WWW.JUSTINS.COM**

# Acknowledgements

For my husband, Jim, who is my ultimate champion and biggest fan. Thank you for taking this wild ride with me. To my littles, Iris and Elliott—everything I do in this life is for you. Thank you for eating tofu, eggplant, and all this funny healthy stuff all the time. I owe you a few bags of potato chips.

To my mother, Ligia, I cannot thank you enough for your support. Even as a grownup, I literally couldn't do it without you, and I am so grateful that my kids get to spend time with their *avo* when mom is out doing whatever it is she does.

All my love to Svein, Wendy, Bonnie, and Casey. Thank you for all the extra babysitting and for not thinking I am crazy for taking this path.

To Carly Watters, you are the agent with the mostest; I am so thrilled to work with you. You make me feel supported and understood and helped shape the vision for *Eat More Plants* so it could become stronger. Thank you for believing in this project and in my ability to pull it off.

To Andrea Magyar, writing a book is a bit like tearing your heart out and spilling it onto the page. In my critical moments, knowing that I had your knowledge, expertise, and experience supporting me gave me strength. I have felt infinitely more confident knowing that I had your support to make *Eat More Plants* the best it possibly could be. I am so grateful to be working with someone who is so passionate about sharing plant-based nutrition with the world.

A big thank you to all the passionate and creative folks at Penguin Random House for helping shape *Eat More Plants* into what it has become and sharing its message with the world.

To Janis Nicolay, you are such a rock star. Your remarkable talent is inspiring. Thank you for getting it and for spending endless days in my chilly basement creating such exceptional images. To Sophie McKenzie, I am eternally grateful for your creative eye and your easygoing spirit—because my cooking usually does not look like the picture.

To Meg Hubert (Meg Hubert Ceramics) and Grace Lee (Eikcam Ceramics), thank you for the gorgeous tableware. Your beautiful work was an exceptional canvas for all of my plants.

To Melissa Quantz, my friend and frequent collaborator. You are the calm, thoughtful yin to my frenetic, everything-all-at-once yang.

To all of you who have been a source of inspiration, friendship, and support. Thank you for your early support of this project, so it could become a reality: Zach Berman, Pailin Chongchitnant, Abbey Sharp, Leah Garrad-Cole, Allison Day, and Tori Wesszer.

To everyone who tested my recipes and spent time in the kitchen helping with all the dishes, thank you for your time and your honest and thoughtful feedback. I am grateful for it. Thank you to Jason and Michelle Kurtz, Jola and Peter Lekich, Ligia Tomas, Austin Hoff, Catherine Newstead, Jessica Pirnak, Marianne Bloudoff, Naomi Oh, Andraya Avison, and Marilee Pumple.

In addition, to *you*, thank you for making *Eat More Plants* a part of your life.

# Bibliography

## Chapter 1

1. Balandaykin, Mikhail E., and Ivan V. Zmitrovich. "Review on Chaga Medicinal Mushroom, Inonotus obliquus (Higher Basidiomycetes): Realm of Medicinal Applications and Approaches on Estimating Its Resource Potential." International Journal of Medicinal Mushrooms 17, no. 2 (2015).

2. Blasbalg, Tanya L., et al. "Changes in Consumption of Omega-3 and Omega-6 Fatty Acids in the United States during the 20th Century." The American Journal of Clinical Nutrition 93, no. 5 (2011): 950–962.

3. Calder, Philip C. "Feeding the Immune System." Proceedings of the Nutrition Society 72, no. 3 (2013): 299–309.

4. Chin, Kok-Yong. "The Spice for Joint Inflammation: Anti-Inflammatory Role of Curcumin in Treating Osteoarthritis." Drug Design, Development and Therapy 10 (2016): 3029.

5. Conlon, Michael A., and Anthony R. Bird. "The Impact of Diet and Lifestyle on Gut Microbiota and Human Health." Nutrients 7, no. 1 (2014): 17–44.

6. Domínguez, Raúl, et al. "Effects of Beetroot Juice Supplementation on Cardiorespiratory Endurance in Athletes: A Systematic Review." Nutrients 9, no. 1 (2017): 43.

7. Feinman, Richard D., et al. "Dietary Carbohydrate Restriction as the First Approach in Diabetes Management: Critical Review and Evidence Base." Nutrition 31, no. 1 (2015): 1–13.

8. Gandía-Herrero, Fernando, Josefa Escribano, and Francisco García-Carmona. "Biological Activities of Plant Pigments Betalains." Critical Reviews in Food Science and Nutrition 56, no. 6 (2016): 937–945.

9. Guggenheim, Alena G., Kirsten M. Wright, and Heather L. Zwickey. "Immune Modulation from Five Major Mushrooms: Application to Integrative Oncology." *Integrative Medicine: A Clinician's Journal* 13, no. 1 (2014): 32–44.

10. Hadley, Kevin B., et al. "The Essentiality of Arachidonic Acid in Infant Development." *Nutrients* 8, no. 4 (2016): 216.

11. He, Yan, et al. "Curcumin, Inflammation, and Chronic Diseases: How Are They Linked?" *Molecules* 20, no. 5 (2015): 9183–9213.

12. Hewlings, Susan J., and Douglas S. Kalman. "Curcumin: A Review of Its Effects on Human Health." *Foods* 6, no. 10 (2017): 92.

13. Jones, Andrew M. "Dietary Nitrate Supplementation and Exercise Performance." *Sports Medicine* 44, no. 1 (2014): 35–45.

14. Li, Xiaoxia, et al. "A Review of Recent Research Progress on the *Astragalus* Genus." Molecules 19, no. 11 (2014): 18850–18880.

15. Li, Yonghong, et al. "Rhodiola rosea L.: An Herb with Anti-Stress, Anti-Aging, and Immunostimulating Properties for Cancer Chemoprevention." *Current Pharmacology Reports* 3, no. 6 (2017): 384–395.

16. Martin, Kirsty, et al. "Ketogenic Diet and Other Dietary Treatments for Epilepsy." *The Cochrane Library* (2016).

17. Patel, Seema, and Abdur Rauf. "Adaptogenic Herb Ginseng (Panax) as Medical Food: Status Quo and Future Prospects." *Biomedicine & Pharmacotherapy* 85 (2017): 120–127.

18. Pietrzkowski, Zbigniew, et al. "Betalain-Rich Red Beet Concentrate Improves Reduced Knee Discomfort and Joint Function: A Double Blind, Placebo-Controlled Pilot Clinical Study." *Nutrition & Dietetics* Supplement 6 (2014).

19. Pratte, Morgan A., et al. "An Alternative Treatment for Anxiety: A Systematic Review of Human Trial Results Reported for the Ayurvedic Herb Ashwagandha (*Withania somnifera*)." *Journal of Alternative and Complementary Medicine* 20, no. 12 (2014): 901–908.

20. Sales-Campos, Helioswilton, et al. "An Overview of the Modulatory Effects of Oleic Acid in Health and Disease." *Mini Reviews in Medicinal Chemistry* 13, no. 2 (2013): 201–210.

21. Schwingshackl, Lukas, Marina Christoph, and Georg Hoffmann. "Effects of Olive Oil on Markers of Inflammation and Endothelial Function—A Systematic Review and Meta-Analysis." *Nutrients* 7, no. 9 (2015): 7651–7675.

22. Sergeant, Susan, Elaheh Rahbar, and Floyd H. Chilton. "Gamma-linolenic Acid, Dihommo-gamma Linolenic, Eicosanoids and Inflammatory Processes." *European Journal of Pharmacology* 785 (2016): 77–86.

23. Simopoulos, Artemis P., and James J. DiNicolantonio. "The Importance of a Balanced ω-6 to ω-3 Ratio in the Prevention and Management of Obesity." *Open Heart* 3, no. 2 (2016): e000385.

24. Singh, Varun Parkash, et al. "Advanced Glycation End Products and Diabetic Complications." *Korean Journal of Physiology & Pharmacology* 18, no. 1 (2014): 1–14.

25. Slyepchenko, Anastasiya, et al. "Gut Microbiota, Bacterial Translocation, and Interactions with Diet: Pathophysiological Links between Major Depressive Disorder and Non-Communicable Medical Comorbidities." *Psychotherapy and Psychosomatics* 86, no. 1 (2017): 31–46.

26. Sonnenburg, Justin L., and Fredrik Bäckhed. "Diet-Microbiota Interactions as Moderators of Human Metabolism." *Nature* 535, no. 7610 (2016): 56–64.

27. Sorice, Angela, et al. "Ascorbic Acid: Its Role in Immune System and Chronic Inflammation Diseases." *Mini Reviews in Medicinal Chemistry* 14, no. 5 (2014): 444–452.

28. Sun, Qiang, Jia Li, and Feng Gao. "New Insights into Insulin: The Anti-Inflammatory Effect and Its Clinical Relevance." *World Journal of Diabetes* 5, no. 2 (2014): 89.

29. Triantafyllou, Konstantinos, Christopher Chang, and Mark Pimentel. "Methanogens, Methane and Gastrointestinal Motility." *Journal of Neurogastroenterology and Motility* 20, no. 1 (2014): 31.

30. Vela, Guillermo, et al. "Zinc in Gut-Brain Interaction in Autism and Neurological Disorders." *Neural Plasticity* 2015 (2015).

## Chapter 2

1. Blum, Kenneth, Panayotis K. Thanos, and Mark S. Gold. "Dopamine and Glucose, Obesity, and Reward Deficiency Syndrome." Frontiers in Psychology 5 (2014): 919.

2. Byrne, C. S., et al. "The Role of Short Chain Fatty Acids in Appetite Regulation and Energy Homeostasis." International Journal of Obesity 39, no. 9 (2015): 1331–1338.

3. Crofts, Catherine, et al. "Hyperinsulinemia: A Unifying Theory of Chronic Disease." Diabesity 1, no. 4 (2015): 34–43.

4. Crowe, Francesca L., et al. "Source of Dietary Fibre and Diverticular Disease Incidence: A Prospective Study of UK Women." Gut 63, no. 9 (2014): 1450–1456.

5. de Melo, Anderson Sanches, et al. "Pathogenesis of Polycystic Ovary Syndrome: Multifactorial Assessment from the Foetal Stage to Menopause." Reproduction 150, no. 1 (2015): R11–R24.

6. Gallagher, Emily Jane, and Derek LeRoith. "Obesity and Diabetes: The Increased Risk of Cancer and Cancer-Related Mortality." Physiological Reviews 95, no. 3 (2015): 727–748.

7. Grundy, Myriam M.-L., et al. "Re-evaluation of the Mechanisms of Dietary Fibre and Implications for Macronutrient Bioaccessibility, Digestion and Postprandial Metabolism." British Journal of Nutrition 116, no. 5 (2016): 816–833.

8. Hooper, Lee, et al. "Reduction in Saturated Fat Intake for Cardiovascular Disease." The Cochrane Library (2015).

9. Hoy, M. K., and J. D. Goldman. "Fiber Intake of the U.S. Population: What We Eat in America, NHANES 2009- 2010." *Food Surveys Research Group Dietary Data Brief* No. 12 (September 2014).

10. Hutkins, Robert W., et al. "Prebiotics: Why Definitions Matter." *Current Opinion in Biotechnology* 37 (2016): 1–7.

11. Louis, Petra, Georgina L. Hold, and Harry J. Flint. "The Gut Microbiota, Bacterial Metabolites and Colorectal Cancer." *Nature Reviews Microbiology* 12, no. 10 (2014): 661–672.

12. Martin, Michael J., Sapna E. Thottathil, and Thomas B. Newman. "Antibiotics Overuse in Animal Agriculture: A Call to Action for Health Care Providers." *American Journal of Public Health* 105, no. 12 (2015): 2409–2410.

13. Poutanen, Kaisa S., et al. "A Review of the Characteristics of Dietary Fibers Relevant to Appetite and Energy Intake Outcomes in Human Intervention Trials." *The American Journal of Clinical Nutrition* 106, no. 3 (2017): 747–754.

14. Rezapour, Mona, Saima Ali, and Neil Stollman. "Diverticular Disease: An Update on Pathogenesis and Management." *Gut and Liver* 12, no. 2 (2018): 125–132.

15. Rizzo, Nico S., et al. "Nutrient Profiles of Vegetarian and Non Vegetarian Dietary Patterns." *Journal of the Academy of Nutrition and Dietetics* 113, no. 12 (2013): 1610–1619.

16. Stashauna, K., et al. "The Correlation between Diabetes Mellitus Type II and the Increased Risk of Alzheimer's Disease: A Collaborative Treatment Approach." *International Journal of Community & Family Medicine* 1, no. 4 (2017): 00019.

17. Stilling, Roman M., et al. "The Neuropharmacology of Butyrate: The Bread and Butter of the Microbiota-Gut-Brain Axis?" *Neurochemistry International* 99 (2016): 110–132.

18. "How Much Feed and Water Are Used to Make a Pound of Beef?" Beef Cattle Research Council. http://www.beefresearch.ca/blog/cattle-feed-water-use/

19. "Water for Food." Water Footprint Network. http://www.waterfootprint.org

20. "Water—Who Uses How Much?" California Water Blog. https://californiawaterblog.com/2011/05/05/water—who-uses-how-much/

## Chapter 3

*All nutrient calculations and intake claims are from Health Canada/United States Department of Agriculture databases and Institute of Medicine Official National Guidelines and so are not referenced.*

1. Green, Ralph, et al. "Vitamin B12 Deficiency." Nature Reviews Disease Primers 3 (2017): 17040.

2. Hunnicutt, Jacob, Ka He, and Pengcheng Xun. "Dietary Iron Intake and Body Iron Stores Are Associated with Risk of Coronary Heart Disease in a Meta-analysis of Prospective Cohort Studies." The Journal of Nutrition 144, no. 3 (2014): 359–366.

3. Hunt, Alesia, Dominic Harrington, and Susan Robinson. "Vitamin B12 Deficiency." BMJ 349 (2014): g5226.

4. Kortman, Guus A. M., et al. "Nutritional Iron Turned Inside Out: Intestinal Stress from a Gut Microbial Perspective." FEMS Microbiology Reviews 38, no. 6 (2014): 1202–1234.

5. Melina, Vesanto, Winston Craig, and Susan Levin. "Position of the Academy of Nutrition and Dietetics: Vegetarian Diets." Journal of the Academy of Nutrition and Dietetics 116, no. 12 (2016): 1970–1980.

# Index